# DIET QUALITY OF AMERICANS

# NUTRITION AND DIET RESEARCH PROGRESS SERIES

**Diet Quality of Americans**
*Nancy Cole and Mary Kay Fox*
2009. ISBN: 978-1-60692-777-9

# DIET QUALITY OF AMERICANS

## NANCY COLE
### AND
## MARY KAY FOX

**Nova Science Publishers, Inc.**
*New York*

For permission to use material from this book please contact us:
Telephone 631-231-7269; Fax 631-231-8175
Web Site: http://www.novapublishers.com

### NOTICE TO THE READER

LIBRARY OF CONGRESS CATALOGING-IN-PUBLICATION DATA

*Available upon request*

ISBN 978-1-60692-777-9

*Published by Nova Science Publishers, Inc.* ✛ *New York*

# CONTENTS

# Executive Summary[1]

## The Food Stamp Program

The Food Stamp Program is the nation's largest nutrition assistance program, disbursing over $30 billion in benefits in FY2007 to an average monthly caseload of 11.8 million households containing 26.4 million persons (USDA/FNS, 2008). On average, households received $215 in food stamp benefits per month (or $96 per person). Food stamp benefits are designed to permit low-income households to obtain a more nutritious diet through normal channels of trade. To that end, food stamp benefits are accepted as tender for purchase of food and beverages at nearly 164,000 retail outlets throughout the United States (USDA/FNS, 2007a).

In FY2006, the most recent year for which administrative data are available, 54 percent of FSP households contained children, 18 percent included an elderly person, and 23 percent included someone who was disabled. The majority of FSP households lived in metropolitan areas (77 percent); 13 percent lived in metropolitan areas of 10,000 to 50,000 population; and 10 percent lived in rural areas (USDA/FNS, 2007b).

The overarching aim of the Food Stamp Program (FSP) is to ensure that low-income households have enough food to eat. Over time, as evidence has accumulated about the role diet plays in the development of chronic disease, the program's goals have expanded to include an interest in the quality of foods eaten by FSP participants. Interest in diet quality has also been fueled by the on going obesity epidemic in the U.S., the high prevalence of obesity among some segments of the FSP population, and speculation that participation in the FSP and other Federal food assistance programs may be contributing to this problem (Baum, 2007; Ver Ploeg et al., 2007).

The increasing policy interest in the quality of FSP participants' diets over time is reflected in the dramatic expansion of the FSNE program over the past 15 years. In 1992, only seven States participated in FSNE; by 2006, the program had grown to include all 50 States, two territories, and the District of Columbia. Over this period Federal investment in FSNE has almost quadrupled, from $661,076 to $247 million.

While no consistent evidence exists of a relationship between participation in nutrition assistance programs and overweight (USDA/FNS, 2005), some State agencies and health

---

[1] This is an edited, excerpted and augmented edition of USDA Report FSP-08-NH, dated July 2008.

advocates have recommended that the FSP implement more specific strategies to promote healthful food choices among FSP participants. These include strategies that would reward selection of healthful choices, such as increased benefits for the purchase of fruits and vegetables, as well as restrictive strategies that would limit the types of foods and beverages that can be purchased with FSP benefits (USDA/FNS, 2007c; Guthrie et al., 2007). There is no evidence that either of these strategies would be effective in improving the quality of FSP participants' diets or in stemming the tide of obesity. In recognition of this fact, USDA's proposals for the 2007 Farm Bill include strengthening and expanding Food Stamp Nutrition Education (FSNE) through a substantive initiative to develop and evaluate strategies for improving diet quality and decreasing obesity in FSP populations (USDA, 2007).

## FOCUS OF THE RESEARCH

Strategies for improving the diets of FSP participants—whether developed by policy makers, program administrators, nutrition educators, or researchers—should be based on valid and reliable information about the current dietary practices of FSP participants. This chapter uses the most recently available data from the National Health and Nutrition Examination Survey (NHANES 1999-2004) to provide that foundation. The intent is to provide an up-to-date and comprehensive picture of the diets of FSP participants—a reference point that can be used to target efforts to improve participants' diets and as a benchmark for monitoring participants' diets over time. FSP participants are compared to two groups of nonparticipants—those who were income-eligible for the FSP but did not participate and higher-income individuals who were not eligible for the FSP.

*This research was not designed to assess the impact of the FSP or in any way attribute differences observed between FSP participants and nonparticipants to an effect of the program.* Estimation of program impacts requires a randomized experiment or quasi-experimental design to control for selection bias (Hamilton and Rossi, 2002). A quasi-experimental study design was not feasible due to limitations of the NHANES data. In this chapter, data on nonparticipants are presented strictly to provide context for data on FSP participants. For example, it is useful to understand the extent to which patterns observed in the diets of FSP participants mirror those observed in other populations groups.

The research presented in this chapter addresses four basic questions about the diets of FSP participants: Do FSP participants get enough of the right kinds of foods to eat (measured in terms of nutrient intakes and energy sources)? Are FSP participants more likely to be overweight than nonparticipants (are they consuming too many calories)? How does the quality of diets consumed by FSP participants compare with those of nonparticipants? And how do food choices differ for FSP participants and nonparticipants (do different food choices help explain differences in diet quality)?

# Do Food Stamp Program Participants Get Enough of the Right Kinds of Food to Eat?

For this study, we addressed the question of whether FSP participants get "enough food" by examining intakes of 18 essential vitamins and minerals.[2] We also examined intakes of macronutrients (protein, carbohydrates, and fat) as a percent age of energy, and the percentage of energy consumed as solid fats, alcoholic beverages, and added sugars (SoFAAS).

Intakes were examined for the overall population, and comparisons were made for FSP participants and nonparticipants. The main findings are:

- For every vitamin and mineral examined, the prevalence of adequate usual daily intakes was comparable for FSP participants and income- eligible nonparticipants. Intakes of macronutrients as a percentage of energy were comparable for the two groups. On average, FSP participants obtained a significantly larger percentage of their total energy intake from SoFAAS than income-eligible nonparticipants.

- FSP participants were significantly less likely than higher-income nonparticipants to have adequate usual daily intakes of vitamins and minerals. Intakes of macronutrients as a percentage of energy did not differ between groups for children and older adults. However, FSP adults were less likely than higher-income adults to consume more total fat than recommended. For protein and carbohydrate, intakes of FSP adults were less likely than those of higher-income adults to be below recommend levels. On average, FSP participants obtained a significantly larger percentage of their total energy intake from SoFAAS than higher-income nonparticipants.

Detailed findings are discussed below.

## Vitamins and Minerals with Defined Estimated Average Requirements (EARs)

The prevalence of adequate usual daily intakes of vitamins and minerals is assessed by comparing the usual daily intakes of a population group to Estimated Average Requirements (EARs). The prevalence of adequate usual daily intakes is defined as the proportion of the group with usual daily intakes at or above the EAR. Thirteen of the 18 vitamins and minerals examined in this chapter have defined EARs. The NHANES data indicate that:

- Over 90 percent of all persons had adequate usual daily intakes of thiamin, riboflavin, niacin, vitamin B12, folate, iron and phosphorus and nearly 90 percent hade adequate usual daily intakes of vitamin B6 and zinc.

---

[2] Nutrient intake data presented do not include contributions from dietary supplements.

- Usual daily intakes of vitamins A, C, and E, and magnesium need improvement—30 percent or more of the U.S. population had inadequate usual daily intakes.[3]
- For all vitamins and minerals examined, the prevalence of adequate usual daily intakes was consistently higher for children than for adults and older adults.

There were no significant differences between FSP participants and income-eligible nonparticipants in the prevalence of adequate usual intakes. However, for each of the 13 vitamins and minerals examined, the prevalence of adequate usual intakes was significantly lower for FSP participants than for higher-income nonparticipants (shown in Figure 1).

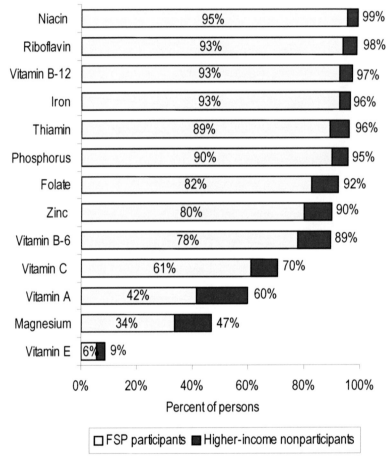

Note: Bars for FSP participants overlay bars for higher-income nonparticipants. All differences between
    FSP participants and higher income nonparticipants are statistically significant at the .05 level or
    better. Estimates are age adjusted.

Figure 1. Percent of FSP Participants and Higher Income Nonparticipants with Adequate Usual Intakes
of Vitamins and Minerals

---

[3] The prevalence of adequate usual daily intakes of vitamin E was especially low (7.5 percent), consistent with most recent studies of vitamin E intake. Devaney and colleagues have pointed out that vitamin E deficiency is rare in the U.S., despite low measured intakes, and that the EARs for vitamin E may need to be reassessed (Devaney et al., 2007).

## Calcium, Potassium, Sodium, and Fiber

It is not possible to assess fully the adequacy of calcium, potassium, sodium, and fiber intakes because EARs have not been defined. Populations with mean usual daily intakes that meet or exceed the Adequate Intake (AI) levels defined for these nutrients can be assumed to have high levels of adequacy. However, no conclusions can be drawn when mean usual daily intakes fall below the AI. For sodium, the major concern is the potential for excessive intakes, so usual daily intakes were compared to the Tolerable Upper Intake Level (UL) which is the maximum intake considered to be safe for long-term consumption.

For the entire U.S. population:

- Mean usual daily intakes of calcium were 100, 88, and 62 percent of the AI for children, adults, and older adults, respectively.
- Mean usual daily intakes of potassium and fiber were 58 and 53 percent of the AI, for all age groups combined, and no age groups had a mean usual daily intake that met or exceeded the AI.
- Sodium intakes were of concern for all age groups. Nearly 90 percent of the population had usual daily intakes that exceeded the Tolerable Upper Intake Level (UL).

Mean usual daily calcium intakes were more than 100 percent of the AI for FSP children and both groups of nonparticipant children, indicating that the prevalence of adequate calcium intakes is likely to be high for all three groups of children. For adults and older adults, mean usual daily intakes of calcium were consistently less than the AI. Although no firm conclusions can be drawn about the adequacy of usual daily calcium intakes of adults and older adults, mean usual daily calcium intakes in both age groups were significantly lower for FSP participants than for higher-income nonparticipants.

For potassium and fiber, mean usual daily intakes were less than the AI for all groups. Among adults and older adults, mean usual daily intakes of FSP participants were significantly lower than those of higher-income nonparticipants.[4]

## Macronutrients

The 2005 DGA and MyPyramid Food Guidance system recommend a particular distribution of calories from energy-providing macronutrients— total fat, saturated fat, carbohydrate, and protein. Usual daily intakes of total fat, protein, and carbohydrate were compared to Acceptable Macronutrient Distribution Ranges (AMDRs) defined in the DRIs (IOM, 2006). Usual daily intakes of saturated fat were compared to the 2005 *Dietary Guidelines for Americans* (DGA) recommendation (USDHHS/ USDA, 2005).

The NHANES data show that, for the overall population:

---

[4] Usual daily fiber intakes of all age groups were low, relative to the AIs. Mean usual intakes were equivalent to about half of the 14 grams of fiber per 1,000 calories standard used to establish the AIs. It has been suggested that the methods used to establish AIs for fiber may need to be reexamined (Devaney et al., 2007).

- Over 95 percent of children consumed protein and carbohydrate within acceptable ranges, but 20 percent of children consumed too much energy from total fat, and 17 percent consumed too much energy from saturated fat.
- Nearly all adults and older adults consumed protein within acceptable ranges, but about 37 percent consumed too much energy from total fat, about 60 percent consumed too much energy from saturated fat, and about 22 percent consumed too little energy from carbohydrates.

Among children and older adults, there were no statistically significant differences in macronutrient intakes (as a percentage of energy) of FSP participants and nonparticipants. Among adults, however, FSP participants were less likely than higher-income nonparticipants to have consumed too much energy from total fat and too little energy from carbohydrate and protein.

## Discretionary Calories from Solid Fats, Alcoholic Beverages, and Added Sugars (SoFAAS)

Dietary patterns recommended in the DGA and *MyPyramid Food Guidance System* include specific discretionary calorie allowances based on energy needs for age and gender groups. Discretionary calories are defined as calories that can be used flexibly after nutrient requirements are met (Britten, 2006). These allowances assume that individuals satisfy nutrient requirements with the fewest possible calories by eating foods in their most nutrient-dense form (fat-free or lowest fat form, with no added sugars) (Basiotis et al., 2006). Discretionary calories may be used to consume additional amounts from the basic food groups or to consume less nutrient-dense foods that provide calories from solid fats, alcoholic beverages, added sugars (SoFAAS).

The most generous allowance for discretionary calories in the *MyPyramid* food intake patterns (based on age, gender, and level of physical activity) is 20 percent of total energy needs (for physically active boys age 14 to 18).

NHANES data show that for all persons, an average of 38 percent of calories were consumed from solid fats, alcoholic beverages, and added sugars (SoFAAS). This percentage was far in excess of the discretionary calorie allowances included in the *MyPyramid* food guidance system. Comparison of FSP participants and nonparticipants is shown in Figure 2:

- On average, FSP adults consumed more energy from SoFAAS than either group of nonparticipant adults: 43 percent versus 40 and 39 percent for income-eligible and higher- income adults, respectively.
- For children and older adults, there were no significant differences between FSP participants and either group of nonparticipants in the mean proportion of usual energy intakes contributed by SoFAAS. Children consumed 39 percent of energy from SoFAAS, while older adults consumed 33 percent of energy from SoFAAS.

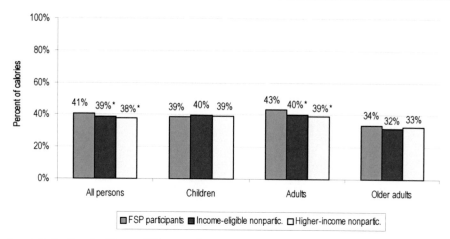

* Denotes statistically significant difference from FSP participants at the .05 level or better. Estimates are age adjusted.
Note: Calories from alcoholic beverages include calories from carbohydrate in beer and wine, and calories from grams of alcohol in all alcoholic beverages except cooking wine.

Figure 2. Average Percent of Energy from Solid Fats, Alcoholic Beverages, and Added Sugars (SoFAAS)

Mean daily energy (calorie) intakes are examined in this chapter (Chapter 3). However, we did not use caloric intakes to assess whether FSP participants obtained "enough food" because there is a wide range of energy requirements for age/gender groups depending on body measurement and activity level.[5] As recommended by the Institute of Medicine (IOM), we assess the adequacy of energy intakes according to the prevalence of healthy weight, overweight, and obesity (IOM, 2005b).

## ARE FOOD STAMP PROGRAM PARTICIPANTS MORE LIKELY TO BE OVERWEIGHT THAN NONPARTICIPANTS?

Measures of Body Mass Index (BMI) and BMI for-age (for children) were used to assess the appropriateness of usual daily energy intakes. A BMI in the healthy range indicates that usual daily energy intake is consistent with requirements; a BMI below the healthy range indicates inadequate usual daily energy intake; and a BMI above the healthy range indicates that usual daily energy intake exceeds requirements. Fewer than 3 percent of all persons have BMI below the healthy range.

The percent of FSP participants and nonparticipants with BMI above the healthy range is shown in Figure 3. The trend for all groups is an increase in overweight until middle age and then a leveling off or decline. The difference between FSP participants and nonparticipants varies by gender:

- Female FSP participants of all ages were more likely to have BMI above the healthy range than either income-eligible or higher-income nonparticipants.

---

[5] Activity levels are not adequately measured by most surveys, including NHANES 1999-2002.

- Overall, male FSP participants were no more likely than income-eligible nonparticipants to have BMI above the healthy range, but male FSP participants were more likely than higher- income nonparticipants to be overweight at young ages and less likely to be overweight as adults.

## HOW DOES DIET QUALITY COMPARE FOR FSP PARTICIPANTS AND NONPARTICIPANTS?

In this research we used two measures to assess overall diet quality.

- We used the Healthy Eating Index (HEI)-2005, developed by the USDA Center for Nutrition Policy and Promotion (CNPP), to assess compliance with the diet-related recommendations of the 2005 DGA and the MyPyramid food guidance system.

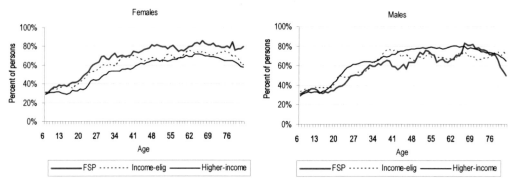

Note: Graphs display smoothed trend lines produced by moving averages. Estimates for specific ages should not be read off graphs.

Figure 3. Percent of FSP Participants and Nonparticipants with BMI Above the Healthy Range

- We used a composite measure of nutrient density to assess the nutrient content of foods relative to their energy content. We assessed nutrient density of overall diets and individual meals and snacks. "Nutrient-dense" foods are defined as "low-fat forms of foods in each food group and forms free of added sugar."

### The Healthy Eating Index-2005 (HEI-2005)

The HEI-2005 consists of 12 component scores that measure consumption of food and nutrients relative to *MyPyramid* recommendations and the DGA. Eight components are food-based and assess intakes of *MyPyramid* food groups and subgroups. The four remaining components assess intakes of oils; saturated fat; sodium; and calories from SoFAAS.

HEI-2005 component scores are assigned based on a density approach that compares intakes per 1,000 calories to a reference standard. This approach reflects the overarching recommendation of the DGA and *MyPyramid* that individuals should strive to meet food group and nutrient needs while maintaining energy balance. Scores for the food- based and oils components reward greater consumption, up to a maximum score of 5 or 10 points per component. Scores for saturated fat, sodium, and calories from SoFAAS reward low consumption. Scores on the 12 components are summed for the Total HEI Score, worth a maximum of 100 points.

Results show that the diets of all groups fell considerably short of the diet recommended in the DGA and *MyPyramid*. The overall average score on the HEI-2005 was 58 out of a possible 100. On average, FSP participants scored below income- eligible and higher-income nonparticipants (52 vs. 56 and 58 points, respectively) (Figure 4).

HEI-2005 component scores are shown in Figure 5, expressed as a percentage of the maximum score per component. FSP participants and both groups of nonparticipants achieved maximum scores on 2 components (Total Grains and Meat and Beans), but all three groups scored below 50 percent on 4 components: Dark Green and Orange Vegetables and Legumes; Whole Grains; Saturated Fat; and Calories from SoFAAS.

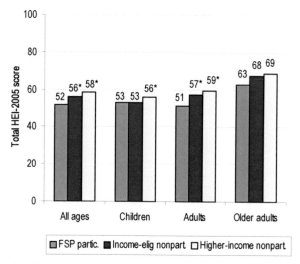

* Denotes statistically significant difference from FSP participants at the .05 level or better. Estimates are age adjusted.

Figure 4. Healthy Eating Index-2005: Total Scores

The HEI-2005 component scores point to the following key concerns in the diets of all age groups and all participant/nonparticipant groups:

- Very low intakes of whole grains and dark green and orange vegetables and legumes.
- High intakes of saturated fat and discretionary calories from SoFAAS.

In addition, all groups scored below 75 percent of the maximum scores for Total Fruit, Whole Fruit, Total Vegetables, Milk, and Oils; indicating low intake relative to the con-centrations needed to meet nutrient requirements without exceeding calorie requirements. These findings indicate that the diets of FSP participants suffer from the same shortcomings of the diets consumed by other groups of Americans, including those with higher incomes.

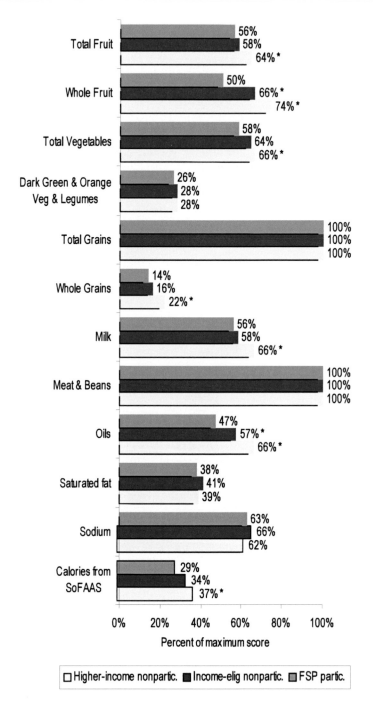

* Denotes statistically significant difference from FSP participants at the .05 level or better. Estimates are age adjusted.

Figure 5. Healthy Eating Index-2005: Component Scores

FSP participants scored significantly below higher- income nonparticipants on 7 HEI-2005 component scores (Figure 5), although there were some differences by age group:

- Results for adults mirrored those for the overall population: FSP adults scored significantly below higher-income adults on 7 components.
- FSP children scored below higher income children on 4 components: Whole Fruit, Whole Grains, Milk, and Saturated Fat.
- FSP older adults scored below higher income older adults on 3 components: Total Vegetables, Milk, and Oils.

## Nutrient Density of Overall Diets, Meals, and Snacks

To assess nutrient density, we used a modified version of the Naturally-Nutrient-Rich (NNR) score developed by Drewnowski (2005). The NNR is a nutrients-to-calories ratio that considers nutrients commonly included in efforts to define healthy diets. The NNR, as initially conceived, excludes fortified foods. For our analysis, we used a modified NNR—the NR (Nutrient-Rich) score— that includes fortified foods because these foods make important contributions to nutrient intakes. The NR score measures the contributions of 16 nutrients (see Chapter 4).[6] The NR score is difficult to interpret on its own, but provides a metric for comparing foods, meal, or overall diets.

Overall diets of FSP participants and income- eligible nonparticipants comparable in nutrient density, as measured using the NR score. Compared with higher-income nonparticipants, FSP adults adults had overall diets that were lower in nutrient density, indicating in these age groups, diets consumed by FSP participants provide fewer nutrients on a per-calorie basis than the diets consumed by higher-income nonparticipants (Figure 6).

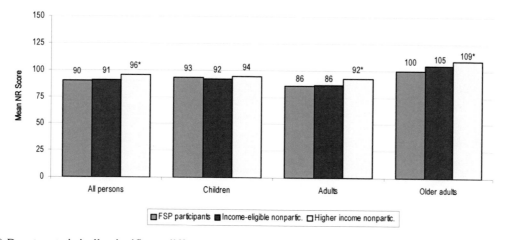

* Denotes statistically significant difference from FSP participants at the .05 level or better. Estimates are age adjusted.

Figure 6. Nutrient-Rich (NR) Scores for All Meals and Snacks Combined

---

[6] The NR score for a food is constructed as the weighted average of the contributions of 16 nutrients, with nutrient contributions measured as a percent of daily value (DV) contributed per 2000 kcal of the food. The NR score for a meal or the full complement of meals and snacks is similarly constructed, after aggregating the nutrient contributions of all foods consumed.

To understand the source of differences in overall nutrient density of foods consumed, we examined the nutrient density of individual meals and snacks. Differences between FSP participants and nonparticipants varied by meal and by age group.

Compared with higher income nonparticipants:

- Adult FSP participants had significantly lower NR scores for all three meals and for snacks;
- FSP children had lower NR scores for breakfast; and
- Older adult FSP participants had lower NR scores for breakfast and lunch.

Differences in NR scores for adults and older adults were attributable to differences among females.

## In What Ways Do FSP Participants Make Different Food Choices than Nonparticipants?

Analyses of food choices helps us to understand the avenues by which FSP participants and nonparticipants obtain different nutrient intakes and levels of diet quality. It can also reveal dietary behaviors that can be targeted by FSP nutrition education efforts.

We used two different approaches to compare food choices of FSP participants and nonparticipants based on a single 24-hour recall:

- Supermarket aisle approach—This approach looks at the percentage of FSP participants and nonparticipants who consumed foods from broad food groups and the choices made within food groups.
- Nutritional quality approach—This approach examines the percentage of foods consumed by FSP participants and nonparticipants within three broad groups based on nutritional characteristics—foods suggested for frequent, selective, or occasional consumption.

### Supermarket Aisle Approach

We examined the proportions of FSP participants and nonparticipants consuming foods from each of 10 major food groups (food groups are shown in Figure 7). Compared with income-eligible nonparticipants, FSP participants were less likely to consume any vegetables or fruit, but were equally likely to consume foods from all other major food groups.[7] Figure 7 shows results for FSP participants compared with higher-income nonparticipants: FSP participants were less likely to consume foods from 8 of the 10 food groups, suggesting that FSP participants as a group have less variety in their diet.[8]

---

[7] For children and older adults, there were no significant differences between FSP participants and income-eligible nonparticipants.

[8] Comparisons of energy intakes (Chapter 3) showed no significance differences between FSP adults and higher-income adults; however, FSP older adults had significantly lower energy intakes than higher-income older adults

Comparison of FSP adults and higher-income adults were consistent with the overall findings shown in Figure 7. For children and older adults, however, there were fewer between-group differences: FSP children were less likely to consume from 2 of the 10 food groups (grains; added fats and oils); and FSP older adults were less likely to consume from 5 of the 10 food groups (grains; vegetables; fruits; milk and milk products; and added fats and oils).

- less likely to choose whole grains
- less likely to consume raw vegetables (including salads)
- less likely to consume reduced-fat milk and more likely to consume whole milk
- less likely to consume sugar-free sodas and more likely to consume regular sodas.

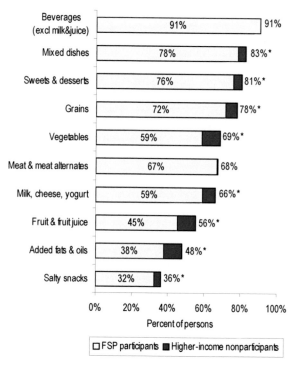

* Denotes statistically significant difference from FSP participants at the .05 level or better. Estimates are age adjusted. Bars for FSP participants overlay bars for higher-income nonparticipants.

Figure 7. Percent of FSP Participants and Higher income Nonparticipants Consuming Foods from 10 Major Food Groups

Examination of food choices within food group identified some common food choice patterns across all age groups. Compared with higher- income nonparticipants, FSP participants in all age groups made the following less healthful food choices:

On the other hand, FSP adults made healthier choices than higher-income adults in the following categories:

suggesting that, for older adults, differences in food group consumption may be due to a combination of less variety and lower overall food intake.

- less likely to consume alcoholic beverages
- less likely to consume sweets and desserts
- less likely to consume salty snacks.

## Nutritional Quality of Food Choices

Our second method for examining food choices was based on the radiant pyramid/power calories concept, as described by Zelman and Kennedy (2005) (Figure 8). The idea is that foods within a food group are ranked by nutrient density, with the most nutrient-dense food choices at the bottom of the pyramid to be enjoyed frequently; foods with lower nutrient density in the middle of the pyramid to be enjoyed selectively; and the least nutrient- dense foods at the top of the pyramid to be enjoyed only occasionally. We classified foods into these three categories based on characteristics encouraged in the DGAs and MyPyramid Food Guidance System; for example, forms that are fat- free, low-fat, and/or have no added sugar are at the bottom of the pyramid. For some foods, data on total fat content and calories from SoFAAS was used to categorize foods within food group.

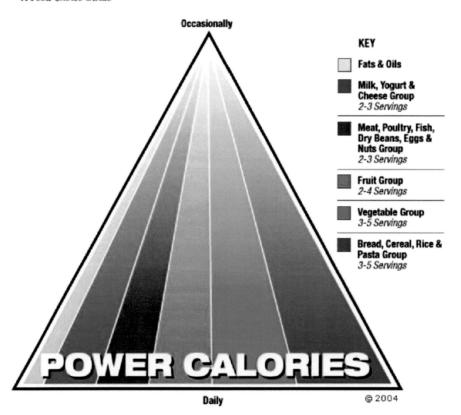

Figure 8. Radiant Pyramid Concept

Analyses of the nutritional quality of foods consumed showed that:

- Over half of the foods consumed by FSP participants and both groups of nonparticipants were foods suggested for occasional consumption (top of the radiant pyramid).
- Overall, FSP participants were somewhat more likely than either group of nonparticipants to consume foods suggested for occasional consumption, and a little less likely to consume foods suggested for selective or frequent consumption (Figure 9).

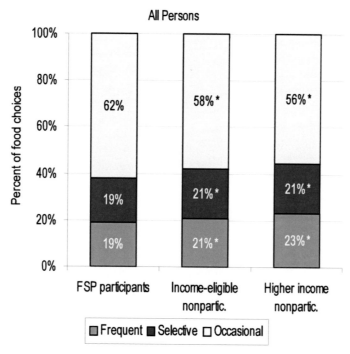

\* Denotes statistically significant difference from FSP participants at the .05 level or better. Estimates are age adjusted.

Figure 9. Percent of Food Choices From Foods Suggested for Frequent, Selective, and Occasional Consumption

## CONCLUSIONS AND IMPLICATIONS FOR FSP NUTRITION EDUCATION

This chapter describes the adequacy and quality of diets consumed by FSP participants and two groups of nonparticipants in three age groups (children, adults, and older adults). Primary conclusions are:

1.  HEI-2005 scores indicate that the following issues are of concern for all age groups and all participant/nonparticipant groups:

- Low intakes of vegetables and oils, relative to the concentrations needed to meet nutrient requirements without exceeding calorie requirements.
- Very low intakes of the most nutritious vegetables—dark green and orange vegetables and legumes.
- Very low intakes of whole grains.
- High intakes of saturated fat, sodium, and calories from solid fats, alcoholic beverages, and added sugars (SoFAAS).

2.  Dietary adequacy and quality vary with income, age, and gender:

- FSP participants and income-eligible nonparticipants had nutrient intakes that were not significantly different, while higher income nonparticipants were significantly more likely to have adequate usual daily intakes of vitamins and
- minerals.
- Overall diets of FSP participants and income-eligible nonparticipants had comparable levels of nutrient density, while higher-income nonparticipants consumed diets with significantly higher nutrient density.
- The total HEI-2005 score of FSP participants was less than that of both income-eligible and higher-income nonparticipants. However, component scores revealed greater differences between FSP participants and higher-income nonparticipants (7 of 12 components) than between FSP participants and income- eligible nonparticipants (2 components).
- Differences between FSP participants and nonparticipants were more often observed for adults (19 to 59 years) and older adults (60 years and older) than for children (1 to 18 years).

3.  Several factors point up the critical need for improvements in diets of FSP participants:

- FSP participants did not achieve the levels of nutritional adequacy achieved by higher- income nonparticipants.
- FSP children and adult/older adult females exhibited higher levels of overweight and obesity than either group of nonparticipants.
- Foods consumed by adult female FSP participants and older adult FSP participants of both genders were lower in nutrient density than foods consumed by comparable higher-income nonparticipants.
- Foods consumed by adult FSP participants of both genders provided, on average, more calories from SoFAAS that foods consumed by adult nonparticipants (both income-eligible and higher-income).
- FSP participants were significantly more likely than either group of nonparticipants to consume foods recommended for occasional consumption and less likely to consume foods recommended for selective or frequent consumption.

## Implications for FSP Nutrition Education

In addition to the dietary concerns noted above for all age groups and all participant/ nonparticipant groups, our analyses revealed specific issues that may prove to be useful targets for Food Stamp Nutrition Education (FSNE) efforts:

- Use of whole milk. In all three age groups, FSP participants were more likely than either income-eligible or higher-income nonparticipants to consume whole milk and less likely to consume reduced-fat or skim milks. Whole milk is less nutritionally desirable than reduced-fat/skim versions because it is less nutrient-dense, contributing more calories from saturated/solid fat.
- Low overall consumption of dairy products. FSP children and adults consumed fewer dairy products, on a cups-per-1,000 calories basis (as measured in the HEI-2005) than higher-income nonparticipants. This pattern is reflected in lower calcium intakes, on average, among FSP participants. In addition to switching from whole milk to reduced-fat and skim milks, FSP participants could benefit from consuming more milk and other low-fat dairy products. (FSP participants in all age groups were less likely than higher-income nonparticipants to consume yogurt).
- Low consumption of whole fruit. FSP participants in all three age groups consumed less whole fruit, on a cups-per-1,000 calorie basis, than higher-income nonparticipants. Among adults, this difference extended to 100 percent fruit juices as well.
- Consumption of regular (not sugar-free) sodas. In all three age groups, regular sodas accounted for a larger share of the added sugars consumed by FSP participants than higher-income nonparticipants. Among older adults, this was also true for income-eligible nonparticipants.
- Consumption of potato chips. FSP adults and children were more likely than higher-income adults and children to consume potato chips. FSP participants were less likely to consume popcorn or pretzels, which are generally lower-fat salty snacks (children only).

Targeting specific food choices, such as those cited above, may be an effective way to affect behavioral change that results in improved diet quality outcomes.

# Chapter 1

# INTRODUCTION

The overarching aim of the Food Stamp Program (FSP) is to ensure that low-income households have enough food to eat. Over time, as evidence has accumulated about the role diet plays in the development of chronic disease, the program's goals have expanded to include an interest in the *quality* of foods eaten by FSP participants. Interest in diet quality has also been fueled by the ongoing obesity epidemic in the U.S., the high prevalence of obesity among some segments of the FSP population, and speculation that participation in the FSP and other Federal food assistance programs may be contributing to this problem (Baum, 2007; Ver Ploeg et al., 2007).

While no consistent evidence exists of a relationship between participation in nutrition assistance programs and overweight (USDA/FNS, 2005), some State agencies and health advocates have recommended that the FSP implement more specific strategies to promote healthful food choices among FSP participants. These include strategies that would reward selection of healthful choices, such as increased benefits for the purchase of fruits and vegetables, as well as restrictive strategies that would limit the types of foods and beverages that can be purchased with FSP benefits (USDA/FNS, 2007c; Guthrie et al., 2007). There is no evidence that either of these strategies would be effective in improving the quality of FSP participants' diets or in stemming the tide of obesity. In recognition of this fact, USDA's proposals for the 2007 Farm Bill include strengthening FSNE and making a $100 million investment over a five-year period to develop and evaluate strategies for improving diet quality and decreasing obesity in FSP populations (USDA, 2007).

Strategies for improving the diets of FSP participants—whether developed by policy makers, program administrators, nutrition educators, or researchers—should be based on valid and reliable information about the current dietary practices of FSP participants. This chapter uses the most recently available data from the National Health and Nutrition Examination Survey (NHANES 1999– 2004) to provide that foundation. The intent is to provide an up-to-date and comprehensive picture of the diets of FSP participants—a reference point that can be used to target efforts to improve participants' diets and as a benchmark for monitoring participants' diets over time.

This chapter examines dietary patterns from multiple perspectives—nutrient intakes, food choices, and diet quality. Information is presented for FSP participants and two groups of nonparticipants— those who were income-eligible for food stamps but did not report that they participated in the program, and higher-income individuals who were not eligible for the program.

*This chapter was not designed to assess the impact of the FSP or in any way attribute differences observed between FSP participants and nonparticipants to an effect of the program.* Estimation of program impacts requires a randomized experiment or quasi-experimental design to control for selection bias (Hamilton and Rossi, 2002). A quasi-experimental study design was not feasible due to limitations of the NHANES data. In this chapter, data on nonparticipants are presented strictly to provide context for data on FSP participants. For example, it is useful to understand the extent to which patterns observed in the diets of FSP participants mirror those observed in other populations

The chapter provides data on the adequacy of usual nutrient intakes of FSP participants and nonparticipants measured relative to accepted nutrition standards. Diet quality is measured in terms of the Healthy Eating Index-2005, based on 24-hour recalls. The chapter also presents data on the appropriateness of long-run energy intakes, as measured by Body Mass Index. We provide context for these findings by examining the food choices reported in 24-hour recalls from a number of different perspectives:

- Meal and snacking patterns;
- Consumption of discretionary calories from solid fats, alcoholic beverages, and added sugars;
- Energy density and nutrient density of meals, snacks, and overall diets;
- Proportions of persons consuming foods from major food groups (for example, grains, vegetables, and milk/milk products);
- Proportions of persons consuming specific types of food within major food groups (for example, whole grains or skim milk);
- Average amounts of foods consumed from each of the major MyPyramid food groups and the relative contributions of specific types of food to intakes.

This introductory chapter provides an overview of the FSP as well as a brief description of the data and methods used in this study. The five chapters that follow present findings on usual daily intakes of vitamins, minerals, and fiber (Chapter 2), energy intakes (Chapter 3), meal and snack patterns (Chapter 4), food choices (Chapter 5), and MyPyramid intakes and the Healthy Eating Index- 2005 (Chapter 6).[1]

## THE FOOD STAMP PROGRAM

The Food Stamp Program (FSP) is the nation's largest nutrition assistance program, disbursing $33 billion in benefits in FY2007 to an average monthly caseload of 11.8 million households containing 26.4 million persons (USDA/FNS, 2008). On average, households received $215 in food stamp benefits per month (or $96 per person). Food stamp benefits are designed to permit low-income households to obtain a more nutritious diet through normal

---

[1] Chapter 3 includes an assessment of the appropriateness of long-run usual energy intakes, based on Body Mass Index (BMI) and the prevalence of overweight and obesity.

channels of trade. To that end, food stamp benefits are accepted as tender for purchase of food and beverages at nearly 164,000 retail outlets throughout the United States (USDA/FNS, 2007a).

In FY2006, the most recent year for which administrative data are available, 54 percent of FSP households contained children, 18 percent included an elderly person, and 23 percent included someone who was disabled. The majority of FSP households lived in metropolitan areas (77 percent); 13 percent lived in metropolitan areas of 10,000 to 50,000 population; and 10 percent lived in rural areas (USDA/FNS, 2007b).

## FSP Eligibility and Benefits

Eligibility for FSP benefits is determined primarily on the basis of monthly household income. Households must have gross income below 130 percent of the federal poverty level, and net income below the poverty level (households with elderly or disabled persons are exempt from the gross income test). Households must also meet a "resource test"— they are permitted up to $2,000 in countable resources ($3,000 if a household member is age 60 or older or disabled). Countable resources include most assets easily converted to cash, but exclude homes and most vehicles. Households are categorically eligible, and not subject to the income and resource tests, if all members received assistance from one or more of the following programs: Temporary Assistance for Needy Families (TANF), Supplemental Security Income (S SI), General Assistance, or TANF funded in-kind benefits. In addition to income and resource limits, there are non-financial eligibility restrictions, including work registration requirements, and restrictions related to citizenship, residency, and immigration status.

Food stamp benefit levels are based on the estimated cost of the USDA Thrifty Food Plan (TFP)—the cost of an adequate diet—and the expectation that households contribute 30 percent of their income to the food budget.[2] In other words, the maximum allotment amount (for households with zero net income) is equal to the cost of the TFP, and the maximum is reduced by 30 cents for every dollar of household net income. In theory, food stamp allotments assure a food budget sufficient to purchase an adequate diet.

Maximum monthly benefit levels in FY2008 were $162 for one-person households, $298 for two- person households, $426 for three-person households, and $542 for four-person households (allotments are specified for household size up to 8 persons, and $122 for each additional person thereafter). These benefit levels correspond to average weekly per-person food expenditures of $37 for a one-person household, $33 for a three- per person household, and $31 for a four-person household.

---

[2] The TFP specifies quantities of food needed for an adequate diet for a family of four with two children. The cost of the TFP was estimated using prices paid by households surveyed in the 1977-78 USDA Nationwide Food Consumption Survey, and annually are updated using the "CPI Detailed Report." The costs of the TFP for families of different sizes are obtained by applying "economies-of-scale adjustment factors" to the basic cost for a family of four.

## Nutrition Education

Under FSP regulations, States have the option to provide nutrition education to FSP participants as part of their administrative operations, through the Food Stamp Nutrition Education (FSNE) program. A major goal of the FSNE program is to increase the likelihood that FSP participants will make healthful food choices within the constraints of a limited budget, and choose physically active lifestyles.

Because State FSP agencies are primarily designed to perform the administrative functions associated with food stamp benefits, most State agencies delegate FSNE activities, through formal contracts, to other agencies that routinely provide nutrition education (Bell et al., 2006). State Cooperative Extension Services are the major providers of FSNE services; other providers include public health departments, public assistance agencies, and universities. State-level FSNE agencies generally use local organizations to deliver nutrition education to FSP participants.

State agencies that obtain FSNE funding must submit an annual plan to FNS that describes the nutrition education activities to be conducted and provides a budget for those activities. Nutrition education provided through FSNE must be compatible with the dietary advice provided in the *Dietary Guidelines for Americans* and in USDA's *MyPyramid* food guidance system. Approved FSNE plans are reimbursed at the level of 50 percent of the allowable costs expended; States are expected to contribute the remaining 50 percent.

The increasing policy interest in the quality of FSP participants' diets over time is reflected in the dramatic expansion of the FSNE program over the past 15 years. In 1992, only seven States participated in FSNE; by 2006, the program had grown to include all 50 States, two territories, and the District of Columbia. Over this period, Federal investment in FSNE has almost quadrupled, from $661,076 to $247 million.

A comprehensive review of FSNE in fiscal year (FY) 2004 showed that the program had a broad reach but was not universally available—about 80 percent of U.S. counties had some FSNE activities, but the breath and depth of services varied (Bell et al., 2006). Nutrition education was largely targeted toward children and women; FSNE providers cited difficulties in reaching other populations such as working adults and seniors.

## THE NATIONAL HEALTH AND NUTRITION EXAMINATION SURVEY

This chapter is based on data from the National Health and Nutrition Examination Survey (NHANES, 1999-2004), supplemented by data from the *MyPyramid Equivalents Database* which is compiled by USDA's Agricultural Research Service (ARS).

NHANES is conducted by the National Center for Health Statistics (NCHS) and is designed to provide national estimates of the health and nutrition status of the civilian, non-institutionalized population in the 50 United States. The survey includes interviews, physical examinations, and laboratory tests. Beginning in 1999, NHANES is a continuous annual survey with data released in public data files every two years. Most of the analyses in this chapter are based on six years of survey data from NHANES 1999-2004.

## NHANES Dietary Interview Data

This study relies primarily on data from the NHANES 24-hour dietary recall interview, which collects quantitative data on foods and beverages consumed during the preceding 24 hours. The NHANES dietary interview is conducted in-person using a computer-assisted dietary interview (CADI) system with a "multiple pass" approach to facilitate respondent recall of all foods and beverages consumed in the past 24 hours.[3],[4]

In survey years 1999-2002, NHANES conducted a single 24-hour recall for each respondent. Beginning in 2003, NHANES conducts a second follow-up dietary interview, by telephone, 3-10 days after the initial dietary interview. The "second day recall" provides data needed to estimate usual dietary intakes, thus controlling for within person day-to-day variance in nutrient intakes.

Beginning in 2003, NHANES dietary recall data are processed using a separate nutrient database program known as Survey Net, which incorporates data on nutrient values from USDA's Food and Nutrient Database for Dietary Studies (FNDDS). The NHANES public data release includes a food level file (containing one record for each food item reported by each respondent) and a total nutrient file (containing one record per respondent with total nutrient intakes for the day).

## NHANES Interview and Examination Data

In addition to dietary recall data, this study uses data collected through the NHANES household interview, examination survey, and physical examination. This includes information on person characteristics (FSP program participation, age, and sex), dietary supplement use, and body measurements (height and weight). These data are described in Appendix A.

## MYPYRAMID EQUIVALENTS DATABASE
## FOR USDA SURVEY FOOD CODES

Data from the MyPyramid Equivalents Database were used to estimate scores on the Healthy Eating Index-2005 (HEI-2005) and to assess sources of MyPyramid food group intakes. The HEI-2005 was developed by the USDA Center for Nutrition Policy and Promotion (Guenther, et al., in press). HEI-2005 is a measure of diet quality with 12 component scores that assess intakes of food groups and selected nutrients relative to dietary patterns recommended in the MyPyramid Food Guidance System (USDA, CNPP, 2005) and the 2005 Dietary Guidelines for Americans (USDHHS/ USDA, 2005).

---

[3] In 1999-2000 a small subsample of respondents completed dietary interviews via telephone as part of a methodological study (the Dietary Interview Mode Evaluation Study (DIMES)) of the operational feasibility of the telephone interview mode.

[4] The multiple passes include: a) quick list of foods, without interviewer interruption; b) reporting of the time, place, and eating occasion for each food; c) specific probes about food details; and d) a final review of reported foods in chronological order.

MyPyramid, which replaced the Food Guide Pyramid introduced in 1992, provides recommendations for the types and quantities of foods individuals age 2 and older should eat from different food groups (grains, vegetables, fruits, milk, meat and beans), tailored to individuals' age, gender, and activity level. MyPyramid also specifies discretionary calorie allowances based on energy needs for age and gender groups. Discretionary calories are defined as calories that can be used flexibly after nutrient requirements are met by foods consumed in the most nutrient dense form (fat-free or lowest fat form, with no added sugars) (Britten, 2006).

The *MyPyramid Equivalents Database Version 1.0* contains files corresponding to the 1999-2002 NHANES individual food files (one record per food) and NHANES total nutrient files (one record per person, with total daily intake). MyPyramid data are expressed in cups or 'cup equivalents' for vegetables, fruit, and milk products; in ounces or 'ounce equivalents' for grains, and meat and beans; in grams for discretionary fats, teaspoons for added sugars, and in drinks for alcoholic beverages.

MyPyramid data are available for single day intakes for respondents age 2 and above, corresponding to NHANES survey years 1999-2002. Data corresponding to NHANES 2003-04 were not available at the time of this study. As a result, all analyses of HEI-2005 and sources of MyPyramid food group intakes in this chapter are limited to persons age 2 and older for the 4-year period 1999-2002.

## NHANES SAMPLES FOR TABULATION

This chapter contains tabulations of dietary measures for FSP participants and nonparticipants. FSP participants were self-identified by response to the survey question, "[In the last 12 months], were {you/you or any members of your household} authorized to receive Food Stamps [which includes a food stamp card or voucher, or cash grants from the state for food]?" Those who did not report food stamp receipt in the last 12 months were considered nonparticipants.[5] Nonparticipants were further subdivided into those who were income-eligible for the FSP (household income at or below 130 percent of poverty) and those whose income exceeded the eligibility standard (income above 130 percent of poverty).

All analyses in this chapter are based on NHANES respondents with complete dietary recalls. Pregnant and lactating women and infants are excluded because the dietary reference standards are different for these groups, and many of the food choice and diet quality measures used for this chapter do not apply to infants Sampling weights for this sub sample of the NHANES population are discussed in Appendix A. Tabulations of FSP participants and nonparticipants are provided for three age groups: children (age 1-18), adults (age 19-59), and older adults (age 60 and over). In addition, most of detailed tables included in appendices include separate estimates by age group and gender. Sample sizes and weighted population counts for the groups of FSP participants and nonparticipants are shown in Table 1-1.

---

[5] NHANES asked about current food stamp participation at the time of the survey, but computer programming problems during data collection resulted in substantial missing data for that item. See Appendix A.

**Table 1-1. HANES Respondents with Complete Dietary Recalls,
1999-2004: Sample Sizes and Weighted Population Counts**

| | Total Persons | Food Stamp Program Participants | Income-eligible Nonparticipants | Higher-income Nonparticipants |
|---|---|---|---|---|
| **Sample sizes** | | | | |
| All persons | 25,170 | 4,020 | 5,370 | 13,934 |
| Males | 12,747 | 1,936 | 2,702 | 7,201 |
| Females | 12,423 | 2,084 | 2,668 | 6,733 |
| Children (age 1-18) | 11,878 | 2,644 | 2,738 | 5,727 |
| Males | 6,000 | 1,343 | 1,389 | 2,867 |
| Females | 5,878 | 1,301 | 1,349 | 2,860 |
| Adults (age 19-59) | 8,570 | 1,022 | 1,629 | 5,313 |
| Males | 4,424 | 441 | 854 | 2,837 |
| Females | 4,146 | 581 | 775 | 2,476 |
| Older adults (age 60+) | 4,722 | 354 | 1,003 | 2,894 |
| Males | 2,323 | 152 | 459 | 1,497 |
| Females | 2,399 | 202 | 544 | 1,397 |
| **Weighted population counts** | | | | |
| All persons | 270,972,483 | 29,729,988 | 42,720,308 | 180,968,320 |
| Males | 134,995,707 | 13,134,300 | 20,498,269 | 92,853,551 |
| Females | 135,976,776 | 16,595,688 | 22,222,039 | 88,114,769 |
| Children (age 1-18) | 71,868,995 | 12,400,555 | 13,323,512 | 42,417,281 |
| Males | 36,928,736 | 6,297,009 | 7,232,866 | 21,553,756 |
| Females | 34,940,259 | 6,103,546 | 6,090,646 | 20,863,526 |
| Adults (age 19-59) | 150,408,066 | 14,636,446 | 21,624,625 | 105,100,358 |
| Males | 76,763,406 | 5,814,180 | 10,652,766 | 55,660,530 |
| Females | 73,644,660 | 8,822,266 | 10,971,859 | 49,439,827 |
| Older adults (age 60+) | 48,695,423 | 2,692,987 | 7,772,171 | 33,450,681 |
| Males | 21,303,565 | 1,023,111 | 2,612,637 | 15,639,265 |
| Females | 27,391,857 | 1,669,876 | 5,159,535 | 17,811,416 |

Notes: Weighted population is based on NHANES examination weights, recalibrated to account for nonresponse to the dietary recall and to proportionately weight weekday and weekend recalls (See Moshfegh et al., 2005). Six percent of the NHANES examination sample did not have complete dietary recalls. NHANES is weighted by year 2000 U.S. Census population totaling 281 million persons. Table excludes pregnant women, breastfeeding women, and infants (population weight of 10 million).

Source: NHANES 1999–2004 dietary recalls. Excludes pregnant and lactating women. "Total Persons" includes persons with missing Food Stamp Program participation or income.

## Characteristics of FSP Participants and Nonparticipants

Table 1-2 presents demographic data for FSP participants, income-eligible nonparticipants, and higher-income nonparticipants. Compared with higher-income nonparticipants, FSP participants were more likely to come from a racial/ethnic minority group, had significantly less education, were less likely to be married, and were more likely to be widowed, divorced, separated, never married, or cohabitating.

## Table 1-2. Demographic Characteristics of Food Stamp Participants
## and Nonparticipants

| | Total Persons | | Food Stamp Program Participants | | Income-eligible Nonparticipants | | Higher-income Nonparticipants | |
|---|---|---|---|---|---|---|---|---|
| | Percent | Standard Error | Percent | Standard Error | Percent | Standard Error | Percent | Standard Error |
| **Race/Ethnicity** | | | | | | | | |
| All persons | | | | | | | | |
| White, Non-Hispanic ....... | 68.9 | (1.67) | 46.2 | (3.81) | † 55.1 | (3.51) | † 76.3 | (1.28) |
| Black, Non-Hispanic ....... | 11.9 | (1.08) | 28.1 | (2.97) | 13.5 | (1.76) | 8.5 | (0.84) |
| Mexican American .......... | 8.6 | (0.99) | 10.0 | (1.99) | 14.9 | (2.03) | 6.7 | (0.77) |
| Other Hispanic ............. | 5.6 | (1.07) | 11.3 | (2.78) | 9.4 | (2.30) | 3.9 | (0.71) |
| Other race ................. | 5.0 | (0.44) | 4.5 | (1.12) | 7.1 | (1.03) | 4.6 | (0.42) |
| Children (age 1-18) | | | | | | | | |
| White, Non-Hispanic ....... | 61.0 | (1.96) | 38.3 | (4.28) | † 48.0 | (4.06) | † 72.1 | (1.64) |
| Black, Non-Hispanic ....... | 14.6 | (1.39) | 33.4 | (3.14) | 14.8 | (1.99) | 8.7 | (1.00) |
| Mexican American .......... | 12.3 | (1.33) | 12.9 | (2.29) | 21.4 | (2.65) | 8.8 | (1.03) |
| Other Hispanic ............. | 5.9 | (1.09) | 8.7 | (2.28) | 8.5 | (1.64) | 4.5 | (0.90) |
| Other race ................. | 6.2 | (0.68) | 6.7 | (1.41) | 7.3 | (1.47) | 6.0 | (0.78) |
| Adults (age 19-59) | | | | | | | | |
| White, Non-Hispanic ....... | 68.8 | (1.71) | 46.3 | (4.50) | † 55.0 | (3.35) | † 74.9 | (1.37) |
| Black, Non-Hispanic ....... | 11.8 | (1.04) | 27.2 | (3.22) | 13.6 | (1.90) | 9.1 | (0.87) |
| Mexican American .......... | 8.5 | (0.95) | 9.5 | (2.00) | 14.2 | (2.00) | 7.1 | (0.80) |
| Other Hispanic ............. | 5.9 | (1.15) | 13.0 | (3.58) | 9.6 | (2.32) | 4.4 | (0.79) |
| Other race ................. | 5.0 | (0.53) | 4.0 u | (1.39) | 7.7 | (1.32) | 4.6 | (0.51) |
| Older adults (age 60+) | | | | | | | | |
| White, Non-Hispanic ....... | 82.0 | (1.70) | 58.1 | (4.00) | † 66.6 | (5.45) | † 87.9 | (1.08) |
| Black, Non-Hispanic ....... | 8.0 | (1.03) | 22.7 | (3.82) | 11.4 | (1.92) | 6.0 | (0.82) |
| Mexican American .......... | 3.3 | (0.76) | 7.0 u | (2.62) | 7.1 | (1.82) | 2.1 | (0.46) |
| Other Hispanic ............. | 3.9 | (1.14) | 9.2 u | (3.05) | 10.1 u | (4.06) | 1.5 | (0.44) |
| Other race ................. | 2.8 | (0.38) | 2.9 u | (1.44) | 4.8 | (1.34) | 2.4 | (0.46) |
| **Country of Birth** | | | | | | | | |
| All persons | | | | | | | | |
| U.S. ................................. | 88.0 | (0.96) | 85.7 | (2.07) | † 80.4 | (2.35) | 90.3 | (0.74) |
| Mexico ........................... | 3.5 | (0.31) | 3.6 | (0.75) | 8.1 | (1.05) | 2.4 | (0.20) |
| Elsewhere ...................... | 8.2 | (0.86) | 10.1 | (1.91) | 11.4 | (1.93) | 7.2 | (0.69) |
| Children (age 1-18) | | | | | | | | |
| U.S. ................................. | 94.0 | (0.47) | 92.3 | (1.74) | † 89.8 | (1.12) | 96.0 | (0.38) |
| Mexico ........................... | 1.9 | (0.19) | 1.5 | (0.39) | 5.3 | (0.74) | 0.8 | (0.11) |
| Elsewhere ...................... | 4.0 | (0.44) | 5.9 | (1.69) | 4.7 | (0.89) | 3.1 | (0.39) |
| Adults (age 19-59) | | | | | | | | |
| U.S. ................................. | 84.9 | (1.20) | 84.1 | (2.33) | † 75.4 | (2.88) | 87.2 | (1.06) |
| Mexico ........................... | 4.9 | (0.41) | 4.8 | (0.98) | 10.6 | (1.40) | 3.6 | (0.30) |
| Elsewhere ...................... | 10.0 | (1.07) | 10.6 | (2.16) | 13.8 | (2.31) | 9.1 | (0.98) |
| Older adults (age 60+) | | | | | | | | |
| U.S. ................................. | 89.5 | (1.29) | 80.9 | (3.97) | 82.7 | (3.52) | † 92.1 | (0.85) |
| Mexico ........................... | 1.4 | (0.29) | 3.0 u | (1.16) | 3.8 | (0.96) | 0.7 | (0.12) |
| Elsewhere ...................... | 8.8 | (1.18) | 15.0 | (3.72) | 13.5 | (3.18) | 6.9 | (0.81) |

## Table 1-2. (Continued)

| | Total Persons | | Food Stamp Program Participants | | Income-eligible Nonparticipants | | Higher-income Nonparticipants | |
|---|---|---|---|---|---|---|---|---|
| | Percent | Standard Error | Percent | Standard Error | Percent | Standard Error | Percent | Standard Error |
| **Education** | | | | | | | | |
| All adults | | | | | | | | |
| Less than H.S. ............... | 20.7 | (0.72) | 48.0 | (1.92) | † 39.2 | (1.80) | † 13.3 | (0.65) |
| H.S. diploma or GED ...... | 26.2 | (0.77) | 26.0 | (1.71) | 27.2 | (1.26) | 25.8 | (0.90) |
| More than H.S. .............. | 52.9 | (1.05) | 25.7 | (1.97) | 33.4 | (1.95) | 60.8 | (1.01) |
| Adults (age 19-59) | | | | | | | | |
| Less than H.S. ............... | 18.0 | (0.68) | 43.4 | (2.16) | † 34.4 | (2.01) | † 11.0 | (0.72) |
| H.S. diploma or GED ...... | 25.6 | (0.91) | 28.1 | (2.21) | 26.7 | (1.45) | 24.7 | (1.03) |
| More than H.S. .............. | 56.4 | (1.12) | 28.4 | (2.32) | 38.8 | (2.43) | 64.2 | (1.12) |
| Older adults (age 60+) | | | | | | | | |
| Less than H.S. ............... | 30.0 | (1.53) | 64.3 | (3.80) | † 55.4 | (2.72) | † 21.1 | (1.25) |
| H.S. diploma or GED ...... | 28.6 | (1.01) | 18.5 | (3.08) | 28.7 | (1.91) | 29.7 | (1.13) |
| More than H.S. .............. | 41.1 | (1.39) | 16.3 | (3.08) | 15.5 | (1.71) | 49.0 | (1.31) |
| **Marital Status** | | | | | | | | |
| All adults | | | | | | | | |
| Married ........................... | 52.9 | (1.21) | 29.9 | (2.29) | † 39.8 | (1.73) | † 58.5 | (1.43) |
| Widowed, divorced, separated ...................... | 18.1 | (0.67) | 32.9 | (2.28) | 27.1 | (1.18) | 15.0 | (0.63) |
| Never married ................ | 19.3 | (0.70) | 24.4 | (2.24) | 22.0 | (1.42) | 17.5 | (0.76) |
| Cohabitating ................... | 5.6 | (0.41) | 8.0 | (1.59) | 8.0 | (0.94) | 4.9 | (0.45) |
| Not reported ................... | 4.1 u | (1.26) | 4.8 u | (2.55) | 3.2 u | (1.22) | 4.1 | (1.20) |
| Adults (age 19-59) | | | | | | | | |
| Married ........................... | 51.4 | (1.36) | 29.9 | (2.84) | † 39.4 | (1.88) | † 56.7 | (1.63) |
| Widowed, divorced, separated ...................... | 13.4 | (0.62) | 25.6 | (2.34) | 20.3 | (1.41) | 11.0 | (0.58) |
| Never married ................ | 24.0 | (0.86) | 30.0 | (2.81) | 26.7 | (1.58) | 22.0 | (0.95) |
| Cohabitating ................... | 6.9 | (0.52) | 9.6 | (1.96) | 10.1 | (1.23) | 6.0 | (0.58) |
| Not reported ................... | 4.3 u | (1.31) | 4.9 u | (2.98) | 3.5 u | (1.47) | 4.3 u | (1.30) |
| Older adults (age 60+) | | | | | | | | |
| Married ........................... | 58.2 | (1.13) | 29.7 | (4.37) | 40.5 | (3.54) | † 64.9 | (1.26) |
| Widowed, divorced, separated ...................... | 34.3 | (1.45) | 58.7 | (4.75) | 50.6 | (3.06) | 28.9 | (1.40) |
| Never married ................ | 2.8 | (0.44) | 4.8 u | (1.76) | 5.5 | (1.60) | 2.0 | (0.35) |
| Cohabitating ................... | 1.0 | (0.20) | 2.4 u | (1.57) | 1.1 u | (0.49) | 0.8 | (0.21) |
| Not reported ................... | 3.7 u | (1.34) | 4.4 u | (2.42) | 2.3 u | (1.13) | 3.3 u | (1.19) |

Note: Significant differences in distributions are noted by †. Differences are tested in comparison to FSP participants using chi-square tests.

U Denotes individual estimates not meeting the standards of reliability or precision due to inadequate cell size or large coefficient of variation.

Source: NHANES 1999-2004 sample of persons with complete dietary recalls. Excludes pregnant and breastfeeding women and infants. 'Total Persons' includes persons with missing food stamp participation or income. Percents are age adjusted to account for different age distributions of Food Stamp participants and nonparticipants

FSP participants also differed from income-eligible nonparticipants in a number of important ways. Income-eligible nonparticipants were more likely than FSP participants to be white or Mexican and, with the exception of older adults, were more likely to be immigrants. In addition, income-eligible nonparticipants had higher levels of education than FSP participants, and were more likely to be married.

Differences in sociodemographic characteristics of FSP participants and higher-income nonparticipants are expected, and are consistent with differences in income used to define the two groups. The differences in sociodemographic makeup of the FSP participant and income-eligible nonparticipant groups are of greater interest because some of these differences, particularly differences in race/ ethnicity and prevalence of immigrants, may influence dietary behaviors (Perez-Escamilla and Putnik, 2007).

## GENERAL ANALYTIC APPROACH[6]

This chapter provides a description of the nutrient intakes and food choices of FSP participants and nonparticipants. Descriptive statistics are provided with tests of statistical significance to indicate differences between FSP participants and each group of nonparticipants. *This research was not designed to assess program impacts or in any way attribute differences observed between FSP participants and either group of nonparticipants to an effect of the program.*

An important consideration in comparing estimates for FSP participants and nonparticipants is that the age composition of these groups is different. FSP participants tend to be younger than both nonparticipant groups (see population counts in Table 1-1). Thus, we present age-adjusted estimates to eliminate between-group differences that are due solely to differences in the age distributions of the groups. Data for children, adults, older adults, and all persons are "built-up" from estimates for smaller age groups, standardized according to the age distribution of the U.S. population in the year 2000.[7]

It is important to understand that age-adjusted estimates do not represent the true or raw estimates for a given population or subgroup. Rather, the age- adjusted estimates should be viewed as constructs or indices that provide information on the relative comparability of two or more populations (in this case, FSP participants and two different groups of nonparticipants) on a particular measure (U.S. DHHS, 2000).

### Statistical Tests

The statistical significance of differences between FSP participants and each group of nonparticipants was tested using t-tests or chi-square tests. Nonetheless, because of the large number of t-tests conducted—comparing FSP participants and nonparticipants, overall and by age group and gender—caution must be exercised in interpreting results. In general, findings discussed in the text are limited to those with strong statistical significance (1 percent level or better) or those that are part of an obvious trend or pattern in the data.

Text discussions generally focus on differences between FSP participants and one or both groups of nonparticipants. Reference may be made to other between-group differences— children vs. adults or males vs. females—when the differences are noteworthy. The statistical significance of these secondary comparisons has not been tested, however, and this fact is

---

[6] A detailed description of data and methods appears in Appendix A.

[7] Age standardization is applied to estimates for the following age groups: 1-3 year, 4-8 years, 9-13 years, 14-18 years, 19-30 years, 31-50 years, 51-59 years, 60-70, and 71 and over.

noted in the text. Statistical tests were not performed on these second-level differences because of the expansive number of statistical tests performed in the main analysis and because these comparisons are not the focus of the report.

Additional information about the analytic approach, including use of NHANES sampling weights, calculation of standard errors, age standardization, and guidelines used to flag point estimates deemed to be statistically unreliable, is provided in Appendix A. Individual point estimates may be deemed statistically unreliable because of small sample size or a large coefficient of variation. In keeping with NHANES reporting guidelines, such estimates are reported in detailed tables and are clearly flagged. Between-group differences may be statistically significant even when one point estimate is statistically unreliable.

The chapters that follow summarize key findings. Graphics are used to illustrate observed differences between FSP participants and nonparticipants. Differences that are statistically significant at the 5 percent level or better are indicated on the graphs. Detailed tables provided in Appendices B and C differentiate three levels of statistical significance (p <.001, .01, and .05).

As noted previously, this research was not designed to measure program impacts. Thus, significant differences that do appear between FSP participants and nonparticipants cannot be attributed to participation in the FSP. At the same time, the absence of a significant difference cannot be interpreted as evidence that participation in the FSP has no effect. Accurate assessment of FSP impacts requires specially designed studies or, at a minimum, complex analytical models that require a variety of measures that are not available in the NHANES data.

# Chapter 2

# USUAL DAILY INTAKES OF VITAMINS, MINERALS, AND FIBER

To assess the nutritional adequacy of diets consumed by FSP participants and nonparticipants, we compared usual daily intakes of vitamins, minerals, and fiber consumed in foods to the Dietary Reference Intakes (DRIs) (IOM 1997-2005).[1] The DRIs, developed by the Food and Nutrition Board of the Institute of Medicine (IOM), are the most up-to- date scientific standards for assessing diets of individuals and population groups. The DRIs define different standards for different types of nutrients (see box).

---

**ESTIMATION OF USUAL NUTRIENT INTAKES**

**Data**
- NHANES 1999-2002: Single 24-hour recalls per person
- NHANES 2003-2004: Two separate 24-hour recalls per person

**Methods\***
- Estimate variance components (average day-to-day variation per person) for each nutrient and subgroup using NHANES 2003-04
- Adjust NHANES 1999-2004 single 24-hour recalls using estimated variance components

\* See Appendix A.

---

## VITAMINS AND MINERALS WITH DEFINED ESTIMATED AVERAGE REQUIREMENTS

Estimated Average Requirements (EARs) are specified for all of the nine vitamins examined in this analysis and for four of the minerals (iron, magnesium, phosphorus, and zinc.) Among all persons, the prevalence of adequate usual daily intakes (usual daily intakes equal to or greater than the EAR) was over 90 percent for 7 of these 13 vitamins and minerals (Figure 2-1 and Table 2-1).

---

[1] Nutrient intake data presented do not include contributions from dietary supplements.

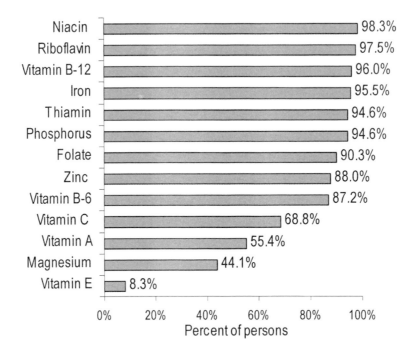

Figure 2-1. Percent of Persons with Adequate Usual Intakes—All Persons

The prevalence of nutrient adequacy was lowest for vitamin E (8.3 percent), followed by magnesium (44.1), vitamin A (55.4) and vitamin C (68.8).

---

**DIETARY REFERENCE INTAKES**

**Estimated Average Requirement (EAR):**
   The usual daily intake level that is estimated to meet the requirement of half the healthy individuals in a life stage and gender group. The proportion of a group with usual daily intakes greater than or equal to the EAR is an estimate of the prevalence of adequate daily intakes in that population group. *[Used to assess usual daily intakes of most vitamins and minerals.]*

**Adequate Intake (AI):**
   The usual daily intake level of apparently healthy people who are maintaining a defined nutritional state or criterion of adequacy. AIs are used when scientific data are insufficient to establish an EAR. When a population group's mean usual daily intake exceeds the AI, the prevalence of inadequate usual daily intakes is likely to be low. However, mean usual daily intakes that fall below the AI do not indicate that the prevalence of inadequacy is high. [Used to assess usual daily intakes of calcium, potassium, sodium, and fiber].

**Tolerable Upper Intake Level (UL):**
   The highest usual daily intake level that is likely to pose no risk of adverse health effects to individuals in the specified life stage group. As usual daily intake increases above the UL, the risk of adverse effects increases. [Used to assess usual daily intakes of sodium. ULs for other nutrients are based on intakes from both food and supplements, and are not examined in this chapter]

See Appendix A for DRI values.

There were no significant differences between FSP participants and income-eligible nonparticipants in the prevalence of adequate usual daily intakes of vitamins and minerals (Table 2-1 ).[2] In contrast, for every vitamin and mineral examined, FSP participants were significantly less likely than higher- income nonparticipants to have adequate usual daily intakes. The magnitude of differences and the absolute levels of adequacy varied across nutrient:

### Table 2-1. Prevalence of Adequate Usual Daily Intakes of Vitamins, Minerals, and Fiber

| | All persons | | | | Children (age 1-18) | | | |
|---|---|---|---|---|---|---|---|---|
| | Total Persons | Food Stamp Program Partic. | Income-eligible Nonpartic. | Higher-income Nonpartic. | Total Persons | Food Stamp Program Partic. | Income-eligible Nonpartic. | Higher-income Nonpartic. |
| **Vitamins** | | | | | | | | |
| Percent > EAR | | | | | | | | |
| Vitamin A | 55.4 | 41.5 | 48.1 | ***59.8 | 75.8 | 69.9 | 70.6 | **78.9 |
| Vitamin C | 68.8 | 60.8 | 64.2 | **70.3 | 87.6 | 87.3 | 89.2 | 86.5 |
| Vitamin B$_6$ | 87.2 | 77.8 | 79.8 | ***89.3 | 96.7 | 93.3 | *96.7 | 97.2 |
| Vitamin B$_{12}$ | 96.0 | 92.5 | 92.2 | **97.0 | 98.6 | 97.3 | 98.0 | 98.9 |
| Vitamin E | 8.3 | 5.5 | 6.8 | **8.9 | 11.9 | 13.1 | 12.1 | 11.4 |
| Folate | 90.3 | 82.4 | 83.8 | ***92.2 | 96.4 | 93.7 | 95.9 | 97.0 |
| Niacin | 98.3 | 94.9 | 95.9 | ***98.8 | 99.4 | 98.1 | 99.3 | *99.5 |
| Riboflavin | 97.5 | 93.4 | 94.6 | ***98.3 | 99.0 | 98.2 | 98.3 | 99.4 |
| Thiamin | 94.6 | 89.0 | 89.8 | ***95.9 | 98.1 | 96.2 | 97.7 | *98.5 |
| **Minerals and Fiber** | | | | | | | | |
| Percent > EAR | | | | | | | | |
| Iron | 95.5 | 92.6 | 93.0 | ***96.4 | 98.0 | 96.7 | 97.6 | **98.3 |
| Magnesium | 44.1 | 33.6 | 38.2 | ***46.8 | 68.0 | 65.5 | 67.3 | 68.4 |
| Phosphorus | 94.6 | 89.9 | 92.2 | ***95.4 | 83.9 | 78.4 | 81.1 | **85.5 |
| Zinc | 88.0 | 80.1 | 80.9 | ***89.8 | 94.3 | 90.7 | 93.0 | *95.0 |
| Mean % AI | | | | | | | | |
| Calcium | 88.1 | 78.2 | 81.1 | ***91.4 | 106.5 | 101.6 | 104.2 | *109.1 |
| Potassium | 57.8 | 52.4 | 54.9 | ***58.9 | 56.3 | 55.7 | 57.7 | 55.7 |
| Sodium | 240.2 | 225.6 | 229.3 | ***244.2 | 230.2 | 230.7 | 233.6 | 227.7 |
| Dietary Fiber | 52.8 | 47.4 | 51.0 | ***53.8 | 46.4 | 44.9 | 47.7 | 46.3 |
| Percent > UL | | | | | | | | |
| Sodium | 86.1 | 78.6 | 80.0 | ***87.9 | 90.6 | 88.6 | 90.7 | 90.4 |

See footnotes on next page.

---

[2] Tables providing detailed data (means, distributions, and comparisons to DRIs) for seven DRI age groups by gender are provided in Appendix D, available on-line at: http:// www.fns.usda.gov.

## Table 2-1. (Continued)

| | Adults (age 19-59) | | | | Older adults (age 60+) | | | |
|---|---|---|---|---|---|---|---|---|
| | Total Persons | Food Stamp Program Partic. | Income-eligible Nonpartic. | Higher-income Nonpartic. | Total Persons | Food Stamp Program Partic. | Income-eligible Nonpartic. | Higher-income Nonpartic. |
| **Vitamins** | | | | | | | | |
| Percent > EAR | | | | | | | | |
| Vitamin A | 45.5 | 27.9 | 37.1 | ***50.7 | 56.1 | 43.8 | 46.4 | **58.6 |
| Vitamin C | 61.4 | 53.6 | 57.4 | 63.7 | 64.3 | 46.5 | 50.8 | **67.6 |
| Vitamin B$_6$ | 87.5 | 78.3 | 79.6 | ***89.8 | 70.3 | 52.0 | 52.8 | **73.9 |
| Vitamin B$_{12}$ | 95.8 | 92.7 | 91.6 | *96.9 | 92.5 | 82.5 | 85.7 | **94.2 |
| Vitamin E | 7.4 | 3.2 u | 5.9 | ***8.8 | 5.6 | 0.5 u | 2.5 u | ***6.0 |
| Folate | 89.1 | 79.9 | 82.9 | ***91.5 | 83.9 | 71.8 | 72.3 | **87.0 |
| Niacin | 98.6 | 95.9 | 97.0 | *99.1 | 95.4 | 88.1 | 88.8 | **96.9 |
| Riboflavin | 97.2 | 92.5 | 93.9 | **98.3 | 96.0 | 87.8 | 91.8 | **97.3 |
| Thiamin | 93.9 | 88.0 | 89.8 | **95.3 | 91.1 | 81.9 | 81.2 | **93.5 |
| **Minerals and Fiber** | | | | | | | | |
| Percent > EAR | | | | | | | | |
| Iron | 93.8 | 88.7 | 89.5 | ***95.3 | 99.6 | 98.1 | 98.8 | 99.7 |
| Magnesium | 38.1 | 24.3 | 30.4 | ***41.9 | 27.1 | 15.3 u | 17.7 | **29.6 |
| Phosphorus | 98.9 | 95.5 | 97.6 | **99.4 | 96.7 | 90.3 | 91.9 | **97.8 |
| Zinc | 88.5 | 83.0 | 80.5 | *90.5 | 74.9 | 56.2 | 61.4 | **78.0 |
| Mean % AI | | | | | | | | |
| Calcium | 87.2 | 75.1 | 79.7 | ***90.9 | 62.0 | 52.1 | 53.6 | ***64.0 |
| Potassium | 59.2 | 52.1 | 55.0 | ***61.2 | 55.4 | 47.0 | 48.6 | ***57.1 |
| Sodium | 247.9 | 228.5 | 232.9 | **253.6 | 229.9 | 207.5 | 211.6 | *235.3 |
| Dietary Fiber | 52.7 | 46.9 | 49.8 | **54.3 | 63.5 | 53.4 | 59.1 | *65.1 |
| Percent > UL | | | | | | | | |
| Sodium | 87.7 | 81.1 | 82.1 | *89.7 | 72.0 | 58.6 | 57.9 | *75.7 |

Notes: Significant differences in means and proportions are noted by * (.05 level), ** (.01 level), or *** (.001 level). Differences are tested in comparison to FSP participants, identified as persons in households receiving food stamps in the past 12 months. See Appendix B for standard errors of estimates.

u Denotes individual estimates not meeting the standards of reliability or precision due to inadequate cell size or large coefficient of variation.

Source: NHANES 1999-2004 dietary recalls. 'Total Persons' includes those with missing FSP participation or income. Data reflect nutrient intake from foods and do not include the contribution of vitamin and mineral supplements. Usual intake was estimated using C-SIDE: Software for Intake Distribution Estimation. Percents are age adjusted to account for different age distributions of FSP participants and nonparticipants.

- Vitamins A, C, and E, and magnesium were the most problematic nutrients for all groups. Nonetheless, the prevalence of adequate usual intakes was consistently and significantly lower for FSP participants than for higher-income nonparticipants (42 percent vs. 60 percent for vitamin A; 61 percent vs. 70 percent for vitamin C; 6 percent vs. 9 percent for vitamin E, and 34 percent versus 47 percent for magnesium).[3]
- For vitamin B6, folate, and zinc, 89 to 92 percent of higher-income nonparticipants had adequate usual intakes, while the percent of FSP participants with adequate intakes was about 10 percentage points lower.
- For Vitamin B12, niacin, riboflavin, thiamin, iron and phosphorus, 90 percent or more of FSP participants and nonparticipants had adequate intake. Nonetheless, FSP participants had somewhat lower prevalence of adequacy compared to higher income nonparticipants.

The prevalence of adequate usual intakes among children was consistently higher, for all vitamins and minerals, relative to adults and older adults. In addition, there are fewer statistically significant differences between FSP children and higher- income children, and between-group differences were smaller. FSP children were less likely than higher-income children to have adequate usual intakes of vitamin A (70 percent vs. 79 percent), vitamin $B_6$ (93 percent vs. 97 percent), iron (97 percent vs. 98 percent), phosphorus (78 percent vs. 86 percent), and zinc (91 percent vs. 95 percent) (Table 2-1).

The results for adults and older adults, assessed separately, are consistent with differences between FSP participants and higher-income nonparticipants for the full sample, except for vitamin C for adults and vitamin A and iron for older adults (Table 2-1).

## NUTRIENTS ASSESSED USING ADEQUATE INTAKE LEVELS

EARs are not defined for calcium, potassium, sodium, or fiber so it is not possible to assess the adequacy of usual daily intakes. Populations with mean usual daily intakes that meet or exceed Adequate Intake (AI) levels defined for these nutrients can be assumed to have high levels of adequacy. However, no firm conclusions can be drawn about levels of adequacy when mean usual daily intakes fall below the AI.

Because excessive sodium intakes may increase risk of hypertension, sodium intakes are also assessed relative to the Tolerable Upper Intake Level (UL). Individuals with usual daily intakes that exceed the UL may be at increased risk of developing hypertension.

## Calcium

There were no significant differences between FSP participants and income-eligible nonparticipants in mean usual daily intakes of calcium expressed as a percentage of the AI

---

[3] The low prevalence of adequate intakes of vitamin E is consistent with most recent studies. Devaney and colleagues pointed out that vitamin E deficiency is rare in the U.S., despite low measured intakes, and suggested that the EARs for vitamin E may need to be reassessed (Devaney et al. 2007).

(Table 2-1). FSP participants, however, had significantly lower intakes of calcium compared with higher-income nonparticipants (78 percent of the AI vs. 91 percent) (Figure 2-2).

Differences between FSP participants and higher-income nonparticipants were observed for all three age groups. Among children, mean usual daily intakes exceeded 100 percent of the AI for FSP participants and both groups of nonparticipants, indicating that the prevalence of adequate usual daily intakes was likely to have been high for all groups of children.

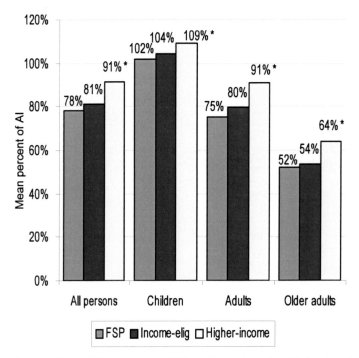

* Denotes statistically significant difference from FSP participants at the .05 level or better. Estimates are age adjusted.

Figure 2-2. Mean Usual Daily Intakes as Percents of Adequate Intake (AI)—Calcium.

## Potassium

FSP participants and income-eligible nonparticipants had comparable mean usual daily intakes of potassium expressed as a percentage of the AI (Table 2-1). FSP participants, however, had significantly lower usual intakes of potassium compared with higher-income nonparticipants (52 percent of the AI vs. 59 percent) (Figure 2-3). This difference was concentrated among adults and older adults. The differences in mean usual daily intakes of potassium do not necessarily imply that FSP participants were less likely than higher- income nonparticipants to have adequate usual intakes.

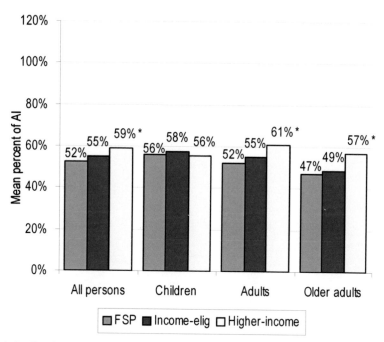

* Denotes statistically significant difference from FSP participants at the .05 level or better. Estimates
  are age adjusted.

Figure 2-3. Mean Usual Daily Intakes as Percents of Adequate Intake (AI)—Potassium

## Sodium

Mean usual daily sodium intakes of both FSP participants and higher-income nonparticipants were more than twice the AI (Table 2.1). In addition, more than three-quarters of both groups had usual daily sodium intakes that exceeded the UL. FSP participants, however, had a lower mean usual sodium intake than higher-income nonparticipants (226 percent of the AI vs. 244 percent) and were less likely to have usual sodium intakes that exceeded the UL (79 percent versus 88 percent) (Table 2-1).

## Fiber

Usual daily fiber intakes were examined in two ways—(1) mean intakes, expressed as a percentage of the AI, and (2) mean intakes, expressed on a gram-per-calorie basis. The standard used to establish AIs for fiber was 14 grams per 1,000 calories, based on the median energy intake of specific age-and-gender subgroups, as reported in the 1994-96, 98 Continuing Survey of Food Intakes by Individuals (CSFII) (IOM, 2005b).

Mean usual daily intakes of fiber for all persons was about 50 percent of the AI (Table 2-1) — about half of the recommended 14 grams per 1,000 calories (Table B-18). On a gram-per-1,000 calorie basis, FSP participants had lower mean usual daily intakes of fiber compared with both income-eligible nonparticipants and higher-income nonparticipants (6.6 vs. 7.2 and 7.3) (Figure 2-4). The between- group differences were significant overall and for adults, but not for children and older adults.

Usual daily fiber intakes of all groups were low, relative to the AIs; even the 95th percentile of the distribution of usual fiber intake was less than the AI. This pattern has been reported by others (Fox and Cole, 2004; Devaney et al., 2007; and Devaney et al., 2005). Part of the discrepancy is due to the fact that the AIs are defined for *total* fiber, but food composition databases are limited to information on *dietary* fiber.[4] However, the magnitude of this discrepancy is relatively small compared to the gap between usual intakes and the AIs. For this reason, some have suggested that the methods used to establish the AIs for fiber may need to be reexamined, especially for children and adolescents (Devaney et al., 2007).[5]

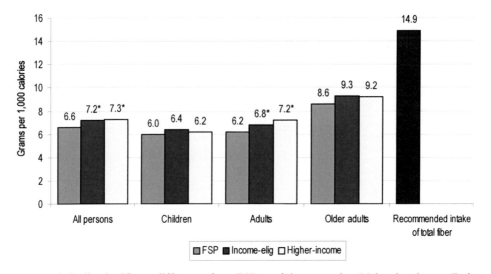

* Denotes statistically significant difference from FSP participants at the .05 level or better. Estimates
   are age adjusted.

Figure 2-4. Mean Usual Daily Intakes of Dietary Fiber (grams per 1,000 calories)

## USE OF DIETARY SUPPLEMENTS

NHANES 1999-2004 collected detailed data about the use of dietary supplements. Respondents were first asked whether they used any dietary supplements during the past 30 days. To help them answer this question, respondents were handed a card defining 13 types of supplements, including single and multiple vitamin or mineral products; antacid taken as a calcium supplement; fiber taken as a dietary supplement; botanicals, herbs, and herbal medicine products; amino acids; and fish oils.6 Respondents who reported supplement use were asked to show the actual bottles or jars to interviewers so the type of supplement and associated dosage information could be recorded.

---

[4] It is estimated that adults consume about 5.1 more grams per day of fiber than estimated from current food composition databases (IOM, 2005a).

[5] The data used to establish AIs are drawn from studies of coronary heart disease risk among adults. Moreover, the AIs for children are 2 to 3 times higher than the standard previously used to assess fiber intake in this age group (Devaney et al., 2007).

[6] NHANES Documentation: Dietary Supplement Data, 1999- 2000, 2001-02, and 2003-04.

Because data on dietary intake and supplement use were collected for different reference periods (preceding 24 hours and preceding month, respectively) combining the two data sets is not straightforward. Consequently NHANES 1999-2004 dietary intake data do not include contributions from dietary supplements.[7] For this reason, estimates of the proportions of individuals with adequate usual daily intakes may be understated. In addition, observed differences in usual daily intakes of FSP participants and higher-income nonparticipants are probably understated because the prevalence of dietary supplement use is different in the two groups. Data about the prevalence and patterns of dietary supplement use can provide useful insights into the potential influence of supplements on the adequacy of usual daily intakes.

Overall, and for all age groups, FSP participants were significantly less likely than higher-income nonparticipants to use dietary supplements (Figure 2-5). Among children and older adults, FSP participants were also significantly less likely to use supplements than income-eligible nonparticipants.

The most commonly reported type of supplement was a vitamin/mineral combination, followed by single vitamins, other types of supplements (for example, fish oils, herbs, and botanicals), single minerals, and multi-vitamins without minerals (Table 2-2). Thirty-four percent of all persons reported a vitamin/mineral combination (73 percent of those using supplements). FSP participants were less likely than nonparticipants to report any supplements, and therefore, less likely to report every type of supplement. The distribution of persons by type of supplement sums to more than 100 because some persons reported multiple types of supplements.

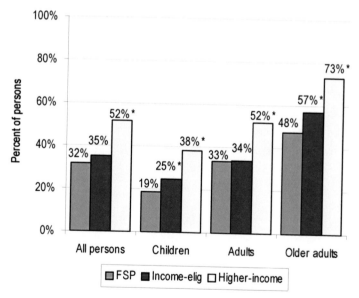

* Denotes statistically significant difference from FSP participants at the .05 level or better. Estimates are age adjusted.

Figure 2-5. Prevalence of Dietary Supplement Use in Past Month

---

[7] Carriquiry (2003) recommends collecting information about supplement use (past 30 days), combined with information about supplement intakes collected during the 24-hour recall. This approach is currently being used in collecting data for NHANES 2007-08.

Among those who used supplements, more than half reported one supplement, 20 percent reported two supplements, and 24 percent reported three or more supplements (Table 2-2).

The distribution of FSP participants by number of supplements was significantly different than higher income nonparticipants for all age groups, and significantly different from older adult income- eligible nonparticipants. FSP participants in all age groups were less likely than higher-income nonparticipants to use three or more supplements.

Since higher income nonparticipants reported greater supplement use than FSP participants, observed differences in the prevalence of adequate usual intakes may be understated. That is, the proportions of higher-income nonparticipants with adequate usual intakes may be larger than estimated. The same is true for the proportions of income-eligible children and older adults.

## SUMMARY

Data from NHANES 1999-2004 were analyzed to examine the prevalence of adequate intakes of 13 vitamins and minerals with defined EARs. The prevalence of adequate intakes cannot be assessed for calcium, potassium, sodium, and fiber; however, mean intakes relative to AIs provide an indication of the levels of adequate intakes. Overall findings include:

- Over 90 percent of the U.S. population receives from their diet adequate usual daily intakes of 7 essential vitamins and minerals.
- Usual intakes of Vitamins A, C, E, and magnesium need improvement.
- Mean usual intake of calcium were 100, 88, and 62 percent of the AI for children, adults, and older adults, respectively. Indicating high prevalence of adequate intakes for children and declining prevalence of adequate intake with age.
- Mean usual intakes of potassium and fiber are only 50 to 60 percent of Adequate Intakes, indicating deficiencies for some portion of the population.
- Sodium intakes are of concern, with nearly 90 percent of the population having usual intake in excess of the UL.
- Fiber intakes are of concern, with mean usual intakes equal to half of the recommended 14 grams of fiber per 1,000 calories.

There were no significant differences between FSP participants and income-eligible nonparticipants in the prevalence of adequate usual intakes of vitamins and minerals, or in mean usual intake of calcium, potassium, sodium, and fiber. In contrast, compared with higher-income nonparticipants, FSP participants had lower prevalence of adequate intake for the 13 vitamins and minerals with defined EARs, and lower mean usual intakes of calcium, potassium, sodium, and fiber, also fewer differences in the prevalence of adequate intakes between FSP participants and higher-income nonparticipants among children.

It is not possible to estimate the contribution of dietary supplements to usual daily intakes using the NHANES data. Nonetheless, NHANES data indicate that supplements are used by 47 percent of the population. Supplement use increases with age. FSP participants and income-eligible nonparticipants are about equally likely to use supplements; but these low-income groups are less likely to use supplements than higher-income nonparticipants.

# Table 2-2. Prevalence of Dietary Supplement Use in Past Month

| | All persons | | | | Children (age 1-18) | | | |
|---|---|---|---|---|---|---|---|---|
| | Total Persons | Food Stamp Program Partic. | Income-eligible Nonpartic. | Higher-income Nonpartic. | Total Persons | Food Stamp Program Partic. | Income-eligible Nonpartic. | Higher-income Nonpartic. |
| Sample size | 25,129 | 4,015 | 5,365 | 13,914 | 11,859 | 2,641 | 2,735 | 5,720 |
| Used supplements last month | 46.5 | 31.9 | 35.3 | ***51.6 | 32.0 | 18.9 | *24.6 | ***38.4 |
| Type of supplements[1] | | | | | | | | |
| None | 53.4 | 68.0 | 64.7 | 48.2 | 67.8 | 81.0 | 75.3 | 61.4 |
| Single vitamin | 16.4 | 9.0 | 11.4 | 18.4 | 4.9 | 1.9 | 3.9 | 6.2 |
| Multiple vitamin | 5.3 | 2.4 | 3.5 | 6.2 | 4.1 | 1.9 | 3.1 | 5.0 |
| Single mineral | 13.0 | 8.7 | 9.8 | 14.1 | 3.4 | 2.5 | 3.5 | 3.6 |
| Vitamin/ mineral combo | 34.1 | 21.2 | 23.5 | 38.7 | 22.7 | 13.7 | 16.3 | 27.9 |
| Other | 14.4 | 8.5 | 10.8 | 15.8 | 3.3 | 0.7 | 3.0 | 3.9 |
| Among those using supplements Number of supplements | | | | | | | | |
| One | 56.1 | 65.8 | †59.2 | †54.6 | 81.6 | 92.0 | 83.2 | †79.6 |
| Two | 20.2 | 18.5 | 20.8 | 20.7 | 13.2 | 7.9 | 10.8 | 14.7 |
| Three+ | 23.7 | 15.7 | 20.0 | 24.7 | 5.2 | 0.2 u | 6.0 u | 5.7 |

| | Adults (age 19-59) | | | | Older adults (age 60+) | | | |
|---|---|---|---|---|---|---|---|---|
| | Total Persons | Food Stamp Program Partic. | Income-eligible Nonpartic. | Higher-income Nonpartic. | Total Persons | Food Stamp Program Partic. | Income-eligible Nonpartic. | Higher-income Nonpartic. |
| Sample size | 8,558 | 1,021 | 1,629 | 5,304 | 4,712 | 353 | 1,001 | 2,890 |
| Used supplements last month | 46.7 | 33.4 | 33.7 | ***51.6 | 68.6 | 47.5 | *57.1 | ***72.9 |
| Type of supplements[1] | | | | | | | | |
| None | 53.2 | 66.6 | 66.3 | 48.3 | 31.4 | 52.4 | 42.8 | 27.0 |
| Single vitamin | 16.2 | 9.2 | 11.1 | 18.1 | 35.4 | 19.7 | 24.0 | 39.1 |
| Multiple vitamin | 4.9 | 1.9 | 3.2 | 5.7 | 8.6 | 5.2 u | 5.6 | 9.9 |
| Single mineral | 13.7 | 10.4 | 9.2 | 15.1 | 25.5 | 12.4 | 21.4 | 27.2 |
| Vitamin/ mineral combo | 34.5 | 22.4 | 21.8 | 39.1 | 50.6 | 28.8 | 40.2 | 54.4 |
| Other | 15.9 | 11.6 | 11.4 | 17.5 | 26.6 | 9.6 | 21.6 | 28.8 |
| Among those using supplements Number of supplements | | | | | | | | |
| One | 50.7 | 56.0 | 53.7 | †49.5 | 35.0 | 58.6 | †40.8 | †33.1 |
| Two | 22.4 | 23.7 | 24.5 | 22.4 | 23.6 | 17.0 | 24.1 | 24.1 |
| Three+ | 27.0 | 20.3 | 21.8 | 28.1 | 41.4 | 24.5 | 35.1 | 42.8 |

Notes: For "Used supplements last month", significant differences between proportions of FSP participants and each group of nonparticipants were identified with t-tests and are noted by * (.05 level), ** (.01 level), or *** (.001 level). For "Number of supplements", significant differences in the distribution of FSP participants and each group of nonparticipants were identified with chi-square tests and are noted by †.

FSP participants are identified as persons in households receiving food stamps in the past 12 months.

1 Significance test not done because categories are not mutually exclusive for persons who take multiple supplements.

u Denotes individual estimates not meeting the standards of reliability or precision due to inadequate cell size or large coefficient of variation.

Source: NHANES 1999–2004 sample of persons with complete dietary recalls. Excludes pregnant and breastfeeding women and infants. 'Total Persons' includes persons with missing food stamp participation or income. Percents are age adjusted to account for different age distributions of Food Stamp participants and nonparticipants

*Chapter 3*

# ENERGY INTAKES

In this chapter, we examine mean usual daily energy (calorie) intakes, and the sources of energy intakes, for FSP participants and nonparticipants. We use several measures to examine the sources of energy intakes. These include usual daily intakes of macronutrients (total fat, saturated fat, carbohydrate, and protein) expressed as percentages of usual energy intakes, and 24-hour intakes of discretionary calories from solid fats, alcoholic beverages, and added sugars. We also examine the energy density (calories per gram of food) of 24- hour intakes.

We conclude the chapter with measures of Body Mass Index (BMI) and BMI-for-age (for children). These measures are used to assess the appropriateness of usual daily energy intakes, as recommended by the Institute of Medicine (IOM, 2005a).[1] Because energy consumed in excess of requirements is stored as body fat, the BMI provides a reliable indicator of the extent to which long-run (usual) energy intakes were consistent with or exceeded energy requirements.

Some of the analyses presented in this chapter exclude children 1 year of age: (1) usual daily intakes of energy from saturated fat, (2) 24-hour intakes of discretionary calories from solid fats, alcoholic beverages, and added sugars, and (3) BMI-for-age. The standards used in these analyses apply only to children 2 years of age and older.

Mean daily energy intakes are shown in Figure 3-1. There were no significant differences between FSP participants and income-eligible nonparticipants in mean daily energy intakes This was true for children, adults, and older adults. FSP participants had a significantly lower mean energy intake than higher-income nonparticipants (2,068 calories vs. 2,186 calories).

This difference in the overall population was due to a difference among older adults (1,583 calories vs. 1,814 calories), which was concentrated among older adult males (Table B-1). Among children and adults, FSP participants and higher-income nonparticipants had comparable mean daily energy intakes.

---

[1] BMI is recommended for assessing usual energy intakes because: (1) energy intakes are often underreported, (2) an individual's estimated energy requirement (EER) is strongly influenced by physical activity, which is not measured precisely in most surveys (including NHANES 1999-2002), and (3) the EER is an estimate of energy requirement but actual energy requirements vary among individuals (IOM, 2005a).

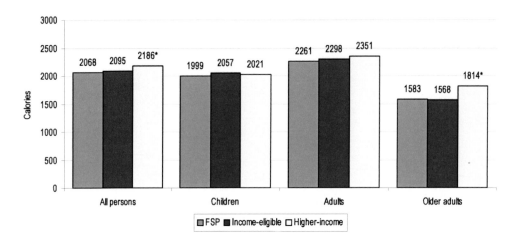

Figure 3-1. Mean Daily Energy Intakes

It is difficult to assess the adequacy of mean daily energy intakes because there is a wide range of energy requirements for age/gender groups depending on body measurement and activity level (Table 3-1). Activity levels are not adequately measured by most surveys, including NHANES 1999-2002. Thus, the IOM recommends that measures of BMI be used to assess the adequacy of energy intakes (IOM, 2005a). Data on BMI are presented later in this chapter.

## MEAN DAILY ENERGY INTAKES

| MEASURES OF ENERGY INTAKES | | |
|---|---|---|
| Measure | Data | Age[a] |
| *Estimates based on 24-hr intakes:* | | |
| 1. Mean daily energy intakes | NHANES 1999-2004 | 1+ |
| 2. Percent of energy from SoFAAS (solid fats, alcoholic beverages, and added sugars) | MyPyramid 1999-2002 | 2+ |
| 3. Energy density of daily intakes | NHANES 1999-2004 | 1+ |
| 4. Weight status (Body Mass Index) as indicator of long run adequacy of energy intakes | NHANES 1999-2004 | 2+ |
| *Estimates based on usual intakes:* | | |
| 5. Percent of energy from: | | |
| • Total fat, protein, carbohydrates (relative to AMDRs) | NHANES 1999-2004 | 1+ |
| • Saturated fat (relative to DGA) | | 2+ |

*The following reference standards apply only to persons age 2 and above: Dietary Guidelines for saturated fat, MyPyramid National growth charts for BMI. recommendations for SoFAAS, and

\* Denotes statistically significant difference from FSP participants at the .05 level or better. Estimates are age adjusted.

# USUAL DAILY INTAKES OF ENERGY FROM MACRONUTRIENTS

To gain insights into the sources of energy in the diets of FSP participants and nonparticipants, we examined energy intakes for macronutrients relative to Acceptable Macronutrient Distribution Ranges (AMDRs) defined in the DRIs (total fat, carbohydrate, and protein) and the 2005 *Dietary Guidelines for Americans* recommendation for saturated fat (IOM, 2005 a and USDHHS/USDA, 2005). We also examined intake of discretionary calories from solid fats, alcoholic beverages, and added sugars.

**Table 3-1. Estimated Energy Requirements for Age/Gender Groups by Activity Level**

| Age | Sedentary | Moderately Active | Active |
|---|---|---|---|
| *Females* | | | |
| 2-3 | 1,000 | 1,000-1,200 | 1,000-1,400 |
| 4-8 | 1,200-1,400 | 1,400-1,600 | 1,400-1,800 |
| 9-13 | 1,400-1,600 | 1,600-2,000 | 1,800-2,200 |
| 14-18 | 1,800 | 2,000 | 2,400 |
| 19-30 | 1,800-2,000 | 2,000-2,200 | 2,400 |
| 31-50 | 1,800 | 2,000 | 2,200 |
| 51+ | 1,600 | 1,800 | 2,000-2,200 |
| *Males* | | | |
| 2-3 | 1,000 | 1,000-1,400 | 1,000-1,400 |
| 4-8 | 1,200-1,400 | 1,400-1,600 | 1,600-2,000 |
| 9-13 | 1,600-2,000 | 1,800-2,200 | 2,000-2,600 |
| 14-18 | 2,000-2,400 | 2,400-2,800 | 2,800-3,200 |
| 19-30 | 2,400-2,600 | 2,600-2,800 | 3,000 |
| 31-50 | 2,200-2,400 | 2,400-2,600 | 2,800-3,000 |
| 51+ | 2,000-2,200 | 2,200-2,400 | 2,400-2,800 |

Source: http://www.mypyramid.gov/downloads/ MyPyramid_Calorie_Levels.pdf

AMDRs define a range of usual daily intakes that is associated with reduced risk of chronic disease while providing adequate intakes of essential nutrients (IOM, 2005a). AMDRs are expressed as a percentage of total energy intake. If an individual's usual daily intake is above or below the AMDR, risks of chronic disease and/or insufficient intake of essential nutrients are increased.[2]

---

[2] Usual intakes of macronutrients as a percent of energy were estimated using the same methods described in Chapter 2 for estimating usual intake distributions.

## Table 3-2. Usual Daily Intakes of Macronutrients Compared to Standards

| | All persons | | | | Children (age 1–18) | | | |
|---|---|---|---|---|---|---|---|---|
| | Total Persons | Food Stamp Program Partic. | Income-eligible Nonpartic. | Higher-income Nonpartic. | Total Persons | Food Stamp Program Partic. | Income-eligible Nonpartic. | Higher-income Nonpartic. |
| **Percent of Persons** | | | | | | | | |
| Total Fat | | | | | | | | |
| % < AMDR | 2.1 | 2.6 | 2.3 | 2.1 | 6.4 | 5.5 | 6.0 | 6.8 |
| % within AMDR | 66.0 | 68.0 | 68.6 | 65.3 | 73.4 | 68.4 | 70.2 | 75.2 |
| % > AMDR | 31.9 | 29.4 | 29.1 | 32.5 | 20.2 | 26.1 | 23.8 | * 18.0 |
| Protein | | | | | | | | |
| % < AMDR | 1.6 | 3.9 | 2.6 | ** 1.2 | 1.3 | 1.9 u | 1.5 u | 1.3 |
| % within AMDR | 98.3 | 96.1 | 97.4 | ** 98.8 | 98.5 | 98.0 | 98.4 | 98.6 |
| % > AMDR | 0.0 u | 0.0 u | 0.0 u | 0.0 u | 0.1 u | 0.1 u | 0.1 u | 0.1 u |
| Carbohydrate | | | | | | | | |
| % < AMDR | 16.4 | 13.0 | 11.6 | * 17.6 | 1.8 | 2.7 | 2.5 | 1.5 |
| % within AMDR | 82.1 | 83.9 | 86.0 | 81.2 | 96.6 | 95.7 | 96.1 | 96.8 |
| % > AMDR | 1.5 | 3.1 | 2.3 | ** 1.2 | 1.6 | 1.6 u | 1.4 u | 1.7 |
| Saturated fat, % < DGA | 31.0 | 32.3 | 37.0 | 29.9 | 16.7 | 14.5 | 15.9 | 18.0 |

| | Adults (age 19–59) | | | | Older adults (age 60+) | | | |
|---|---|---|---|---|---|---|---|---|
| | Total Persons | Food Stamp Program Partic. | Income-eligible Nonpartic. | Higher-income Nonpartic. | Total Persons | Food Stamp Program Partic. | Income-eligible Nonpartic. | Higher-income Nonpartic. |
| **Percent of Persons** | | | | | | | | |
| Total Fat | | | | | | | | |
| % < AMDR | 0.7 | 1.5 u | 1.0 u | 0.6 | 0.6 u | 2.4 u | 0.9 u | 0.5 u |
| % within AMDR | 62.7 | 69.1 | 70.2 | * 60.0 | 60.4 | 62.8 | 61.5 | 60.0 |
| % > AMDR | 36.6 | 29.4 | 28.8 | * 39.4 | 38.9 | 34.8 | 37.6 | 39.5 |
| Protein | | | | | | | | |
| % < AMDR | 2.2 | 6.6 | 4.4 | ** 1.4 | 0.2 u | 0.4 u | 0.2 u | 0.2 u |
| % within AMDR | 97.8 | 93.4 | 95.6 | ** 98.6 | 99.8 | 99.6 | 99.8 | 99.8 |
| % > AMDR | 0.0 | 0.0 | 0.0 | 0.0 | 0.0 | 0.0 | 0.0 | 0.0 |
| Carbohydrate | | | | | | | | |
| % < AMDR | 24.9 | 19.0 | 16.1 | ** 27.6 | 20.7 | 17.1 | 16.7 | 21.6 |
| % within AMDR | 72.6 | 75.6 | 79.2 | 70.8 | 77.5 | 77.8 | 81.0 | 76.8 |
| % > AMDR | 2.4 | 5.4 | 4.7 | ** 1.6 | 1.9 | 5.1 u | 2.3 u | 1.5 |
| Saturated fat, % < DGA | 34.8 | 38.0 | 45.6 | 32.2 | 40.2 | 41.0 | 38.8 | 40.7 |

Notes: Significant differences in means and proportions are noted by * (.05 level), ** (.01 level), or ***
(.001 level). Differences are tested in comparison to FSP participants, identified as persons in
households receiving food stamps in the past 12 months. See Appendix B for standard errors of
estimates.

u Denotes individual estimates not meeting the standards of reliability or precision due to inadequate
cell size or large coefficient of variation.

Source: NHANES 1999–2004 dietary recalls. 'Total Persons' includes those with missing FSP
participation or income. Data reflect nutrient intake from foods and do not include the contribution
of vitamin and mineral supplements. Usual intake was estimated using *C-SIDE: Software for
Intake Distribution Estimation.* Percents are age adjusted to account for different age distributions
of FSP participants and nonparticipants.

Usual daily fat intakes of 66 percent of all persons were consistent with the AMDR (Table 3-2). Overall, there were no significant differences between FSP participants and either group of nonparticipants in the extent to which usual daily intakes of fat exceeded or fell below the AMDR. Adult FSP participants, however, were significantly less likely than higher-income adults to have usual daily fat intakes that exceeded the AMDR (29 percent vs. 39 percent). That is, FSP adults were less likely than higher-income nonparticipant adults to consume more total fat than recommended (Figure 3-2).

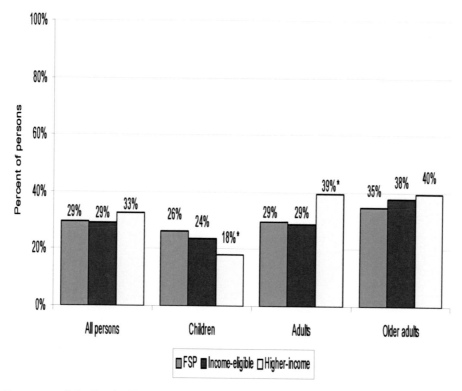

\* Denotes statistically significant difference from FSP participants at the .05 level or better. Estimates are age adjusted.

Figure 3-2. Percent of Persons with Usual Daily Intakes of Total Fat Above the AMDR

We assessed usual daily intakes of saturated fat relative to the 2005 *Dietary Guidelines* recommendation that saturated fat account for less than 10 percent of total calories (USDHHS/USDA, 2005).[3] There were no significant differences between FSP participants and either group of nonparticipants in the percentage of individuals whose usual daily intake of saturated fat met the *Dietary Guidelines* recommendation. In all three participant groups, the percentage of children who met this standard was substantially lower than the percentage of adults (15-18 percent vs. 32 to 46 percent) (Table 3-2).

---

[3] The DRIs do not include quantitative standards for saturated fat. Dietary Guidelines recommendations are intended for adults and children over 2 years of age (USDHHS/USDA, 2005). For this reason, children up to 24 months are excluded from comparisons of usual daily intakes of saturated fat to the Dietary Guidelines standard.

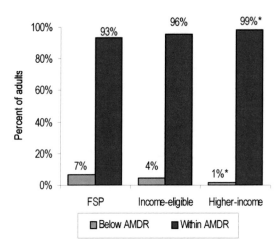

* Denotes statistically significant difference from FSP participants at the .05 level or better. Estimates are age adjusted. Between-group differences for children and older adults were not statistically significant.

Figure 3-3. Percent of Adults with Usual Daily Intakes of Protein Relative to the AMDR

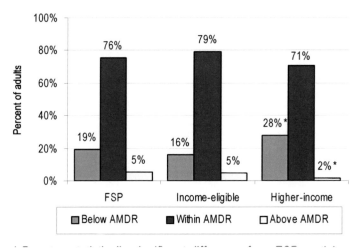

* Denotes statistically significant difference from FSP participants at the .05 level or better. Estimates are age adjusted. Between-group differences for children and older adults were not statistically significant.

Figure 3-4. Percent of Adults with Usual Daily Intakes of Carbohydrates Relative to the AMDR

## 24-HOUR INTAKES OF ENERGY FROM SOLID FATS, ALCOHOLIC BEVERAGES, AND ADDED SUGARS

Dietary patterns recommended in the *Dietary Guidelines for Americans* and *MyPyramid* food guidance system include specific discretionary calorie allowances based on energy needs for age and gender groups. Discretionary calories are defined as calories that can be used flexibly after nutrient requirements are met (Britten, 2006).[4] The allowances are based on estimated energy needs and calories in the most nutrient dense form (fat- free or lowest fat form, with no added sugars) of the various foods needed to meet recommended nutrient intakes (Basiotis et al., 2006).

The most generous allowance for discretionary calories in the *MyPyramid* food intake patterns (based on age, gender, and level of physical activity) is 20 percent of total energy needs (for physically active boys age 14 to 18). Table 3-3 shows discretionary calorie allowances for sedentary individuals by age group.

**Table 3-3. Estimated Discretionary Calorie Allowances for Sedentary Individuals**

| Gender / age group | Estimated daily calorie needs | Estimated discretionary calorie allowance | Discretionary calories as percent of total |
|---|---|---|---|
| Children | | | |
| 2-3 yrs | 1000 | 165 | 16.5% |
| 4-8 yrs | 1300 | 170 | 13.1 |
| Females | | | |
| 9-13 yrs | 1600 | 130 | 8.1 |
| 14-18 yrs | 1800 | 195 | 10.8 |
| 19-30 yrs | 2000 | 265 | 13.3 |
| 31-50 yrs | 1800 | 195 | 10.8 |
| 51+ yrs | 1600 | 130 | 8.1 |
| Males | | | |
| 9-13 yrs | 1800 | 195 | 10.8 |
| 14-18 yrs | 2200 | 290 | 13.2 |
| 19-30 yrs | 2400 | 360 | 15.0 |
| 31-50 yrs | 2200 | 290 | 13.2 |
| 51+ yrs | 2000 | 265 | 13.3 |

*Source:* www.MyPyramid.gov/pyramid/discretionary_calories_amount.html

A method for assessing discretionary energy intake was introduced by USDA's Center for Nutrition Policy and Promotion (CNPP) (Basiotis et al., 2006). CNPP measured discretionary calories from SoFAAS (solid fats, alcoholic beverages, and added sugar) using data from the NHANES Individual Foods Files (energy and grams of alcohol) and MyPyramid Equivalents database (discretionary solid fats and added sugars). Following CNPP, we used these measures to compute the total number of calories provided by SoFAAS for FSP participants and nonparticipants based on 24-hour intakes (see Appendix A). Total calories from SoFAAS should be viewed as lower-bound estimates of discretionary energy intake because discretionary calories may also come from additional amounts of the nutrient-dense foods recommended in the *MyPyramid* food intake patterns.

On average, FSP participants obtained a significantly greater share of their daily energy intake from SoFAAS than either income-eligible or higher- income nonparticipants (Figure 3-5 and Table C-1). On average, 41 percent of FSP participants' daily energy intake was contributed by SoFAAS, compared with 39 and 38 percent for income-eligible and higher-

---

[4] Individuals may satisfy nutrient requirements with the fewest calories by eating nutrient dense foods. Calories remaining in their estimated energy requirement are discretionary.

income nonparticipants, respectively. Differences for the overall populations reflect differences among adults; for children and older adults, there were no significant differences between FSP participants and either group of nonparticipants in the mean proportion of usual energy intakes contributed by SoFAAS (Figure 3-5).

## ENERGY DENSITY

The *Dietary Guidelines* stresses the importance of consuming foods so that individuals stay within their energy needs. In developing the 2005 edition of the Guidelines, the *Dietary Guidelines Advisory Committee* concluded that, while the available scientific data were insufficient to determine the contribution of energy dense foods to unhealthy weight gain and obesity, there was suggestive evidence that consuming energy dense meals may contribute to excessive caloric intake and that, conversely, eating foods of low energy density may be a helpful strategy to reduce energy intake when trying to maintain or lose weight (USDHHS/USDA, 2005).

The energy density of a food is equivalent to the available food energy per unit weight (e.g., calories per gram). The energy density of individual foods depends on the composition of the food: the relative concentration of energy-providing nutrients (fat, carbohydrate, protein), alcohol (which provides almost as many calories per gm as fat), and water. Water content may be the single most influential characteristic in determining energy density (Drewnowski, 2005). For example, whole grains and cereal, which have low water content, are energy dense, while fruits, vegetables, and milk, which have high water content, are energy dilute. Beverages, which are mostly water, may have comparable energy densities despite important differences in nutrient content. For example, orange juice, 1% milk, and regular cola all provide roughly 0.43 kcal per gm (Drewnowski and Specter, 2004).

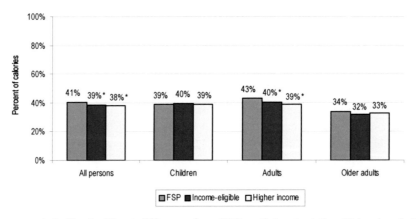

* Denotes statistically significant difference from FSP participants at the .05 level or better. Estimates are age adjusted.
Note: Calories from alcohol include calories from carbohydrate in beer and wine, and calories from grams of alcohol in all alcoholic beverages except cooking wine.

Figure 3-5. Average Percent of Energy from Solid Fats, Alcoholic Beverages, and Added Sugars (SoFAAS)

Assessing the energy density of combinations of foods (the total diet) is not straightforward.[5] There is no scientific consensus about which of several potential approaches should be used. We estimated energy density using a method that considers only foods—solid items and liquid/soft items that are typically consumed as foods, such as soups and ice cream—and excludes all beverages.

For FSP participants and both groups of nonparticipants, energy density of the diet decreased as age increased (Figure 3-6 and Table C-2). This is consistent with general trends in energy requirements—children, whose diets must support ongoing growth and physical development, have greater energy needs than adults.

Overall, there were no significant differences in the mean energy density of foods consumed by FSP participants and income-eligible nonparticipants (Figure 3-6). Adult FSP participants, however, had diets with higher mean energy density, compared with adult higher-income nonparticipants (1.74 calories per gram versus 1.69 calories per gram); this difference was due to a difference among females. Mean energy densities of children and older adults were comparable for FSP participants and higher-income nonparticipants.

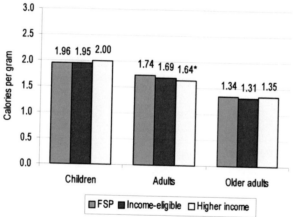

* Denotes statistically significant difference from FSP participants at the .05 level or better. Estimates are age adjusted.

Figure 3-6. Mean Energy Density of Foods

# BODY MASS INDEX AS AN INDICATOR OF THE APPROPRIATENESS OF USUAL DAILY ENERGY INTAKES

BMI is a measure of the relationship between weight and height and is the commonly accepted index for classifying adiposity (fatness) (Kuczmarski and Flegal, 2000).[6] Individuals

---

[5] Ledikwe et al. (2005) compared eight approaches to estimating the energy density of the total diet: one approach included only foods, and seven included foods and various combinations of beverages. They concluded that inclusion of all beverages may result in meaningless measures of energy density if drinking water is not included because persons vary with respect to their source of liquids and energy density will be overstated for persons consuming (unmeasured) drinking water. Dietary surveys (including NHANES 99-02) generally do not collect information on water intake.

[6] BMI = Weight (kg) ÷ Height (m)2.

can be assigned to one of four weight categories based on guidelines from the Centers for Disease Control and Prevention (CDC) (Table 3-4). A BMI in the healthy range indicates that usual daily energy intake is consistent with requirements; a BMI below the healthy range indicates inadequate usual daily energy intake; and a BMI above the healthy range indicates that usual daily energy intake exceeds requirements.

We assigned NHANES sample members to weight categories based on their BMI. Among all persons, 2.3 percent were classified with a BMI below the healthy range, 42 percent were classified with healthy weight, and 56 percent with BMI above the healthy range (Table C-3).

As shown in Table 3-4, adults with BMI above the healthy range are classified as overweight or obese; children are classified as "at risk for overweight" or overweight. CDC does not use the term "obese" for children due to uncertainty in identifying children during critical periods of growth as having true excess body fat, versus lean muscle and large frame, based on BMI.

Among all age groups, the distribution of BMIs for FSP participants was significantly different from the BMI distributions of both income-eligible and higher-income nonparticipants (Figure 3-7 and Table C-3). Data on BMI are presented separately for males and females because findings differed substantially by gender. Differences between FSP participants and income-eligible nonparticipants were largely due to females. Differences between FSP participants and higher income nonparticipants were observed for both males and females, but the nature of the differences was not the same.

### Table 3-4. Weight Categories Based on BMI

|  | Adults | Children[a] |
|---|---|---|
| Underweight | BMI <18.5 | BMI < 5th % |
| Healthy weight | $18.5 \leq BMI <25$ | 5th % $\leq$ BMI < 85th % |
| At risk for overweight | n.a. | 85th % $\leq$ BMI < 95th % |
| Overweight | $25 \leq BMI < 30$ | BMI $\geq$ 95th % |
| Obese | BMI $\geq$ 30 | n.a. |

n.a. Not applicable.

[a] Children are categorized based on comparison of BMI with the percentiles of the CDC BMI-for-age growth chart. The growth charts were developed based on pooled data from past national U.S. health examination surveys (1963-1994) (Kuczmarski, et al., 2000).

Among females, FSP participants were less likely to have healthy weights and more likely to be in the top weight category (overweight for children; obese for adults and older adults) compared with income- eligible nonparticipants. This finding was consistent across age groups (children, adults, and older adults) (Figure 3-7). This same pattern was observed for the comparison of FSP females and higher-income nonparticipant females, but the between-group differences were larger (Figure 3-7).

Male children showed a pattern similar to females: FSP participants were less likely than higher- income nonparticipants to have healthy weights and more likely to be overweight. Among adult and older adult males, however, FSP participants were *more* likely than higher-income nonparticipants to have healthy weights and less likely to be overweight, with little difference in obesity rates (Figure 3-7). The magnitude of the between-group differences was largest for adult males, with a 10 percentage point difference in rates of healthy weight and overweight for FSP participants and higher-income nonparticipants.

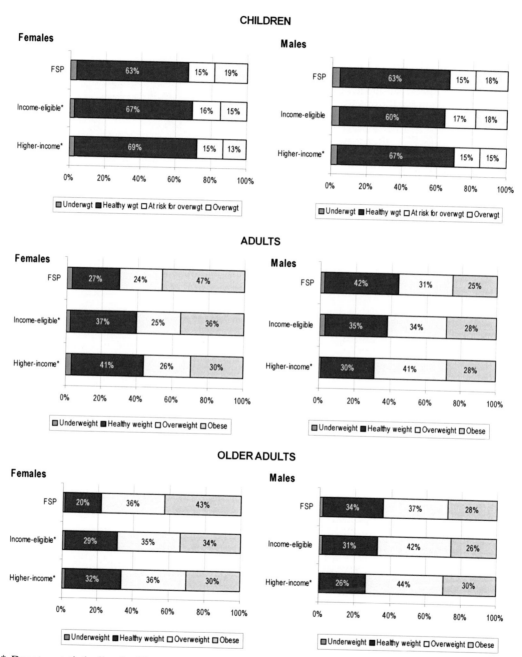

**CHILDREN**

**Females**

**Males**

**ADULTS**

**Females**

**Males**

**OLDER ADULTS**

**Females**

**Males**

* Denotes statistically significant difference from FSP participants at the .05 level or better based on chi-square tests of the distributions of weight status. Estimates are age adjusted.

Note: The percent underweight is 4 percent or less in all age-by-gender groups (Table C-3).

Figure 3-7. Distribution of Food Stamp Participants and Nonparticipants by Weight Status

## Summary

Data from NHANES 1999-2004 show that mean usual energy intakes, by broad age group, were comparable for FSP participants and both income- eligible and higher-income nonparticipants. The only difference was found among older adult males, with FSP participants consuming, on average, 87 percent of the calories consumed by higher-income nonparticipant older adult males.

In contrast, comparison of the adequacy of long run energy intakes, measured by BMI, shows significant differences between FSP participants and both groups of nonparticipants.

- Female FSP participants in all age groups were less likely to have healthy weights and more likely to be in the top weight category (overweight for children; obese for adults and older adults) compared with female nonparticipants.
- Male children showed a pattern similar to females: FSP participants were less likely to have healthy weights and more likely to be in the top weight category.
- Adult and older adult male FSP participants, in contrast, were more likely to have healthy weights and less likely to be overweight, compared with higher-income nonparticipants.

The findings of comparable mean usual energy intakes and different BMI distributions suggest either different levels of physical activity between groups, or different levels of misreporting on dietary recalls. It is beyond the scope of this research to identify the source of the inconsistency.

### Sources of Energy

Usual intakes of macronutrients (protein, carbohydrate, and total fat) were within acceptable ranges for the majority of persons. In contrast, a majority of persons had usual intake of saturated fat above recommended levels. And mean intakes of solid fats, alcoholic beverages, and added sugars (SoFAAS) were in excess of average discretionary calorie allowances. Specific findings include:

- Over 95 percent of children consumed protein and carbohydrate within acceptable ranges, but 20 percent of children consumed too much energy from total fat, and 83 percent consumed too much saturated fat.
- Nearly all adults and older adults consumed protein within acceptable ranges, but about 37 percent consumed too much total fat, about 60 percent consumed too much saturated fat, and about 22 percent consumed too few carbohydrates.
- On average for all persons, 38 percent of calories were consumed from solid fats, alcoholic beverages, and added sugars (SoFAAS). This percentage varied only slightly across age groups. This level is far in excess of the maximum discretionary calorie allowance of 15 percent of calories.

Among children and older adults, there were no statistically significant differences between FSP participants and nonparticipants in sources of energy. Adult FSP participants differed from higher-income nonparticipants on a number of measures: they were less likely to over consume total fat or under consume carbohydrates; they were somewhat less likely to consume enough protein; they consumed more energy from SoFAAS; and they consumed foods with higher mean energy density.

# Chapter 4

# MEAL AND SNACK PATTERNS

In this chapter, we examine meal and snack patterns of FSP participants and nonparticipants. We look first at the proportion of FSP participants and nonparticipants who consumed specific meals, and the average number of snacks consumed per day.[1] We then assess the quality of the meals and snacks consumed by FSP participants and nonparticipants using three measures listed in the box to the right. Energy density and the percentage of energy contributed by SoFAAS were described in Chapter 3. Nutrient density assesses nutrient content relative to energy content, or the amount of nutrients received per calorie consumed. All of the analyses presented in this chapter are based on the single 24-hour recall completed by NHANES respondents, and represent average dietary behaviors for each group.[2]

## MEALS EATEN

NHANES 24-hour dietary recall respondents were asked to report, for every food and beverage, the eating occasion (breakfast, lunch, dinner, or snack) and the time of day at which the food or beverage was consumed. We used these data to determine the proportions of individuals who ate each of the three main meals, the proportion who ate all three main meals, and the total number of snacks eaten. Classifications of eating occasions are self- reported and reflect respondents' perceptions about what constituted a meal vs. a snack. NHANES "cleaned" the meal codes for consistency with respect to meals reported at unusual times. The data contain 16 meal codes corresponding to English and Spanish meal names, and we recoded these as breakfast, lunch, dinner, and snacks, as described in Appendix A.[3]

---

[1] Tables and figures in this chapter focus on estimates by age group. Results by age group and gender are included in Appendix C, and cited where appropriate.

[2] "Usual intakes" are not presented because the focus is on mean intakes, not the percentage of the population above or below a cutoff. Usual intakes are needed to obtain correct estimates of the population distribution, but are not needed for valid estimates of mean intakes.

[3] For snacks, we counted the number of distinct snack times, rather than the number of foods reported as snacks.

---

**MEAL AND SNACK PATTERNS**

**Data**
- NHANES 1999-2004: Single 24-hour recall per person

**Measures**
- Number of meals and snacks eaten
- Nutritional quality of each meal and all snacks
  a) Energy density
  b) Percentage of energy from SoFAAS (solid fat and added sugar)
  c) Nutrient density

---

FSP participants were less likely than either income-eligible nonparticipants or higher-income nonparticipants to have eaten all three main meals (Figure 4-1). The difference between FSP participants and income-eligible nonparticipants in the percent reporting all three main meals was mainly due to older adults (38 percent vs. 51 percent). A difference between FSP participants and higher- income nonparticipants in the percent reporting all three meals was observed for all three age groups, but was smallest for children (60 percent vs. 69 percent) and largest for older adults (38 percent vs. 70 percent).

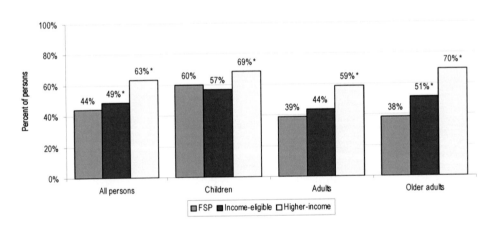

* Denotes statistically significant difference from FSP participants at the .05 level or better. Estimates are age adjusted.

Figure 4-1. Percent of Persons Reporting All Three Main Meals (Breakfast, Lunch, and Dinner)

Data on individual meals show that:

- FSP participants were more likely to skip lunch than income-eligible nonparticipants (Table 4- 1). Only 69 percent of FSP participants reported eating lunch, compared with 75 percent of income-eligible nonparticipants. This difference was not apparent among children—82 percent of children in both groups reported a lunch—but was noted for adults (66 percent vs. 73 percent) and older adults (58 percent vs. 69 percent).

- Roughly equal proportions of FSP participants and income-eligible nonparticipants reported eating breakfast (about 75 percent) and roughly equal proportions reported eating dinner (about 85 percent).

- FSP participants were less likely than higher- income nonparticipants to eat each type of meal. This was true for all three age groups. The between-group differences were largest for lunch among adults (66 percent vs. 80 percent) and older adults (58 percent vs. 80 percent).

## Table 4-1. Percent of Persons Reporting Different Meals and Average Number of Snacks

| | All persons | | | | Children (age 1-18) | | | |
|---|---|---|---|---|---|---|---|---|
| | Total Persons | Food Stamp Program Partic. | Income-eligible Nonpartic. | Higher-income Nonpartic. | Total Persons | Food Stamp Program Partic. | Income-eligible Nonpartic. | Higher-income Nonpartic. |
| Percent eating | | | | | | | | |
| Breakfast | 80.1 | 73.6 | 76.2 | ***81.8 | 81.6 | 78.0 | 78.8 | ***83.0 |
| Lunch | 79.5 | 69.1 | **74.8 | ***82.0 | 85.4 | 82.8 | 82.0 | ***87.3 |
| Dinner | 90.8 | 85.3 | 86.5 | ***92.6 | 91.0 | 88.6 | 87.6 | **92.9 |
| All three | 58.8 | 44.2 | *48.5 | ***63.2 | 64.9 | 59.7 | 56.9 | ***68.6 |
| Average number of snacks | 2.3 | 2.2 | 2.2 | **2.4 | 2.5 | 2.4 | 2.5 | 2.5 |

| | Adults (age 19-59) | | | | Older adults (age 60+) | | | |
|---|---|---|---|---|---|---|---|---|
| | Total Persons | Food Stamp Program Partic. | Income-eligible Nonpartic. | Higher-income Nonpartic. | Total Persons | Food Stamp Program Partic. | Income-eligible Nonpartic. | Higher-income Nonpartic. |
| Percent eating | | | | | | | | |
| Breakfast | 76.0 | 68.4 | 71.4 | ***78.0 | 91.9 | 84.4 | 88.1 | ***93.3 |
| Lunch | 77.5 | 66.0 | *73.2 | ***80.2 | 76.9 | 58.4 | *68.6 | ***80.1 |
| Dinner | 90.6 | 85.0 | 86.0 | ***92.3 | 91.6 | 81.0 | 86.5 | ***93.3 |
| All three | 54.3 | 38.8 | 43.7 | ***58.8 | 64.6 | 38.2 | **51.4 | ***69.6 |
| Average number of snacks | 2.3 | 2.2 | 2.2 | 2.4 | 2.0 | 1.8 u | 1.8 | **2.1 |

Notes: Significant differences in means and proportions are noted by * (.05 level), ** (.01 level), or *** (.001 level). Differences are tested in comparison to FSP participants, identified as persons in households receiving food stamps in the past 12 months.

Source: NHANES 1999-2004 dietary recalls. Estimates are based on a single dietary recall per person. Excludes pregnant and breastfeeding women and infants. 'Total Persons' includes persons with missing food stamp participation or income. Percents are age adjusted to account for different age distributions of FSP participants and nonparticipants.

## SNACKS EATEN

FSP participants and income-eligible nonparticipants had comparable snacking patterns—an average of 2.2 snacks, overall, ranging from 1.8 snacks for older adults to 2.5 snacks for children (Table 4-1). In comparison to higher-income nonparticipants, however, FSP participants consumed significantly fewer snacks, on average (2.2 vs. 2.4). This difference was largely due to older adults (1.8 vs. 2.1).

## ENERGY DENSITY OF MEALS AND SNACKS

Mean energy density was consistently highest for snacks and lowest for breakfast (Figure 4-2), indicating that the mix of foods consumed as snacks provided a higher concentration of energy per gram than foods consumed for breakfast.[4]

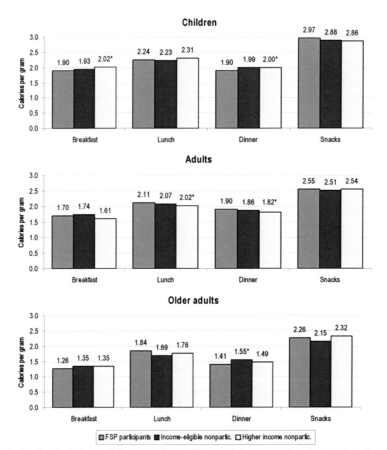

* Denotes statistically significant difference from FSP participants at the .05 level or better. Estimates are age adjusted.

Figure 4-2. Energy Density of Meals and Snacks

---

[4] See Chapter 3 for a description of the energy density measure used in this analysis.

Mean energy densities were consistently higher for lunches than for dinners.

Overall, there were no significant differences between FSP participants and either group of nonparticipants in the energy density of meals and snacks (Table C-2). However, several differences were noted for individual age groups (Figure 4-2).

Among children, the energy density of breakfasts and dinners eaten by FSP children was significantly lower than the energy density of breakfasts and dinners eaten by higher-income nonparticipant children (1.90 vs. 2.00 to 2.02). The same is true of the dinners eaten by older adult FSP participants, relative to income-eligible nonparticipant older adults (1.41 vs. 1.55). In contrast, the energy density of lunch and dinner eaten by FSP adults was significantly higher than that of higher- income nonparticipant adults (2.11 vs. 2.02 and 1.90 vs. 1.82, respectively).

Analysis by gender indicated that the difference among older adults is attributable to a difference among males and the difference among adults is entirely attributable to a difference among females (Figure 4-3).

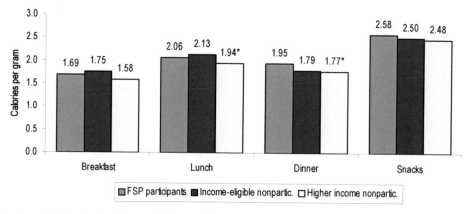

* Denotes statistically significant difference from FSP participants at the .05 level or better. Estimates are age adjusted.

Figure 4-3. Energy Density of Meals and Snacks: Adult Females

## ENERGY FROM SOLID FATS, ALCOHOLIC BEVERAGES, AND ADDED SUGARS IN MEALS AND SNACKS

In Chapter 3 we found that FSP participants obtained a greater share of their energy intake from SoFAAS than either income-eligible or higher-income nonparticipants. This is true of each individual meal and snacks, except dinner (Figure 4-4 and Table C-1). Roughly 30 percent of the calories in the dinners eaten by all three groups came from SoFAAS. In all three groups, SoFAAS calories were highest in snacks (about 50 percent of total calories).

All of the significant differences noted in the overall sample are attributable to differences among adults; no significant differences in the percentage of calories from SoFAAS were noted for either children or older adults.

Differences in SoFAAS intakes for adult FSP participants and higher income nonparticipants are shown by gender in Figure 4-5. Both male and female FSP participants consumed a higher percentage of calories from SoFAAS with breakfast and snack foods; adult female FSP participants also consumed more SoFAAS than their higher income counterparts at lunch and dinner.

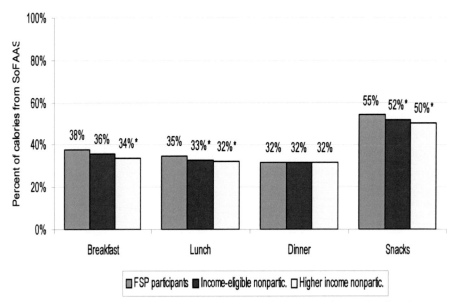

* Denotes statistically significant difference from FSP participants at the .05 level or better. Estimates are age adjusted.

Figure 4-4. Percent of Energy from Solid Fats, Alcoholic Beverages, and Added Sugars (SoFAAS): All Persons

## NUTRIENT DENSITY OF MEALS AND SNACKS

We examined the nutritional quality of individual meals and snacks and of all meals and snacks combined, using a measure of nutrient density. Nutrient density is a ratio that measures the nutrient contribution of a food relative to its energy contribution. This concept has been around for more than 30 years, and has recently received renewed attention because the *Dietary Guidelines for Americans* and *MyPyramid* recommendations emphasize the need for individuals to choose "nutrient-dense" foods to meet nutrient requirements without exceeding energy requirements. "Nutrient-dense" foods are defined as "low-fat forms of foods in each food group and forms free of added sugar."

There is a pressing need to develop a standard definition of nutrient density that can be understood by individuals and used by researchers. Among the several existing approaches, the Naturally-Nutrient-Rich (NNR) score is viewed by some to hold the most promise (Drewnowski, 2005; Zelman and Kennedy, 2005). The NNR is a nutrients-to-calories ratio that considers nutrients commonly included in efforts to define healthy diets (Drewnowski, 2005). The NNR, as initially conceived, excludes fortified foods.

**Adult males**

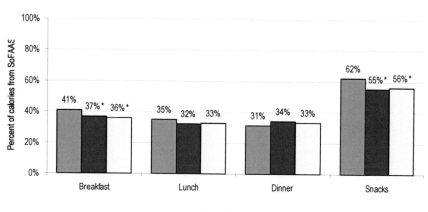

**Adult females**

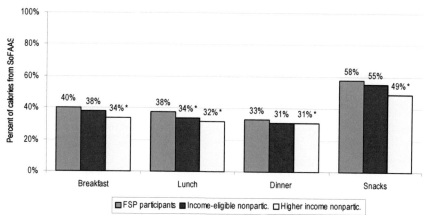

☐ FSP participants  ■ Income-eligible nonpartic.  ☐ Higher income nonpartic.

\* Denotes statistically significant difference from FSP participants at the .05 level or better. Estimates are age adjusted.

Figure 4-5. Percent of Energy from SoFAAS: Adults

For our analysis, we used a modified NNR—the NR (Nutrient-Rich) score—that is not limited to naturally occurring nutrients. We include fortified foods in the analysis because these foods make important contributions to nutrient intakes (Subar et al., 1998a and 1998b). The NR scores presented in this chapter consider the 16 nutrients shown in Table 4-2.[5]

The NR score for a food is constructed as the weighted average of the contributions of 16 nutrients, with nutrient contributions measured as a percent of daily value (DV) contributed per 2000 kcal of the food (DVs are shown in Table 4-2; derivation of the NR score is described in Appendix A). The NR score for a meal or the full complement of meals and snacks is similarly constructed, after aggregating the nutrient contributions of all foods consumed.

---

[5] The nutrients are the same as those used by Drewnowski, with the following exceptions. Vitamin D was not included because it was not available in the NHANES data. Additional nutrients available in NHANES (magnesium, dietary fiber, and the essential fatty acids linoleic acid and alpha-linolenic acid) were added.

The NR score provides a method of assessing multiple key nutrients simultaneously. Mean NR scores must be interpreted with caution. The NR score is not designed to assess nutrient adequacy.

**Table 4-2. Nutrients and Recommended Daily Values (DVs)**
**Used to Calculate Nutrient-Rich Scores[a]**

| Nutrient | Value | Nutrient | Value |
|---|---|---|---|
| Calcium | 1300 mg | Vitamin B$_{12}$ | 2.4 ,g |
| Folate | 400 ,g | Vitamin C | 90 mg |
| Iron | 18 mg | Vitamin E | 15 mg |
| Magnesium | 420 mg | Zinc | 11 mg |
| Potassium | 4.7 g | Dietary Fiber | 38 g |
| Riboflavin | 1.3 mg | Linoleic acid | 17 g |
| Thiamin | 1.2 mg | Linolenic acid | 1. 6 g |
| Vitamin A (RAE) | 900 mg | Protein | 56 g |

· Daily values are the maximum RDA or AI specified for an age group, excluding pregnant and lactating women.

Higher NR scores indicate a higher concentration of nutrients per calorie but, because the score is normalized to 2,000 kcal, it does not provide an absolute measure of nutrient intake relative to DVs. Furthermore, NR scores do not account negatively for excessive concentrations of nutrients such as saturated fat, cholesterol, and sodium, which should be consumed in moderation. And finally, the score weights all nutrients equally. Thus, a person consuming 2000% DV of one nutrient will have a higher NR score from that single nutrient than a person consuming exactly 100% DV of all nutrients.

## Nutrient-Rich (NR) Scores for Individual Meals

Mean NR scores were consistently higher for breakfast (114 to 154; Figure 4-6) and lower for lunch and dinner (range of 86 to 109), indicating that the mix of foods consumed at breakfast meals provided a higher concentration of nutrients per calorie consumed than foods consumed for lunch and dinner.

Differences between FSP participants and nonparticipants in mean NR scores varied by meal and by age group. Where significant differences were noted, FSP participants generally had lower mean scores than nonparticipants, indicating that, on a calorie-per-calorie basis, the meals consumed by FSP participants provide fewer nutrients than the meals consumed by nonparticipants.

Among children, mean NR scores for meals were generally comparable for FSP participants and both groups of nonparticipants (Figure 4-6). The one exception was that FSP children had significantly lower breakfast NR scores, on average, than higher-income nonparticipant children (147 vs. 154).

Among adults, FSP participants had significantly lower NR scores than higher-income nonparticipants for all three meals. For income-eligible nonparticipants, the pattern of differences varied—FSP adults had a significantly higher mean NR score than income-eligible nonparticipants for breakfast (126 vs. 114), but a significantly lower mean NR score for lunch (87 vs. 93).

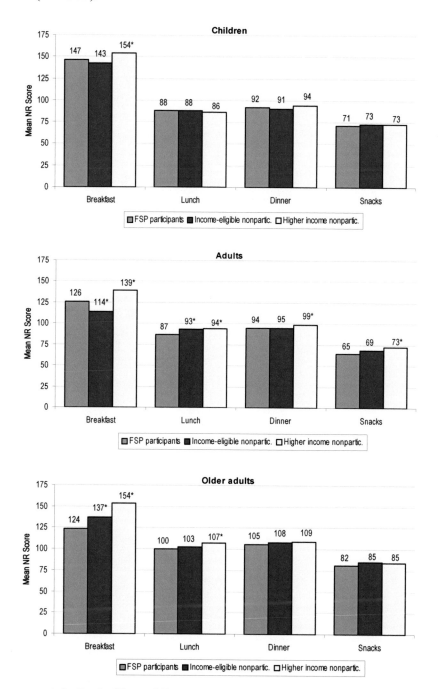

* Denotes statistically significant difference from FSP participants at the .05 level or better. Estimates are age adjusted.

Figure 4-6. Nutrient-Rich (NR) Scores for Meals and Snacks

Among older adults, differences were noted between FSP participants and non-participants for NR scores for breakfast and lunch, but not for dinner. On average, FSP older adults had a significantly lower NR score for breakfast than either income-eligible or higher-income nonparticipant older adults (124 vs. 137 and 154). In addition, FSP older adults had a significantly lower mean NR score for lunch than higher-income nonparticipants (100 vs. 107).

Analysis of data by gender indicated that, as noted previously, many of the differences between FSP adults and higher-income nonparticipant adults were concentrated among females. FSP adult females had lower NR scores than higher-income nonparticipants for every meal: 123 vs. 139 for breakfast; 85 vs. 97 for lunch; and 92 vs. 102 for dinner (Table C-7). Among adult males, there were no significant difference in mean NR scores between FSP participants and higher-income nonparticipants.

## NR Scores for Snacks

Snacks consumed by FSP participants and nonparticipants had lower nutrient density than each type of meal (Figure 4-6). Among children and older adults, the nutrient density of snacks was comparable for FSP participants and both groups of nonparticipants. Adult FSP participants consumed snacks with lower nutrient density than higher- income adults (65 vs. 73), and consistent with the findings for meals.

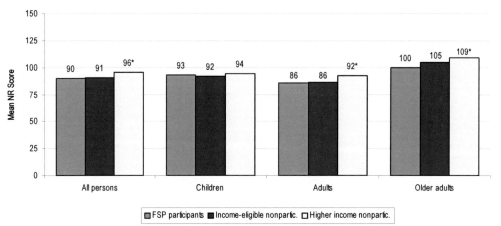

* Denotes statistically significant difference from FSP participants at the .05 level or better. Estimates are age adjusted.

Figure 4-7. Nutrient-Rich (NR) Scores for All Meals and Snacks Combined

## NR Scores for All Meals and Snacks Combined

Mean NR scores for the total daily intakes were comparable for FSP participants and income- eligible nonparticipants, overall and for all the age groups, (Figure 4-7). On the other hand, mean NR scores were significantly lower for the FSP participants than they were for higher-income nonparticipants, except for children. As noted above, differences in NR scores of FSP adults and higher-income nonparticipant adults were entirely concentrated among females (Table C-7).

## SUMMARY

Fewer than half of FSP participants and income- eligible nonparticipants reported all three main meals on the day of the 24-hour recall (44 percent and 49 percent, respectively). In contrast, 63 percent of higher-income nonparticipants reported three meals. Consumption patterns varied by age group and meal:

- About 90 percent of persons in all three age groups ate dinner.

- Children were most likely to skip breakfast (18 percent skipped it), followed by lunch (15 percent). Adults were equally likely to skip breakfast or lunch (23 percent). Older adults were most likely to skip lunch (23 percent) and equally likely to eat breakfast and dinner.

- Meal consumption was comparable for FSP participants and income-eligible nonparticipants, with two exceptions: smaller percentages of adult and older adult FSP participants ate lunch.

- FSP participants were less likely than higher- income nonparticipants to eat each meal. Between-group differences were smallest for children and largest for older adults.

- There were no significant differences between FSP participants and nonparticipants in the number of snacks consumed by children and adults. Older adult FSP participants consumed fewer snacks than higher-income older adults.

Overall, there were no significant differences between FSP participants and either group of nonparticipants in the energy density of meals and snacks (calories per gram of food consumed during the day). Adult FSP participants, however, consumed lunches and dinners with higher energy density than higher-income nonparticipants—perhaps to compensate for eating fewer meals, on average.

For children and older adults, there were no significant differences between FSP participants and either group of nonparticipants in the percent- age of calories consumed from SoFAAS. Adult FSP participants, however, consumed a higher percent-age of calories from SoFAAS than either group of nonparticipants. This was true for overall daily intake (as discussed in Chapter 3) and for each individual meal and snacks, except dinner.

In Chapter 2, we saw that there were no significant differences between FSP participants and income- eligible nonparticipants in the prevalence of adequate usual intakes of vitamins and minerals. Consistent with that finding, FSP participants and income-eligible nonparticipants had overall daily intakes with comparable nutrient density. (Some small offsetting differences were observed for individual meals.)

Also shown in Chapter 2, FSP participants had lower prevalence of adequate usual intakes for most vitamins and minerals, compared with higher- income nonparticipants. Consistent with that finding, FSP participants had overall daily intakes with lower nutrient density compared with higher- income nonparticipants; adult FSP participants had significantly lower NR scores for all three meals; FSP children had lower NR scores for breakfast, and older adult FSP participants had lower NR scores for breakfast and lunch.

# Chapter 5

# FOOD CHOICES

In this chapter, we examine the food choices of FSP participants and nonparticipants. This information provides context for the findings of previous chapters, and for efforts to influence FSP participants' food choices and improve their overall diets.

We examined food choices using two methods. First, a "supermarket aisle" approach compares proportions of FSP participants and nonparticipants consuming specific types of food. We examined food choices at the level of major food groups (fruits, vegetables, milk products, meat, etc.), and subgroups within the major groups (whole milk, 2% milk, cheese, and yogurt in the milk group). This analysis provides a comprehensive picture of the food choices of FSP participants and nonparticipants, and the differences across groups. Some differences in food choice may have important implications for diet quality, while others have less importance or no implications.

The second approach examines food choices across food categories defined by relative nutritional quality. We categorized foods into three groups—foods to be consumed frequently, occasionally, and selectively—based on food descriptions, nutrient content, and the dietary advice provided in the *Dietary Guidelines for Americans (DGA)* or *MyPyramid*. These data provide a picture of the relative quality of the foods eaten by FSP participants and nonparticipants.

## FOOD CHOICES—SUPERMARKET AISLE APPROACH

To describe food choices using a supermarket aisle approach, we assigned all foods in the NHANES data to one of 10 major food groups. The 10 food groups are shown in Figure 5-1, sorted by the percent of persons consuming foods in each group. Beverages (excluding drinking water, milk, and 100% fruit juice) were consumed by 90 percent of all persons. Added fats and oils, and salty snacks were the least common foods, consumed by 35 percent of all persons.

---

### FOOD CHOICE ANALYSES

**Data**

- NHANES 1999-2004: Single 24-hour recall per person

**Measures**

1. Proportion of persons consuming foods from food groups defined by a "supermarket aisle approach": 10 broad food groups and 165 subgroups are defined to correspond to supermarket groupings.

2. Percent of food choices from foods categorized by nutritional quality as:

    - *Food to consume frequently* — high relative nutrient density and low SoFAAS.

    - *Food to consume selectively* — high relative nutrient density and moderate amounts of SoFAAS.

    - *Food to consume occasionally* — low nutrient density and/or high amounts of SoFAAS.

---

The percentages reported throughout this section are of persons consuming one or more foods in a given food group, in any amount, during the preceding 24-hours. Results are based on foods reported as discrete food items. That is, mixed dishes and soups, salads, and sandwiches reported as combination foods were not broken down into their various components (for example, a soup may contain vegetables, chicken, and pasta; a sandwich might contain bread, meat, cheese, and vegetables).[1]

Within the major food groups, we identified 165 subgroups to capture the different types of food available within each group (Table 5-1). We then compared the subgroup choices of FSP participants and nonparticipants who consumed any foods in each of the major groups— for example, the percentage of persons consuming each of the grain subgroups, conditional on consuming any grains. The conditional percents allow us to compare food choices for FSP participants and nonparticipants, while controlling for different overall levels of consumption at the level of major food group.

---

[1] Appendix A discusses the reporting of combination foods in the NHANES food files.

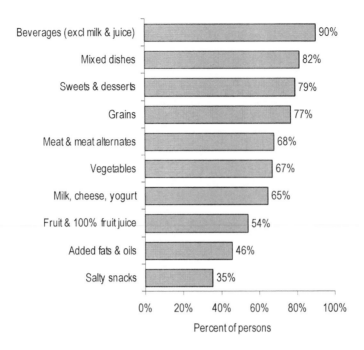

Figure 5-1. Percent of Persons Eating Any Foods from 10 Broad Food Groups

The chapter is organized by major food group. Each section describes the proportions of FSP participants and nonparticipants consuming from the major food group (Figures 5-2 and 5-3), and the differences in food choices for persons choosing any foods in the group.

## Grains

Overall, 77 percent of all people reported eating a grain or a grain-based food that was not part of a mixed dish or combination item such as sandwiches, macaroni and cheese, or pizza (Figure 5-1). There were no significant differences between FSP participants and income-eligible nonparticipants in the proportions eating grains (Figure 5-2). However, FSP participants in all age groups were 6 percentage points less likely than higher-income nonparticipants to eat one or more separate grain- based foods (Figure 5-3).

Consumption of whole grains was low for all groups—overall, only 28 percent of people eating any grains reported eating one or more whole grain foods (Table C-8).[2] FSP participants in all three age groups were less likely to eat whole grain foods, compared with higher income nonparticipants (Figure 5-4).

Among persons eating any grains, bread was the most common grain-based food reported by adults and older adults (32 and 49 percent, respectively). Cold cereals were the most common grain-based food reported by children (51 percent) (Table C-8).

---

[2] The MyPyramid Equivalents database indicates the number of whole grain and non-whole grain ounce equivalents for each food. We coded foods as whole grain if that category had the greater number of ounce equivalents.

**Table 5-1. Food Subgroups Used to Classify Types of Food Eaten by FSP Participants and Nonparticipants**

| | | | |
|---|---|---|---|
| **Grains** | Fresh apple | Hot dogs | **Beverages (excl. milk** |
| Bread | Fresh banana | Cold cuts | **and 100% fruit juice)** |
| Rolls | Fresh melon | Fish | Coffee |
| English muffin Bagels | Fresh watermelon | Shellfish | Tea |
| Biscuits, scones, croissants | Fresh grapes | Bacon/sausage | Beer |
| Muffins | Fresh peach/nectarine | Eggs | Wine |
| Cornbread | Fresh pear | Beans (Dry, cooked) | Liquor |
| Corn tortillas | Fresh berries | Baked/refried beans | Water |
| Flour tortillas | Other fresh fruit | Soy products | Regular soda |
| Taco shells Crackers | Avocado/guacamole | Protein/meal enhancement | Sugar-free soda |
| Breakfast/granola bar | Lemon/lime - any form | Nuts | Noncarbonated |
| Pancakes, waffles, French | Canned or frozen in syrup | Peanut/almond butter | sweetened drinks |
| toast | Canned or frozen, no syrup | Seeds | Noncarbonated low- |
| Cold cereal | Applesauce, canned/frozen | **Mixed Dishes** | calorie/ sugar free drinks |
| Hot cereal | apples | Tomato sauce & meat (no | **Sweets and desserts** |
| Rice | Canned/frozen peaches | pasta) | Sugar and sugar |
| Pasta | Canned/frozen pineapple | Chili con carne | substitutes |
| **Vegetables** | Other canned/frozen | Meat mixtures w/ red meat | Syrups/ sweet toppings |
| Raw lettuce/greens | Non-citrus juice | Meat mixtures w/ | Jelly |
| Raw carrots | Citrus juice | chicken/turkey | Jello |
| Raw tomatoes | Dried fruit | Meat mixtures w/ fish | Candy |
| Raw cabbage/coleslaw | **Milk, cheese, yogurt** | Hamburgers/cheeseburgers | Ice cream |
| Other raw (high nutrients) [a] | Unflavored whole milk | Sandwiches (excl | Pudding |
| Other raw (low nutrients) [a] | Unflavored 2% milk | hamburger) | Ice/popsicles |
| Salads (w/greens) | Unflavored 1% milk | Hot dogs | Sweet rolls |
| Cooked green beans | Unflavored skim milk | Luncheon meat | Cake/cupcakes |
| Cooked corn | Unflavored milk-% fat nfs | Beef, pork, ham | Cookies |
| Cooked peas | Flavored whole milk | Chicken, turkey | Pies/cobblers |
| Cooked carrots | Flavored 2% milk | Cheese (no meat) | Pastries |
| Cooked broccoli | Flavored 1% milk | Fish | Doughnuts |
| Cooked tomatoes | Flavored skim milk | Peanut butter | **Salty snacks** |
| Cooked mixed | Flavored milk-% fat nfs | Breakfast sandwiches | Corn-based salty snacks |
| Cooked starchy | Soymilk | Pizza (no meat) | Pretzels/party mix |
| Other cooked deep yellow | Dry or evaporated milk | Pizza w/ meat | Popcorn |
| Other cooked dark green | Yogurt | Mexican entrees | Potato chips |
| Other cooked (high | Cheese | Macaroni & cheese | **Added fats and oils** |
| nutrients)[a] | **Meat and meat** | Pasta dishes, Italian style | Butter |
| Other cooked (low | **alternatives** | Rice dishes | Margarine |
| nutrients)[a] | Beef | Other grain mixtures | Other added fats |
| Other fried | Ground beef | Meat soup | Other added oils |
| Cooked potatoes-not fried | Pork, | Bean soup | Salad dressing |
| Cooked potatoes-fried | Ham | Grain soups | Mayonnaise |
| Vegetable juice | Lamb and misc. meats | Vegetables mixtures (inc | Gravy |
| **Fruit & 100% fruit juice** | Chicken | soup) | Cream cheese |
| Fresh orange | Turkey | | Cream / sour cream |
| Fresh other citrus | Organ meats | | |

[a] "Other raw" and "Other cooked" vegetables include all vegetables not categorized separately. Within these two groups, vegetables in the top quartile of the distribution of Vitamins A or C per 100 grams were categorized as "high in nutrients"; all others are "low in nutrients." Raw vegetables, high in nutrients include peppers (sweet and hot), broccoli, cauliflower, green peas, seaweed, and snow peas. Raw vegetables, low in nutrients include onions, cucumbers, celery, radishes, and mushrooms. Cooked vegetables, high in nutrients include cabbage, peppers, asparagus, cauliflower, brussel sprouts, snow peas, and squash. Cooked vegetables, low in nutrients include artichokes, onions, mushrooms, eggplant, beets, and yellow string beans.

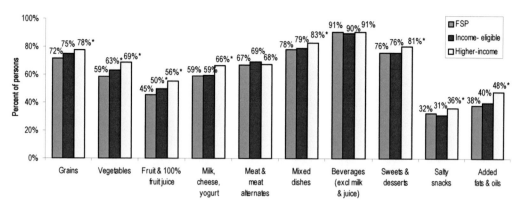

* Denotes statistically significant difference from FSP participants at the .05 level or better. Estimates are age adjusted.

Figure 5-2. Percent of FSP Participants and Nonparticipants Eating Any Foods from 10 Broad Food Groups

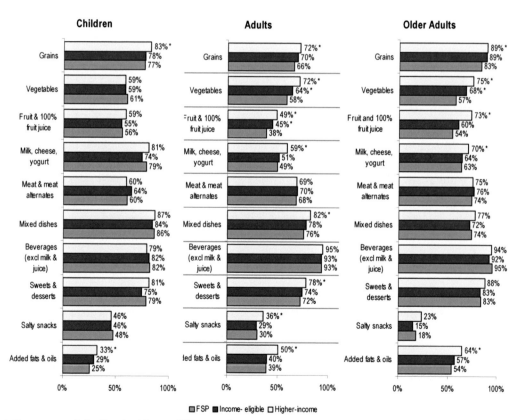

* Denotes statistically significant difference from FSP participants at the .05 level or better. Estimates are age adjusted.

Figure 5-3. Percent of FSP Participants and Nonparticipants Eating Any Foods from 10 Broad Food Groups: By Age Group

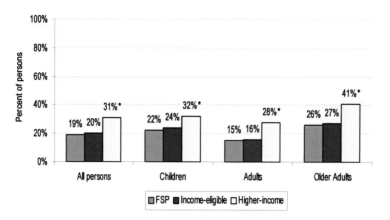

* Denotes statistically significant difference from FSP participants at the .05 level or better. Estimates
  are age adjusted.

Figure 5-4. Percent of Persons Eating Whole Grain Foods, Among those Eating Any Grains

There were relatively few differences between FSP participants and income-eligible nonparticipants in the specific types of grain foods eaten.

There were, however, several differences between FSP participants and higher-income nonparticipants in the types of grain-based foods eaten (Table 5-2). Many differences were related to the types of grain foods chosen as alternatives to bread. For example, FSP participants were less likely than higher-income nonparticipants to choose rolls, bagels, and English muffins and were more likely to choose corn-bread, which is a higher-fat bread alternative. In addition, adult and older adult FSP participants were less likely than higher-income nonparticipants to eat cold cereals and FSP children and older adults were less likely than higher-income nonparticipants to eat pancakes, waffles, or French toast.

**Table 5-2. Grain Choices of FSP Participants Compared
with Higher Income Nonparticipants**

|  | **FSP participants were** | |
|  | **less likely to eat ...** | **more likely ...** |
|---|---|---|
| Children | Crackers; Breakfast/ granola bar; Pancakes/ waffles/French toast | Cornbread; Corn tortillas; Taco shells |
| Adults | Bagels; Muffins; Breakfast/ granola bars; Cold cereal | Cornbread; Rice |
| Older adults | Rolls; English muffin; Muffins; Pancakes/ waffles/ French toast; Cold cereal | Corn tortillas |

Note: Food groups with significant between-group differences are included if reported by at least 2 percent of persons. See Table C-8.

# Vegetables

Overall, 67 percent of people reported eating at least one vegetable as a discrete food item (Figure 5-1). Adult and older adult FSP participants were significantly less likely than either income-eligible or higher-income nonparticipants to eat vegetables (58 percent of adult FSP participants compared with 64 and 72 percent of income-eligible and higher-income, respectively) (Figure 5-3). There were no significant between-group differences for children.

Among persons eating any vegetables, FSP participants in all three age groups were about two-thirds as likely to choose raw vegetables compared with higher-income nonparticipants (Figure 5-5). These differences were largely due to differences in the proportions who reported eating salads or salad greens—higher-income adults were more than twice as likely as FSP adults to eat a salad (11 percent vs. 27 percent) (Table C-8).

In addition to salads/salad greens, FSP participants in one or more age groups were less likely than nonparticipants to eat raw lettuce/greens (not part of a salad), raw carrots, cooked tomatoes (including tomato sauce), and a variety of other cooked vegetables; and more likely to eat corn and cooked potatoes other than french fries (Table 5-3).

### Table 5-3. Vegetable Choices of FSP Participants Compared with Higher Income Nonparticipants

| | FSP participants were | |
| | less likely to eat ... | more likely ... |
| --- | --- | --- |
| Children | Raw carrots; Salads (w/greens); Cooked tomatoes | Cooked corn |
| Adults | Raw lettuce/greens; Raw carrots; Salads (w/greens); Cooked "low nutrient" vegetables[a] | Cooked potatoes |
| Older adults | Raw carrots; Raw cabbage/coleslaw; Salads (w/greens); Cooked "high nutrient" vegetables[b] | |

[a] Includes onions, summer squash, mushrooms, and eggplant.
[b] Includes cabbage, peppers, asparagus, cauliflower, and beets.
Note: Food groups with significant between-group differences are included if reported by at least 2 percent of persons. See Table C-8.

# Fruit

Only 54 percent of all people reported eating fruit or 100% fruit juice during the preceding 24 hours (Figure 5-1). Among children, there were no significant differences between FSP participants and nonparticipants in the proportions who consumed fruit or juice (Figure 5-3). Adult FSP participants were less likely than both income- eligible and higher-income nonparticipants to eat fruit or juice (38 percent vs. 45 and 49 percent), while older adult FSP participants were less likely than higher-income nonparticipants to consume fruit or juice (54 vs. 73 percent) (Figure 5-3).

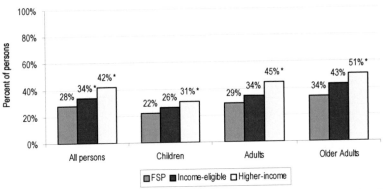

* Denotes statistically significant difference from FSP participants at the .05 level or better. Estimates are age adjusted.

Figure 5-5. Percent of Persons Eating Raw Vegetables, Among those Eating Any Vegetables

Among persons eating any fruit, FSP participants were less likely than higher-income nonparticipants to choose any whole fruit (fresh, canned, or dried), and less likely than both groups of nonparticipants to choose fresh fruit (Figure 5-6). These differences were not significant for older adults. For children, only the between-group difference for any whole fruit was significant, and for adults only the between-group difference for fresh fruit was significant.

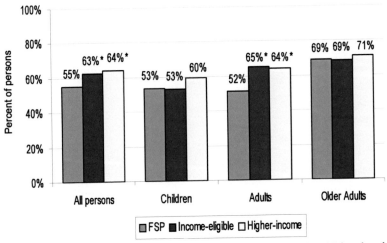

* Denotes statistically significant difference from FSP participants at the .05 level or better. Estimates are age adjusted.

Figure 5-6. Percent of Persons Eating Fresh Fruit, Among those Eating Any Fruit

Table 5-4 lists the fruits and fruit juices accounting for differences in food choices between FSP participants and higher-income nonparticipants.

### Table 5-4. Fruit Choices of FSP Participants Compared with Higher Income Nonparticipants

| | **FSP participants were** | |
|---|---|---|
| | **less likely to eat ...** | **more likely ...** |
| Children | Fresh grapes; Fresh berries; Applesauce, canned/frozen apples | Fresh orange; Citrus juice |
| Adults | Fresh apple; Fresh berries; Lemon/lime | Non-citrus juice |
| Older adults | Fresh melon; Fresh pear; Fresh berries; Canned or frozen peaches; Canned or frozen pineapple; Dried fruit | |

Note: Food groups with significant between-group differences are included if reported by at least 2 percent of persons. See Table C-8.

There were no differences between FSP participants and income-eligible nonparticipants in the proportions who reported eating yogurt or cheese. However, FSP participants in all three age groups were less likely than higher-income nonparticipants to consume either of these foods (Table C-8).

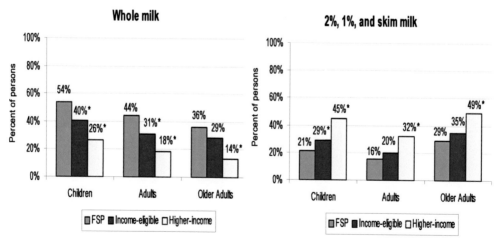

Notes: Graphs show percent of persons consuming unflavored white milk. Persons may report both whole milk and non-whole milk during the preceding 24 hours.
* Denotes statistically significant difference from FSP participants at the .05 level or better. Estimates are age adjusted.

Figure 5-7. Percent of Persons Consuming Whole Milk and Non-Whole Milk, Among those Consuming Any Milk Products

## Milk and Milk Products

Overall, 65 percent of people reported consuming milk or milk products (cheese or yogurt) in the preceding 24 hours (Figure 5-1). Among children, there were no significant differences between FSP participants and either group of nonparticipants in this regard. However, adult and older adult FSP participants were less likely to consume milk products compared with higher-income nonparticipants (Figure 5-3).

Among persons consuming milk products, FSP participants in all three age groups were significantly more likely than higher-income nonparticipants to consume whole milk and less likely to consume reduced-fat or nonfat milk (Figure 5-7). FSP children and adults were also more likely than income-eligible children and adults to consume whole milk, and FSP children were less likely than income-eligible children to consume non-whole milk.

## Meats and Meat Alternates

Roughly 70 percent of all people reported eating a meat or meat alternate that was not part of a mixed dish (Figure 5-1).[3] There were no significant differences between FSP participants and either group of nonparticipants in this regard (Figure 5-2 and 5-3).

Among persons who ate meat and meat alternates, there were relatively few differences in food choices between FSP participant and nonparticipant children and adults (Table 5-5). Among older adults, however, there were many significant differences between FSP participants and one or both groups of nonparticipants (Table 5-5 and C8). FSP older adults were less likely than higher income older adults to eat beef, ham, fish, baked/ refried beans, nuts, and protein/meal replacements, and more likely to eat eggs and legumes.

**Table 5-5. Meat Choices of FSP Participants Compared
with Higher Income Nonparticipants**

|  | **FSP participants were** | |
|---|---|---|
|  | less likely to eat ... | more likely ... |
| Children | Cold cuts; Nuts | Eggs; Beans (dry, cooked) |
| Adults | Nuts; Peanut/ almond butter | Chicken |
| Older adults | Beef; Ham; Fish; Baked/refried beans; Protein/meal enhancement; Nuts | Eggs; Beans (dry, cooked) |

Note: Food groups with significant between-group differences are included if reported by at least 2 percent of persons. See Table C-8.

---

[3] Findings for cold cuts were comparable in analyses that considered sandwich components separately (data not shown). Sandwiches are considered mixed dishes and are discussed in the next section.

## Mixed Dishes

More than 80 percent of all people reported one or more mixed dishes, and sandwiches were the most commonly reported type of mixed dish (Figure 5-1 and Table C-8). Among children and older adults, about equal proportions of FSP participants and nonparticipants consumed mixed dishes. Mixed dishes were less commonly reported by FSP adults than higher-income adults (Figure 5-3).

There was little consistency across age groups in differences noted between FSP participants and nonparticipants for specific types of mixed dishes (Table 5-6).

## Beverages, Excluding Milk and 100% Fruit Juice

Almost everyone reported drinking a beverage other than milk; however, the types of beverages varied by age group (Table C-8). Among children, the leading beverages were regular (not sugar- free) sodas (65 percent) and other sweetened beverages, such as fruit drinks (46 percent). Among adults, regular sodas and coffee were the two leading beverages (53 and 48 percent), and among older adults, the predominant beverage was coffee (76 percent).[4]

### Table 5-6. Mixed Dish Choices of FSP Participants Compared with Higher Income Nonparticipants

| | FSP participants were | |
| | less likely to eat ... | more likely ... |
|---|---|---|
| Children | Peanut butter sandwiches; Breakfast sandwiches; Pizza (no meat) | Meat mixtures w/ red meat; Grain soups |
| Adults | Beef,pork,or ham sandwiches; Chicken or turkey sandwiches | Grain soups |
| Older adults | Beef,pork,or ham sandwiches; Chicken or turkey sandwiches; Cheese sandwiches; Fish sandwiches; Mexican entrees | |

Note: Food groups with significant between-group differences are included if reported by at least 2 percent of persons. See Table C-8.

There were no differences between FSP participants and either group of nonparticipants in the proportions who consumed one or more beverages (Figure 5-2). There were also no significant differences in the types of beverages consumed by FSP children and nonparticipant children. However, there were noteworthy differences between groups of adults in the prevalence of specific types of beverages.

---

[4] NHANES dietary recalls did not collect data on water intake.

For both adults and older adults, FSP participants were significantly less likely than higher-income nonparticipants to consume coffee, tea, or wine; adult FSP participants were also less likely to consume beer (Table 5-7). There were no significant differences in the proportions of FSP participants and nonparticipants who chose any soda (Table C-8), however, FSP adults and older adults were more likely to choose regular (not sugar- free) soda (Figure 5-8).

**Table 5-7. Beverage Choices of FSP Participants Compared
with Higher Income Nonparticipants**

|  | FSP participants were | |
|---|---|---|
|  | less likely to eat ... | more likely ... |
| Children | n.a. | n.a. |
| Adults | Coffee; Tea; Beer; Wine; Sugar-free soft drinks | Regular soft drinks; Sweetened beverage |
| Older adults | Coffee; Tea; Wine; Liquor | Regular soft drinks |

n.a. Not applicable

Note: Food groups with significant between-group differences are included if reported by at least 2 percent of persons. See Table C-8.

## Sweets and Desserts

Overall, about eight in ten people reported eating at least one type of sweet or dessert during the preceding 24 hours (Figure 5-1). Older adults reported these foods somewhat more frequently than other adults or children. Candy, sugar and sugar substitutes, cookies, and ice cream were the most commonly reported foods in this group.

There were no differences between FSP participants and income-eligible nonparticipants in the proportions who reported eating sweets or desserts (Figure 5-2 and 5-3). However, FSP adults were significantly less likely than higher-income adults to eat these foods (72 percent vs. 78 percent) (Figure 5-3).

**Table 5-8. Sweets Choices of FSP Participants Compared
with Higher Income Nonparticipants**

| | FSP participants were less likely to eat ... |
|---|---|
| Children | Syrups & sweet toppings; Ice cream; Pastries |
| Adults | Syrups & sweet toppings; Ice cream; Cookies |
| Older adults | Syrups & sweet toppings; Jelly; Candy; Ice cream; Cookies; Pies & cobblers |

Notes: Food groups with significant between-group differences are included if reported by at least 2 percent of persons. See Table C-8.

There are no food groups for which FSP participants were more likely to eat foods, compared with higher income nonparticipants

FSP participants in all three age groups were significantly less likely than higher-income nonparticipants to report ice cream or syrup and other sweet toppings (which is consistent with the previously reported differences in frequency of pancakes, waffles, and French toast) (Table 5-8). In addition, adult and older adult FSP participants were less likely than higher-income nonparticipants to report jelly, candy, or cookies.

## Salty Snacks

Overall, slightly more than a third (35 percent) of all people reported eating a salty snack food (Figure 5-1). Salty snacks were most commonly reported by children, and were more common among adults than older adults (46 percent vs. 34 percent vs. 21 percent) (Table C-8).

There were no differences between FSP participants and income-eligible nonparticipants in the proportions who reported a salty snack (Figure 5- 2). However, FSP adults were significantly less likely to consume salty snacks, compared with higher-income adults (30 percent vs. 36 percent) (Figure 5-3).

Among persons eating salty snacks, FSP children and adults were more likely to eat potato chips and less likely to eat popcorn, compared with higher income nonparticipants. FSP children were also less likely to eat pretzels/party mix, compared to higher income children (Table C-8).

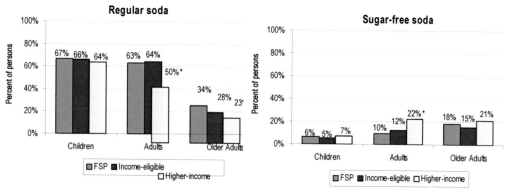

Notes: Persons may report both regular and sugar-free soft drinks during the preceding 24 hours.
* Denotes statistically significant difference from FSP participants at the .05 level or better. Estimates are age adjusted.

Figure 5-8. Percent of Persons Consuming Regular and Sugar-free Soda, Among those Consuming Any Beverages (other than milk and 100% fruit juice)

## Added Fats and Oils

Overall, 46 percent of persons reported adding butter, margarine, salad dressings, or other added fats to the foods they consumed (Figure 5-1). (This does not include fat that may have been added in cooking). There were no differences between FSP participants and income-eligible nonparticipants in the proportions of people reporting adding fats and oils. In comparison with higher-income nonparticipants, however, FSP participants in all three age groups were significantly less likely to have added fat to their foods (Figure 5-3).

There were no differences in types of added fats/ oils used by FSP children and nonparticipant children. FSP adults were less likely than higher income adults to use salad dressings (this is consistent with the difference in the proportion eating salads) and cream cheese; and older adult FSP participants were less likely to use butter (Table C-8).

## FOOD CHOICES—NUTRITIONAL QUALITY APPROACH

Our second method for examining food choices is to examine the nutritional quality of foods consumed by FSP participants and nonparticipants. This approach is based on the radiant pyramid/ power calories concept, as described by Zelman and Kennedy (2005). As shown in Figure 5-9, the radiant pyramid concept was presented as an idea to the committee developing the 2005 edition of the DGAs, and the basic concept was incorporated into the *MyPyramid* food guidance system. The expanded radiant pyramid, described by Zelman and Kennedy and illustrated on the right side of Figure 5-9, uses data on nutrient density to identify "power calorie" foods. The idea is that, within each food group, the most nutrient-dense food choices provide "power calories" and should be enjoyed frequently; foods with lower nutrient density should be enjoyed selectively; and the least nutrient-dense foods in a food group should be enjoyed only occasionally. Choosing foods according to these guidelines makes it easier to obtain recommended levels of nutrients while maintaining energy balance.

### Implementation of the Radiant Pyramid Concept

Categorizing foods into groups corresponding to the radiant pyramid is not straightforward. We explored the idea of using NR scores (described in Chapter 4) to sort foods into the three categories. However, we found this approach less than satisfactory for several reasons.

First, highly fortified foods have higher NR scores than their less-fortified counterparts, leading to some classifications that are not consistent with the basic nutrient density message. For example, highly fortified breakfast cereals, even those containing substantial amounts of sugar and/or fat, ranked much higher than whole wheat bread and unprocessed oatmeal, foods that should certainly be included in the "enjoy frequently" section of a radiant grain group.

Second, foods that provide relatively few nutrients but are very low in calories may be ranked higher than foods that provide substantially more nutrients but are also higher in calories. For example, in the vegetable group, raw iceberg lettuce has an NR score of 466.9, compared with 255.8 for cooked carrots (no fat added).

Finally, because the NR score does not include a 'penalty' for fat or sugar, foods that are concentrated sources of one or more nutrients may be ranked substantially higher than foods that are lower in calories and generally recommended as more optimal choices. For example, in the meat group, the items that received the highest NR scores (506.7 to 636.2) were livers, most of which were fried. Moreover, many beef items that included fat or were prepared with added fat scored higher than chicken items (NR of 130.4 for broiled steak, lean and fat eaten vs. NR of 91.1 for broiled, skinless chicken breast).

1) Radiant Pyramid Concept recommended to the DGA Committee.

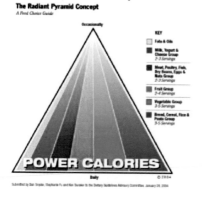

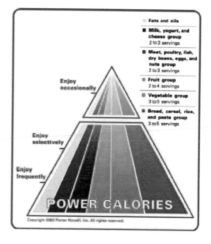

2) MyPyramid adoption of the radiant pyramid concept.

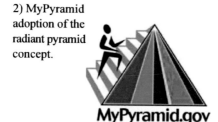

3) Expanded radiant pyramid to emphasize food choices within food groups (Zelman and Kennedy, 2005)

Figure 5-9. Radiant Food Pyramid: Basic and Expanded Concepts

Because of the inherent limitations of NR scores for individual foods, we used an iterative process that used food descriptions and information about SoFAAS and total fat content to categorize foods into the three categories corresponding to the radiant pyramid concept of foods to consume frequently, selectively, and occasionally. We categorized foods within each of the 165 food subgroups listed in Table 5-1. Decision rules were informed by general dietary guidance provided in the *Dietary Guidelines for Americans* and *MyPyramid* which encourage consumption of nutrient-dense foods—foods in their lowest-fat form with no added sugar. For example, whole grains, fruits and vegetables without added fat or sugar, fat-free and low-fat (1%) milk, and lean meat, fish, and poultry were all classified as foods to consume frequently. For other foods, data on calories from SoFAAS and/or total fat were used to divide foods within a food subgroup so that foods with the lowest proportion of calories from SoFAAS/total fat content were included in the "consume frequently" category and foods with the highest proportion of calories from SoFAAS/total fat content were included in the "consume occasionally" category. The rules used in assigning foods to the three consumption categories are summarized in Table 5-2. Table A-4 shows the number and percent of foods in the NHANES individual food files that were assigned to each category, by major food group and subgroups.

## Table 5-9. Categorization of Foods Suggested for Frequent, Selective, and Occasional Consumption

| Food Group | Consume frequently | Consume selectively | Consume occasionally |
|---|---|---|---|
| Grains | All breads, rolls, bagels etc. with 100% wheat, other "wheat", oatmeal, oat bran, or multi-grain description (USDA food code series 512, 513, 515, and 516); other 100% whole wheat/high-fiber breads; whole wheat, high-fiber pancakes and waffles; whole wheat pasta and noodles cooked without added fat; brown rice cooked without added fat; cold cereals with SoFAAS 20; wheat bran, raw oats, wheat bran; oatmeal, whole wheat, and bran hot cereals cooked w/o added fat | Other breads, rolls, bagels, tortillas, crackers, etc. unless fat per 100 gm > 8.0; whole wheat pasta or noodles cooked with added fat; brown rice cooked with added fat; other pasta, noodles, and rice cooked without added fat; cold cereals with SoFAAS 20 but < 35; oatmeal, whole wheat, and bran hot cereals cooked with added fat; other hot cereals cooked w/o added fat | Stuffing, bread sticks, croutons, croissants, biscuits (unless low-fat); other breads, rolls, etc. with fat per 100 gm > 8.0; other pasta, noodles, and rice cooked with added fat; chow mein noodles; cold cereals with SoFAAS 35; other hot cereals cooked with added fat |
| Vegetables | All raw and cooked vegetables without added fat, except potatoes and other starchy vegs; spaghetti sauce w/o meat | Cooked vegetables with added fat, except fried; mashed potatoes; other cooked starchy vegs without added fat; spaghetti sauce w/ meat | All fried vegetables; cooked starchy vegs with added fat (other than mashed potatoes); veg salads with cream, dressing; vegs w/ cheese or cheese sauce; creamed vegs; glazed vegs |
| Fruit and 100% fruit juice | All fresh fruits w/o added sugar; other types of fruits and juice: fruits canned in water or juice w/ no added sugar; frozen fruits w/o added sugar; dried papaya; unsweetened citrus juices (incl. blends); other unsweetened juices with added vitamin C; fruits and juices with NS as to sweetener and SoFAAS = 0 | Fresh fruits with added sugar; other types of fruits and juice: fruits canned in light or medium syrup; unsweetened dried fruit other than papaya; fruits with NS as to sweetener/syrup and SoFAAS > 0; unsweetened (SoFAAS = 0) non-citrus juices w/o added vitamin C; | Fruits canned in heavy syrup; fruits with dressing, cream, marshmallows, chocolate, or caramel; guacamole; all pickled or fried fruits; maraschino cherries; pie filling; fruit soups; frozen juice bars; fruit smoothies; sweetened (SoFAAS > 0) juices; fruit nectars |
| Food Group | Consume frequently | Consume selectively | Consume occasionally |
| Milk and milk products | Unflavored nonfat, skim, 1%, or lowfat fluid/dry milks; NFS unflavored fluid/dry milks with SoFAAS unflavored 1% milk (21.1)<br>All plain yogurt, except from whole milk; fruited or flavored nonfat or lowfat yogurt with low-cal sweetener<br>Non-fat and low-fat cheeses that meet gm fat criteria; cottage cheese except with added fruit/gelatin | Flavored/malted nonfat, skim, 1%, or lowfat fluid milks; unflavored 2% or reduced fat fluid milks; NFS fluid/dry milks and other milk-based beverages/mixtures with SoFAAS > unflavored 1% milk but unflavored 2% milk.<br>Fruited or flavored nonfat and lowfat yogurts with added sugars, with SoFAAS 48.9.<br>Low-fat cheeses that meet gm fat criteria; cottage cheese with added fruit/gelatin | Flavored/malted 2% or reduced fat fluid/dry milks; all types of whole fluid/dry milks; NFS fluid/dry milks and other milk-based beverages/mixtures with SoFASS > unflavored whole milk (33.3)<br>All whole milk yogurts; other yogurt with SoFAAS 48.9.<br>All regular cheeses; cheese sauces, dips, fondues |
| Meat and meat alternates | Meat and poultry with fat per 100 gm 9.28 unless fried and (for chicken) skin eaten; Fish with fat per 100 gm 9.28 and SoFAAS = 0 unless fried.<br>Egg whites | Meat and poultry with fat per 100 gm > 9.28 but 18.56 unless fried and (for chicken) skin eaten; fish that meet gm fat criteria and SoFAAS 0 unless fried.<br>Cooked whole eggs or egg substitutes with no added fat, cheese, or bacon/sausage; other egg/egg substitute mixtures with total fat < 11.21 (max for whole egg cooked w/o fat) | All fried meat, fish, and poultry with skin; meat and poultry with fat per 100 gm > 18.56; fish that meet gm fat criteria and SoFAAS 0.<br><br>Cooked whole eggs with added fat, cheese, or bacon/sausage; egg yolks only; other egg/egg substitute mixtures with total fat 11.21 (max. for whole egg cooked w/o fat) |

## Table 5-9. (Continued)

| | | | |
|---|---|---|---|
| Meat and meat alternates (continued) | Legumes cooked without added fat[a] | Legumes cooked with added fat; peanut butter; nuts and seeds; soy-based meat subs[a] | Soy-based meal replacements, supplements; legumes with cheese or meat; peanut butter with jelly; nuts with dried fruits; soy-based desserts[a] |
| Mixed dishes | Mixed dishes with gm fat/ 100 gm 4.64 or gm fat 9.28 and SoFAAS = 0 | Unless SoFAAS = 0, mixed dishes with fat per 100 gm > 4.64 but 9.28 | All mixed dishes with fat per 100 gm > 9.28 |
| Beverages, excl. milk and 100% fruit juice | Sugar free and low-calorie beverages | Sweeten | ed beverages, alcoholic beverages |
| Sweets and desserts | | Pudding, frozen yogurt, light/non-fat ice cream (excl novelties), sugar-free candy, sugar-free gelatin | All else |
| Salty snacks | | Lowfat/nonfat/baked chips, unflavored pretzels, air-popped popcorn w/o butter | All else |
| Added fats, oils, and condiments | Fat-free. Sugar-free versions, with SoFAAS < 20 and fat per 100 gm < 10 | Low-fat, low-sugar versions, SoFAAS > 20 but < 90 and fat per 100 gm > 10 | Regular versions, SoFAAS > 90 |

[a] Legumes are counted as meat until a person's meat intake reaches 2.5 ounce equivalents per 1000 kcal, then legumes count as vegetables (HEI-2005).

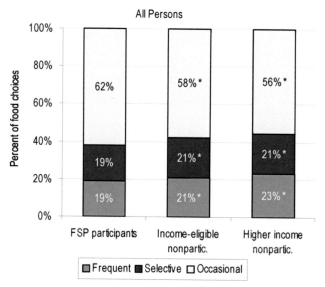

* Denotes statistically significant difference from FSP participants at the .05 level or better. Estimates are age adjusted.

Figure 5-10. Percent of Food Choices From Foods Suggested for Frequent, Selective, or Occasional Consumption

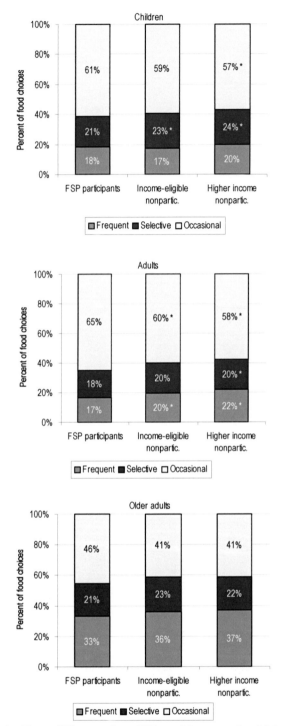

* Denotes statistically significant difference from FSP participants at the .05 level or better. Estimates
   are age adjusted.

Figure 5-11. Percent of Food Choices from Foods Suggested for Frequent, Selective, or Occasional
Consumption, By Age Group

## Food Choices within Food Groups

The only food group for which a majority of food choices came from the 'consume frequently' category was the fruit group (Figure 5-12 and Table C-9). This was true for all three age groups in all three participant groups. In our classification, all fruits without added sugar, all citrus juices, and all non-citrus juices were included in the consume frequently category.

In all three age groups, significant differences were noted between FSP participants and one or both groups of nonparticipants in the relative nutritional quality of food choices in the milk group. FSP participants were generally more likely to consume milk and milk products from the 'consume occasionally' group and less likely to consume milk and milk products from the 'consume selectively' and 'consume frequently' groups. This is consistent with the finding reported in the preceding section that FSP participants in all age groups are more likely than one or both groups of nonparticipants to consume whole milk and less likely to consume low fat or skim milks.

Significant differences were also noted for all three age groups in the nutritional quality of food choices in the meat and meat alternate group. Among adults and older adults, FSP participants were less likely than higher-income nonparticipants to choose meats and meat alternates from the 'consume frequently' category (19 percent vs. 26 percent and approximately 16 percent vs. 30 percent, respectively).[5] This indicates that FSP adults and older adults were less likely than higher-income nonparticipants to choose lean meats, and lower-fat versions of poultry and fish. For older adults, this pattern is also observed for FSP participants and income-eligible nonparticipants.

Among children, FSP participants were more likely than higher-income nonparticipants to choose meats and meat alternates from the 'consume occasionally' group (58 percent vs. 49 percent) and less likely than either income-eligible or higher-income nonparticipants to choose foods from the 'consume selectively' group (22 percent vs. 29 percent and 31 percent). This indicates that FSP children tended to choose higher-fat/fried meat and fish more often than nonparticipant children.

FSP participants in all three age groups were less likely than higher-income nonparticipants to choose salty snacks from the 'consume selectively' group and more likely to choose snacks from the 'consume occasionally' group. For children and adult FSP participants, this pattern was also observed relative to income-eligible nonparticipants. This is consistent with the previous finding that FSP participants are more likely to consume potato chips and less likely to consume popcorn.

Among adults and older adults, FSP participants were less likely than higher-income nonparticipants to choose beverages (other than milk) that were recommended for frequent consumption (18 percent vs. 24 percent and 61 percent vs. 69 percent) and more likely to choose beverages recommended for occasional consumption (83 percent vs. 76 percent and 40 percent vs. 31 percent). This is consistent with the previous finding that FSP participants are more likely to consume regular soft drinks and less likely to consume sugar free soft drinks.

---

[5] The point estimate for older adults is statistically unreliable, but the difference between groups is statistically significant.

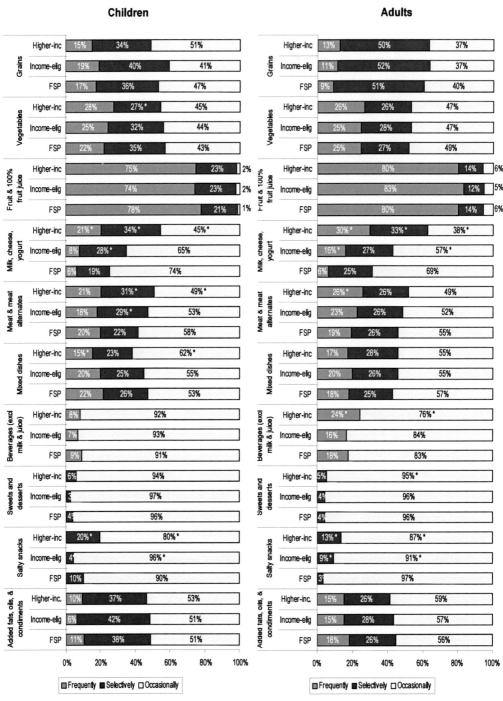

* Denotes statistically significant difference from FSP participants at the .05 level or better. Estimates are age adjusted.

Figure 5-12. (Continued)

## Older Adults

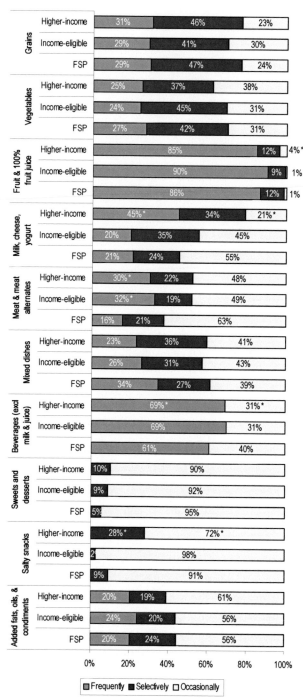

* Denotes statistically significant difference from FSP participants at the .05 level or better. Estimates are age adjusted.

Figure 5-12. Percent of Food Choices Within Food Groups: Foods Suggested for Frequent, Selective, or Occasional Consumption

# SUMMARY

In this chapter, we used two different approaches to compare the food choices of FSP participants and nonparticipants:

- Supermarket aisle approach—What percentage of FSP participants and nonparticipants consumed at least one food item from each food group on the intake day, and what choices were made within food groups?
- Nutritional quality approach—What percentage of foods consumed by FSP participants and nonparticipants were foods suggested for frequent, selective, or occasional consumption?

These analyses focused on food choice without regard to quantities of food consumed, which are examined in the next chapter.


## Supermarket Aisle Approach

We examined the proportions of FSP participants and income-eligible nonparticipants consuming foods from each of 10 major food groups. The main findings were:

- FSP participants were less likely than income- eligible nonparticipants to consume any vegetables or fruit, but were equally likely to consume foods from all other major food groups.
- FSP participants were less likely than higher- income nonparticipants to consume foods from 8 of the 10 food groups, and equally likely to consume meat/meat alternates and beverages other than water, milk, and 100% fruit juice.

Findings varied somewhat by age group. Between- group differences for adults reflected the overall differences listed above. For children and older adults, there was only one significant difference between FSP participants and income-eligible nonparticipants (older adult FSP participants were less likely than income-eligible older adults to consume vegetables).

Compared with higher income nonparticipants, FSP children were less likely to consume from 2 of the 10 food groups (grains; added fats and oils); and FSP older adults were less likely to consume from 5 of the 10 food groups (grains; vegetables; fruits; milk and milk products; and added fats and oils).

There are two possible interpretations for the differences observed between adult and older adult FSP participants and nonparticipants: FSP participants eat less, and therefore are less likely to consume from each food group; or FSP participants as a group have less variety in their diet. Comparisons of energy intakes in Chapter 3 showed no significance differences between FSP adults and higher-income adults, while, FSP older adults had significant lower energy intakes than higher-income older adults. This suggests that, for adults, the observed differences between groups are attributable to less variety in the diets of FSP participants. For older adults, the differences may be due to a combination of less variety and lower overall food intake.

## Food Choices among Subgroups

There were no significant differences between FSP participants and income-eligible nonparticipants in the proportions consuming 165 different subgroups. Compared with higher-income nonparticipants, FSP participants in all age groups made the following less healthful food choices:

- Less likely to choose whole grains
- Less likely to consume raw vegetables (including salads) and more likely to consume potatoes
- Less likely to consume reduced-fat milk and more likely to consume whole milk
- Less likely to consume sugar-free sodas and more likely to consume regular sodas.

## Nutritional Quality of Food Choices

Over half of the foods consumed by FSP participants and both groups of nonparticipants were foods that should be consumed only occasionally (top of the radiant pyramid). Overall, FSP participants were:

- More likely than either income-eligible or higher- income nonparticipants to consume foods suggested for occasional consumption (62% of all food choices vs. 58% and 56%, respectively)
- Less likely to consume foods suggested for selective consumption (19% vs. 21% and 21%)
- Less likely to consume foods suggested for frequent consumption (19% vs. 21% and 23%).

FSP participants make less nutritious choices (more "top-heavy" choices) than higher-income nonparticipants in the following food groups:

- Milk, cheese, yogurt (all ages) – due to greater consumption of whole milk and less reduced-fat milk
- Beverages (other than milk and fruit juice) (adults and older adults) – due to greater consumption of regular sodas and less sugar- free sodas
- Salty snacks (all ages) – due to greater consumption of potato chips and less popcorn.

*Chapter 6*

# THE HEALTHY EATING INDEX-2005 AND SOURCES OF *MYPYRAMID* INTAKES

In this chapter, we examine the overall quality of the diets consumed by FSP participants and nonparticipants using the Healthy Eating Index (HEI)-2005. The HEI-2005 was developed by the USDA Center for Nutrition Policy and Promotion (CNPP) to measure compliance with the diet- related recommendations of the 2005 *Dietary Guidelines for Americans* (DGA) and the *MyPyramid* food guidance system (Guenther et al., in press).

The *MyPyramid* food guidance system translates the DGA into simple messages about the types and amounts of food to consume in five major food groups (grains, vegetables, fruits, milk, meat and beans), based on energy needs. Recommendations are provided for 12 food intake patterns—specific to gender, age, and activity level—based on calorie needs, nutrient goals, nutrient content of foods in each group, and food consumption patterns. *MyPyramid* also provides guidance about intakes of oils and discretionary calories (see box).

The DGA encourages consumption of oils, within recommended calorie allowances, because they provide essential polyunsaturated fatty acids and other nutrients, such as vitamin E. Moderation of saturated fat and sodium intakes is recommended because excess consumption may contribute to cardiovascular disease and high blood pressure. Consumption of solid fats, alcoholic beverages, and added sugars (SoFAAS) should be within discretionary calorie allowances, which reflect the balance of calories remaining in a person's energy allowance after accounting for the calories in the most nutrient-dense (fat-free or lowest fat form, with no added sugars) form of the various foods needed to meet recommended nutrient intakes (Basiotis et al., 2006).

Analyses in this chapter are limited to persons 2 years and older because the DGAs and *MyPyramid* do not apply to younger children. In addition, analyses are limited to data from NHANES 1999-

---

**MyPyramid Intakes and the
Healthy Eating Index (HEI-2005)**

**Data**

- NHANES 1999-2002: Single 24-hour recall per person
- MyPyramid Equivalents Database for USDA Survey Food Codes, 1994-2002, version 1.0

**Measures**

- Average HEI-2005 component scores
- Average number of MyPyramid Equivalents per child

---

2002 because *MyPyramid* data for 2003-2004 were not available at the time the analyses were completed.


# THE HEALTHY EATING INDEX-2005

The HEI-2005 is comprised of 12 component scores that measure consumption of food and nutrients relative to *MyPyramid* recommendations and the DGA (Table 6-1). Eight components are food-based and assess intakes of *MyPyramid* food groups and subgroups. The four remaining components assess intakes of oils, saturated fat, sodium, and calories from SoFAAS. The HEI–2005 scoring gives higher scores for greater consumption of food-based components and oils; but high scores for sodium, saturated fats, and calories from SoFAAS are obtained with low consumption.

---

**MyPyramid Food Groups**

➤**Grains**          **Make Half Your Grains Whole**

➤**Vegetables**     **Vary Your Veggies**

➤**Fruits**

➤**Milk**

➤**Meat & Beans**

**Oils & Discretionary Calories**

Consume oils for essential fatty acids.
Use discretionary calorie allowance to:

- Eat more foods from any food group,
- Eat foods in non-lean forms,
- Add fat or sweeteners to foods, or
- Consume foods that are mostly fats, caloric sweeteners, or alcohol (such as candy, soda, or alcoholic beverages).

## Table 6-1. Healthy Eating Index-2005 (HEI 2005) Scoring System

| Component | Max Score | Criteria for: Zero Score | Criteria for: Maximum Score |
|---|---|---|---|
| 1. Total Fruit | 5 |  | 0.8 cup equiv. per 1,000 kcal |
| 2. Whole Fruit | 5 |  | 0.4 cup equiv. per 1,000 kcal |
| 3. Total Vegetables | 5 |  | 1.1 cup equiv. per 1,000 kcal |
| 4. Dark Green & Orange Vegetables and Legumes | 5 |  | 0.4 cup equiv. per 1,000 kcal |
| 5. Total Grains | 5 | No intake | 3.0 oz equiv. per 1,000 kcal |
| 6. Whole Grains | 5 |  | 1.5 oz equiv. per 1,000 kcal |
| 7. Milk | 10 |  | 1.3 cup equiv. per 1,000 kcal |
| 8. Meat and Beans | 10 |  | 2.5 oz equiv. per 1,000 kcal |
| 9. Oils | 10 |  | 12 grams per 1,000 kcal |
| 10. Saturated fat[a] | 10 | 15% | 7% of energy |
| 11. Sodium[a] | 10 | 2.0 gms | 0.7 grams per 1,000 kcal |
| 12. Calories from SoFAAS | 20 | 50% | 20% of energy |

[a] Saturated Fat and Sodium get a score of 8 for the intake levels that reflect the 2005 Dietary Guidelines, <10% of calories from saturated fat and 1.1 grams of sodium/1,000 kcal, respectively.
*Source:* Guenther, et al., in press.

HEI-2005 component scores are assigned based on a density approach that compares intakes per 1,000 calories to a reference standard. This approach reflects the overarching recommendation of the DGA and *MyPyramid* that individuals should strive to meet food group and nutrient needs while maintaining energy balance. The per- 1,000 calorie reference standards used in the HEI2005 are based on the assumptions that underlie the recommended *MyPyramid* eating patterns, properly reflecting goals for intakes over time and the recommended mix of food groups.

Table 6-1 shows the intake criteria corresponding to minimum and maximum scores for each HEI2005 component. The scoring is linear for all components except saturated fat and sodium. For example, an intake that is halfway between the criteria for the maximum and minimum scores yields a score that is half the maximum score. Saturated fat and sodium are scored on a nonlinear scale, with criteria specified for scores of 0, 8, and 10. A total HEI-2005 score, with a range from 0 to 100, is obtained by summing the component scores.

The source data for calculation of HEI-2005 scores is NHANES 1999-2002 Individual Food Files (IFF) and the *MyPyramid Equivalents Database for USDA Survey Food Codes* (MPED), developed by USDA's Agricultural Research Service (ARS) (see Appendix A). (The analysis is limited to NHANES 1999-2002 because MPED data for NHANES 2003-2004 were not available at the time the analysis was completed.) Both the IFF and MPED files contain one record for each food item reported by respondents. The IFF files contain measures of energy, saturated fat, sodium, and alcoholic beverages. The MPED contains, for every food reported in the IFF, measures of *MyPyramid* food group intakes in cups/cup equivalents (vegetables, fruits, and milk/milk products) or ounce (oz.)/oz. equivalents (grains and meat/beans). Data are also provided for intakes of oils (in grams (gm.), solid fats (gm.), and added sugars (in teaspoons (tsp.)).

We followed CNPP guidance in the *HEI–2005 Technical Report* (Guenther, et. al, 2007) and the CNPP SAS program for HEI–2005 population scores, to apply the HEI–2005 scoring system to population groups.[1] As noted by CNPP, it is preferable to calculate HEI-2005 scores based on *usual* intakes of a population group. When this is not possible because, for example, intake data are available for only one day, usual intake scores can be approximated by applying the HEI-2005 scoring system to the ratio of a group's mean food (or nutrient) intake to the group's mean energy intake. Additional information about methods used in computing HEI-2005 scores is provided in Appendix A.

## HEI-2005 SCORES FOR FSP PARTICIPANTS AND NONPARTICIPANTS

The HEI-2005 score for all persons was 58 out of a possible 100 (Table C-10). Children ages 2-18 and adults scored 55 and 58, respectively, while older adults scored 68 out of 100. On average, FSP participants scored below income-eligible and higher-income nonparticipants (52 vs. 56 and 58 points, respectively) (Figure 6-1). These results, however, indicate that the diets of all age groups and participant/nonparticipant groups fell considerably short of the diet recommended in the DGA and *MyPyramid*.

Scores for the individual HEI-2005 components are shown in Figures 6-2 through 6-4. Adult and older adult FSP participants and both groups of nonparticipants achieved maximum scores on 2 components: Total Grains and Meat and Beans. Children in all three groups also achieved the maximum score on Total Grains, and scores of 8 out of 10 on Meat and Beans. However, in all age groups, FSP participants and nonparticipants scored below 50 percent of the maximum score on 3 components: Dark Green and Orange Vegetables and Legumes; Whole Grains; and Saturated Fat.

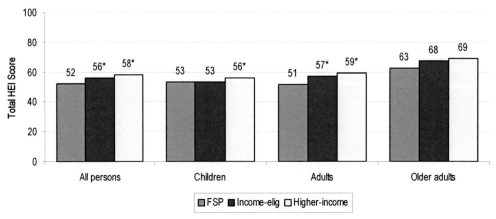

* Denotes statistically significant difference from FSP participants at the .05 level or better. Estimates are age adjusted.

Figure 6-1.Healthy Eating Index-2005 Total Scores

---

[1] HEI guidance is found at http://www.cnpp.usda.gov/ HealthyEating IndexSupportFiles.htm.

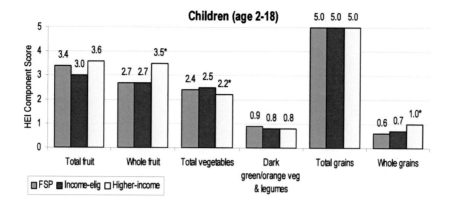

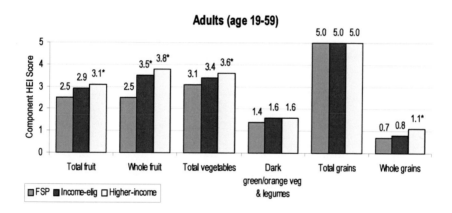

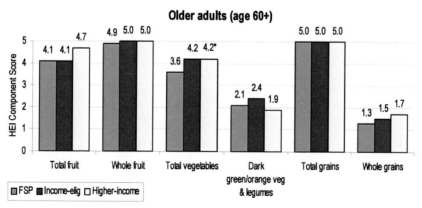

* Denotes statistically significant difference from FSP participants at the .05 level or better. HEI component scores are based on the ratio of group mean food intake to group mean energy intake. Estimates are age adjusted.

Figure 6-2. Healthy Eating Index-2005 (HEI-2005) Component Scores Worth 5 Points

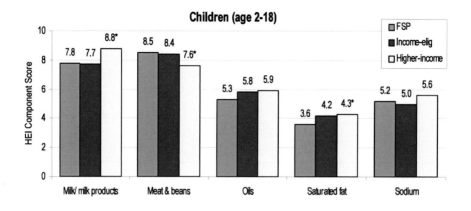

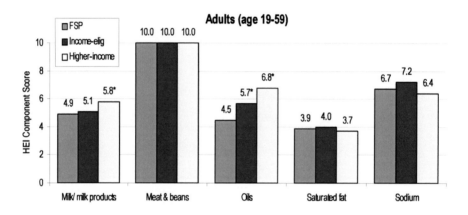

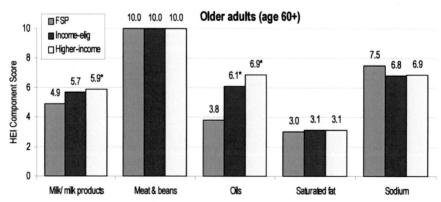

\* Denotes statistically significant difference from FSP participants at the .05 level or better. HEI component scores are based on the ratio of group mean food intake to group mean energy intake. Estimates are age adjusted.

Figure 6-3. Healthy Eating Index-2005 (HEI-2005) Component Scores Worth 10 Points

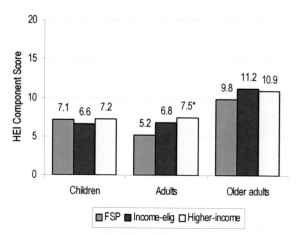

* Denotes statistically significant difference from FSP participants at the .05 level or better. HEI
  component scores are based on the ratio of group mean food intake to group mean energy intake.
  Estimates are age adjusted.

Figure 6-4. HEI-2005 Component Score for Calories from SoFAAS (Max score is 20)

## HEI-2005 COMPONENTS AND UNDERLYING FOOD AND NUTRIENT INTAKES

In this section we discuss each HEI-2005 component score separately. The estimates of
food group intakes that underlie HEI-2005 scores are based at the component or ingredient
level rather than at the whole food level used in the Chapter 5 analyses.[2] Thus, a single food
in the Chapter 5 analysis may contribute to several of the *MyPyramid* food groups considered
in the HEI-2005. For example, pizza contributes to intakes in the grain (crust), vegetable
(tomato sauce and any vegetable toppings), milk (cheese), and, if applicable, meat and bean
(meat toppings, if any) groups. Similarly, fruits canned in heavy syrup are broken down into
fruit and added sugars; and cookies, cakes, and pies are broken down into grains, oils and/or
solid fats, added sugars, and, where appropriate, fruit.

To gain insight into factors that contribute to HEI2005 scores, we also present data on the
specific foods that contributed to total intakes in each population subgroup (Tables 6-2 to 6-
11). For each group of participants and nonparticipants, we ask the question: "Which specific
foods contributed most to consumption in this food group?" For these analyses, we revert
back to the food grouping scheme used in Chapter 5 so that the focus is on foods as they were
eaten. For example, hamburgers or cheeseburgers that included lettuce and tomatoes may

---

[2] Data on total intakes within each MyPyramid food group are presented in Table C-11. Significant differences
between FSP participants and nonparticipants for HEI-2005 component scores are not always be consistent
with differences observed in average intakes of the respective MyPyramid food groups. This can occur
because the HEI-2005 component scores measure food group intake per- 1,000 calories, while average
MyPyramid intakes are not standardized per 1,000 calories.
Where findings for a particular *MyPyramid* group are inconsistent, the HEI-2005 findings should be given
more weight. Comparison of HEI-2005 scores answer the question that is most important in judging overall
diet quality of FSP participants and nonparticipants—that is: Are there differences between FSP participants
and nonparticipants in the extent to which the mix of foods/nutrients in their diets conform to DGA/
*MyPyramid* guidelines?

show up as contributors to vegetable intakes; and pizza, cheeseburgers, and other mixed dishes that contain cheese may show up as contributors to intakes of milk and milk products.

Results of these "food sources" analyses are presented in tables that list all foods that provided two percent or more of total intake for any group (all persons, FSP participants, income-eligible nonparticipants, and higher-income nonparticipants). Foods are listed in rank order, from largest contributor to smallest contributor, based on results for all persons. In discussing results, we focus on significant differences that involved foods that were among the top five contributors to total intakes and differences that were observed for all three age groups.

## Total Fruit and Whole Fruit

Scores on the Total Fruit component of the HEI2005 were highest for older adults (4.6 out of 5), followed by children (3.4) and adults (3.0) (Table C-10). For all age groups, there were no statistically significant differences in the Total Fruit scores of FSP participants and income-eligible nonparticipants (Figure 6-2). The Total Fruit score for FSP adults was significantly below that of higher-income adults (2.5 vs. 3.1).

Older adults as a group scored 5 out of 5 on the Whole Fruit component of the HEI-2005 (Table C10). Whole Fruit scores for FSP children and adults were about 2.5, and both FSP children and adults scored significantly below higher-income nonparticipants.

Citrus juice was the leading contributor to fruit intakes for all three age groups, accounting for roughly one-quarter of total fruit intake overall (Table 6-2). Other leading sources varied across age groups. Among children, non-citrus juice, fresh apples, fresh bananas, and noncarbonated sweetened drinks rounded out the top five contributors to fruit intake. Together with citrus juice, these sources accounted for more than 70 percent of total fruit intake, overall. There were no significant differences between FSP children and either group of nonparticipant children in the relative contributions of these foods to total fruit intakes.

Among adults, there was more variation across groups in the leading sources of fruit intake. FSP adults obtained a significantly larger share of their total fruit intake from non-citrus juices and noncarbonated sweetened drinks than either income- eligible or higher-income nonparticipants: 20 percent vs. 13 and 10 percent (non-citrus juices) and 12 percent vs. 6 and 7 percent (non-carbonated sweetened drinks). In addition, FSP adults obtained a significantly smaller share of their total fruit intake from fresh apples, relative to both groups of nonparticipants (6 vs. 11 percent).

Among older adults, only one significant difference was noted for a food that was a leading contributor to total fruit intakes—fresh apples made a significantly smaller contribution to the fruit intakes of FSP older adults than higher-income older adults (5 vs. 10 percent).

Of the other scattered significant differences shown in Table 6-2, only one was observed for all three age groups. FSP participants consistently obtained significantly smaller shares of their total fruit intakes from fresh berries than higher-income nonparticipants. Among adults, this difference was also significant for FSP participants and income-eligible nonparticipants.

## Table 6-2. Food Sources of MyPyramid Intakes: Fruit

| | All Persons | | | | Children (age 2-18) | | | |
|---|---|---|---|---|---|---|---|---|
| | Total Persons | Food Stamp Program Partic. | Income-eligible Nonpartic. | Higher-income Nonpartic. | Total Persons | Food Stamp Program Partic. | Income-eligible Nonpartic. | Higher-income Nonpartic. |
| Sample size | 16,419 | 2,303 | 3,577 | 9,094 | 7,583 | 1,495 | 1,801 | 3,682 |
| 1. Citrus juice | 24.4 | 25.3 | 22.9 | 24.7 | 23.9 | 25.8 | 25.6 | 22.4 |
| 2. Non-citrus juice | 12.8 | 19.1 | *14.0 | ***11.7 | 21.8 | 24.3 | 22.5 | 20.4 |
| 3. Fresh apple | 11.2 | 7.4 | *10.8 | ***11.8 | 13.0 | 12.7 | 10.1 | 14.5 |
| 4. Fresh banana | 10.8 | 9.7 | 10.4 | 10.7 | 6.1 | 6.6 | 7.0 | 5.8 |
| 5. Noncarbonated sweetened drink | 6.1 | 8.8 | *5.4 | *6.0 | 6.7 | 6.5 | 6.6 | 6.7 |
| 6. Fresh watermelon | 4.5 | 4.6 | 5.7 | 4.0 | 4.4 | 4.1 | 3.8 u | 4.8 |
| 7. Fresh melon | 3.5 | 1.9 | 3.8 | *3.7 | 2.1 | 2.2 u | 0.9 | 2.3 |
| 8. Fresh grapes | 3.0 | 2.4 | 2.6 | 3.0 | 2.6 | 2.3 | 1.8 | 2.8 |
| 9. Fresh orange | 2.6 | 2.0 | *3.5 | 2.3 | 2.7 | 2.8 | *5.4 | 1.9 |
| 10. Other fresh fruit | 2.6 | 3.2 | 1.9 | 2.7 | 1.9 | 1.5 | 1.8 | 2.3 |
| 11. Fresh peach/nectarine | 2.3 | 1.7 | ***2.7 | **2.4 | 1.5 | 1.3 | 1.7 u | ***1.6 |
| 12. Fresh berries | 1.8 | 0.3 | ***0.9 | **2.2 | 1.7 | 0.2 | 0.5 | ***2.4 |
| All other food groups | 14.5 | 13.6 | 15.4 | 14.8 | 11.7 | 9.7 | 12.1 | 12.0 |

| | Adults (age 19-59) | | | | Older Adults (age 60+) | | | |
|---|---|---|---|---|---|---|---|---|
| | Total Persons | Food Stamp Program Partic. | Income-eligible Nonpartic. | Higher-income Nonpartic. | Total Persons | Food Stamp Program Partic. | Income-eligible Nonpartic. | Higher-income Nonpartic. |
| Sample size | 5,775 | 593 | 1,124 | 3,587 | 3,061 | 215 | 652 | 1,825 |
| 1. Citrus juice | 24.9 | 24.2 | 20.9 | 26.2 | 23.2 | 28.6 | 25.0 | 23.1 |
| 2. Non-citrus juice | 10.9 | 20.4 | *12.6 | **9.7 | 5.8 | 6.9 | 6.1 | 5.5 |
| 3. Fresh apple | 10.9 | 5.7 | *10.8 | **11.0 | 9.7 | 5.2 | 11.1 | *10.4 |
| 4. Fresh banana | 11.5 | 8.6 | 10.8 | 11.7 | 15.2 | 17.6 | 14.1 | 14.5 |
| 5. Noncarbonated sweetened drink | 6.7 | 12.0 | *5.7 | *6.5 | 3.2 | 2.0 | 2.7 | 2.9 |
| 6. Fresh watermelon | 4.5 | 3.2 u | 6.4 | 3.8 | 4.7 | 9.6 u | 5.9 u | 3.8 |
| 7. Fresh melon | 3.4 | 1.5 u | *4.2 | *3.5 | 6.2 | 3.0 u | 6.9 | 6.4 |
| 8. Fresh grapes | 2.9 | 2.5 u | 3.3 | 2.8 | 3.6 | 2.3 u | 1.7 | 4.1 |
| 9. Fresh orange | 2.4 | 1.8 | 2.9 | 2.4 | 2.7 | 1.8 u | 2.8 | 2.8 |
| 10. Other fresh fruit | 2.8 | 3.3 | 2.1 | 2.9 | 2.6 | 4.5 u | 1.2 | 2.6 |
| 11. Fresh peach/nectarine | 2.4 | 1.7 u | 2.5 | 2.6 | 3.1 | 2.2 u | 4.5 u | ***3.0 |
| 12. Fresh berries | 1.9 | 0.4 u | *1.1 | ***2.2 | 1.9 | 0.1 u | 1.2 u | **2.2 |
| All other food groups | 14.8 | 14.6 | 16.7 | 14.8 | 18.0 | 16.2 | 16.9 | 18.6 |

Notes: Table shows the percent of MyPyramid equivalents contributed by each food source for each population subgroup (column). Food sources are ranked by their contribution to overall (Total persons, all ages) intake. Food sources shown separately are those contributing at least 2 percent to the Pyramid intake of any population subgroup. Significant differences in means and proportions are noted by * (.05 level), ** (.01 level), or *** (.001 level). Differences are tested in comparison to FSP participants, identified as persons in households receiving food stamps in the past 12 months.

u Denotes individual estimates not meeting the standards of reliability or precision due to inadequate cell size or large coefficient of variation.

Sources: NHANES 1999-2002 dietary recalls and MyPyramid Equivalents Database for USDA Survey Food Codes, 1994-2002, Version 1.0, October2006. Estimates are based on a single dietary recall per person. Excludes pregnant and breastfeeding women and infants. 'Total Persons' includes persons with missing food stamp participation or income. Percents are age adjusted to account for different age distributions of Food Stamp participants and nonparticipants.

## Total Vegetables, Dark Green and Orange Vegetables and Legumes

There were no significant differences in the Total Vegetables scores for FSP participants and income- eligible nonparticipants, in all three age groups (Figure 6-2). Compared with higher-income nonparticipants, FSP children scored significantly higher on Total Vegetables (2.4 vs. 2.2 out of 5), while FSP adults and older adults scored significantly lower (3.1 vs. 3.6 for adults; 3.6 vs. 4.2 for older adults).

Scores for Dark Green and Orange Vegetables and Legumes were low for all groups, with no statistically significant differences between FSP participants and nonparticipants (Figure 6-2). Adults and older adults had somewhat higher scores than children (statistical significance not tested).

The three leading contributors to vegetable intakes varied by age group but not for FSP participants and nonparticipants. The top contributors to vegetable intakes, by age group, were (Table 6-3):

- Children—fried potatoes; potato chips; other types of cooked potatoes
- Adults—salads; cooked potatoes that were not fried; fried potatoes
- Older adults—salads/salad greens; cooked potatoes that were not fried

There were some differences between FSP participants and higher-income nonparticipants in specific items contributing to vegetable intakes below the top three:

- FSP children obtained significantly smaller shares of their total vegetables intake from salads and pizza with meat, compared with higher-income nonparticipant children.
- FSP adults, compared with higher-income nonparticipants, obtained a significantly smaller share of their total vegetable intake from salads/salad greens (7 vs. 16 percent) and a significantly larger share from cooked potatoes that were not fried (13 vs. 9 percent).
- FSP older adults obtained a significantly smaller share of their vegetable intake from salads/salad greens than higher-income nonparticipant older adults (10 vs. 18 percent).

There were several scattered differences between FSP participants and one or both groups of nonparticipants in the relative contributions of specific foods to total vegetable intakes, but none of these differences was observed for all three age groups.

## Table 6-3. Food Sources of MyPyramid Intakes: Vegetables

| | All Persons | | | | Children (age 2-18) | | | |
|---|---|---|---|---|---|---|---|---|
| | Total Persons | Food Stamp Program Partic. | Income-eligible Nonpartic. | Higher-income Nonpartic. | Total Persons | Food Stamp Program Partic. | Income-eligible Nonpartic. | Higher-income Nonpartic. |
| Sample size | 16,419 | 2,303 | 3,577 | 9,094 | 7,583 | 1,495 | 1,801 | 3,682 |
| 1. Salad (greens) | 12.9 | 7.0 | 8.7 | ***14.1 | 6.9 | 5.0 | 5.0 | *7.8 |
| 2. Cooked potatoes-not fried | 9.7 | 11.1 | 9.7 | 9.7 | 8.5 | 7.7 | 9.0 | 8.3 |
| 3. Cooked potatoes-fried | 8.5 | 9.2 | 8.6 | 8.4 | 12.6 | 13.4 | 11.3 | 13.0 |
| 4. Potato chips | 5.4 | 6.1 | 5.7 | 5.1 | 9.3 | 10.6 | 11.7 | 8.1 |
| 5. Sandwiches (excl. burgers) | 4.0 | 3.4 | 3.5 | 4.3 | 3.2 | 3.3 | 3.4 | 3.2 |
| 6. Pizza w/ meat | 3.4 | 3.5 | 3.2 | 3.5 | 5.0 | 3.7 | 5.1 | *5.3 |
| 7. Meat mixtures w/ red meat | 3.0 | 4.2 | 2.9 | 2.9 | 2.5 | 3.4 | 2.8 | 2.5 |
| 8. Vegetables mixtures (inc soup) | 2.9 | 3.5 | 3.4 | 2.6 | 2.3 | 2.2 u | 4.1 | 1.6 |
| 9. Pasta dishes, italian style | 3.1 | 4.0 | *1.9 | 3.2 | 4.8 | 6.6 | *3.2 | 4.9 |
| 10. Cooked corn | 2.9 | 3.1 | 2.8 | 3.0 | 4.0 | 5.1 | 3.7 | 3.8 |
| 11. Cooked tomatoes | 2.5 | 1.3 | *2.7 | **2.8 | 2.4 | 0.7 | ***2.7 | ***2.7 |
| 12. Cooked green beans | 2.4 | 3.4 | 2.7 | *2.2 | 2.2 | 3.2 | 1.7 | 2.1 |
| 13. Hamburgers/cheeseburgers | 2.4 | 2.6 | 2.3 | 2.3 | 2.8 | 3.3 | 2.4 | 2.8 |
| 14. Other cooked (high nutrients) footnote c | 1.9 | 1.8 | 2.4 | 1.8 | 0.7 | 1.0 | 1.0 | 0.5 |
| 15. Rice dishes | 1.8 | 1.5 | 2.1 | 1.8 | 1.8 | 1.0 | **2.4 | 1.8 |
| 16. Meat mixtures w/ chicken/turkey | 1.8 | 2.8 | 1.6 | 1.6 | 1.8 | 2.8 | 2.2 | 1.0 |
| 17. Meat soup | 1.6 | 2.4 | 2.5 | 1.3 | 1.5 | 0.8 u | **2.4 | 1.2 |
| 18. Beans | 1.5 | 1.8 | *3.0 | 1.2 | 1.0 | 1.0 | 2.0 | **0.5 |
| 19. Raw tomatoes | 1.5 | 1.0 | *2.2 | 1.4 | 1.0 | 0.4 u | 0.9 | **1.2 |
| 20. Chili con carne | 1.4 | 3.1 | 2.3 | 1.3 | 1.2 | 2.0 u | 0.7 u | 1.2 |
| 21. Cooked mixed | 1.4 | 1.0 | *2.3 | 1.3 | 1.1 | 1.2 | 1.7 | 0.8 |
| 22. Catsup, mustard, relish, etc | 1.6 | 1.9 | 1.7 | 1.5 | 2.5 | 2.4 | 2.4 | 2.6 |
| All other food groups | 22.3 | 20.4 | 21.9 | 22.8 | 21.0 | 18.9 | 18.2 | 23.0 |

| | Adults (age 19-59) | | | | Older Adults (age 60+) | | | |
|---|---|---|---|---|---|---|---|---|
| | Total Persons | Food Stamp Program Partic. | Income-eligible Nonpartic. | Higher-income Nonpartic. | Total Persons | Food Stamp Program Partic. | Income-eligible Nonpartic. | Higher-income Nonpartic. |
| Sample size | 5,775 | 593 | 1,124 | 3,587 | 3,061 | 215 | 652 | 1,825 |
| 1. Salad (greens) | 14.1 | 7.0 | 9.0 | ***15.6 | 17.8 | 10.0 | 12.6 | *18.1 |
| 2. Cooked potatoes-not fried | 9.4 | 12.8 | 9.4 | *9.3 | 12.6 | 10.5 | 11.8 | 13.2 |
| 3. Cooked potatoes-fried | 8.2 | 9.0 | 8.7 | 7.8 | 3.5 | 3.7 u | 4.2 | 3.4 |
| 4. Potato chips | 4.6 | 4.5 | 4.2 | 4.7 | 2.1 | 4.8 u | 2.1 | 1.9 |
| 5. Sandwiches (excl. burgers) | 4.5 | 3.4 | 4.0 | *4.9 | 3.5 | 3.2 u | 2.0 | 3.8 |
| 6. Pizza w/ meat | 3.4 | 4.1 | 3.1 | 3.4 | 0.9 | 1.0 u | 0.6 u | 1.0 |
| 7. Meat mixtures w/ red meat | 2.9 | 3.6 | 2.4 | 2.7 | 4.3 | 7.4 u | 4.7 | 4.4 |
| 8. Vegetables mixtures (inc soup) | 2.5 | 2.3 | 2.6 | 2.4 | 5.2 | 9.8 u | 4.7 | 5.0 |
| 9. Pasta dishes, italian style | 2.6 | 3.0 | *0.9 | 2.8 | 2.2 | 3.2 u | 2.8 | 2.0 |
| 10. Cooked corn | 2.5 | 2.9 | 2.6 | 2.5 | 2.8 | 1.1 u | 2.2 | *3.5 |
| 11. Cooked tomatoes | 3.0 | 1.4 | 3.0 | **3.3 | 1.1 | 2.0 u | 1.9 u | 0.9 |
| 12. Cooked green beans | 1.9 | 3.4 | 2.2 | *1.8 | 4.0 | 3.5 | 5.7 | 3.6 |
| 13. Hamburgers/cheeseburgers | 2.6 | 2.8 | 2.8 | 2.4 | 1.0 | 1.1 u | 1.0 u | 1.0 |
| 14. Other cooked (high nutrients) footnote c | 2.0 | 1.7 | 2.6 | 2.0 | 3.6 | 3.2 u | 4.2 | 3.3 |
| 15. Rice dishes | 2.1 | 2.0 | 2.2 | 2.1 | 1.0 | 0.5 u | 1.0 | 1.0 |
| 16. Meat mixtures w/ chicken/turkey | 1.8 | 2.5 | 1.3 | 1.8 | 1.5 | 3.6 u | 1.4 | 1.6 |
| 17. Meat soup | 1.7 | 3.1 | 2.9 | 1.4 | 1.5 | 2.2 u | 1.7 | 1.4 |
| 18. Beans | 1.7 | 2.1 | 3.0 | 1.4 | 1.8 | 1.7 u | *4.7 | 1.3 |
| 19. Raw tomatoes | 1.5 | 1.0 u | 2.8 | 1.3 | 2.1 | 1.4 u | 2.0 | 2.3 |
| 20. Chili con carne | 1.5 | 3.3 u | 2.7 u | 1.2 | 1.8 | 4.1 u | 2.8 u | 1.6 |
| 21. Cooked mixed | 1.3 | 0.5 u | *2.6 | 1.1 | 2.3 | 2.2 u | 2.0 | 2.4 |
| 22. Catsup, mustard, relish, etc | 1.5 | 2.2 | 1.6 | 1.4 | 0.6 | 0.4 u | *1.2 u | 0.5 |
| All other food groups | 22.8 | 21.3 | 23.5 | 22.7 | 22.6 | 19.5 | 22.6 | 22.7 |

## Table 6-4. Food Sources of MyPyramid Intakes: Grains

| | All Persons | | | | Children (age 2-18) | | | |
|---|---|---|---|---|---|---|---|---|
| | Total Persons | Food Stamp Program Partic. | Income-eligible Nonpartic. | Higher-income Nonpartic. | Total Persons | Food Stamp Program Partic. | Income-eligible Nonpartic. | Higher-income Nonpartic. |
| Sample size | 16,419 | 2,303 | 3,577 | 9,094 | 7,583 | 1,495 | 1,801 | 3,682 |
| 1. Sandwiches (excl. burgers) | 15.5 | 15.5 | 14.6 | 15.8 | 14.4 | 16.0 | 15.0 | 14.0 |
| 2. Bread | 8.6 | 8.0 | 9.8 | 8.1 | 6.3 | 5.9 | 8.8 | 5.6 |
| 3. Cold cereal | 5.8 | 4.7 | 4.8 | 6.1 | 7.4 | 7.1 | 6.3 | 7.8 |
| 4. Pizza w/ meat | 5.4 | 5.3 | 4.8 | 5.6 | 7.1 | 5.8 | 7.8 | 7.2 |
| 5. Hamburgers/cheeseburgers | 4.6 | 4.9 | 4.3 | 4.6 | 4.5 | 5.2 | 4.4 | 4.3 |
| 6. Rice | 4.0 | 5.8 | 5.8 | 3.3 | 3.4 | 5.1 | 4.8 | 2.6 |
| 7. Cookies | 3.8 | 4.0 | 3.8 | 3.8 | 4.4 | 4.6 | 4.5 | 4.4 |
| 8. Corn-based salty snacks | 3.6 | 3.2 | 3.3 | 3.7 | 5.2 | 5.1 | 4.9 | 5.2 |
| 9. Crackers | 3.0 | 2.4 | 3.1 | 3.1 | 3.2 | 2.5 | 2.2 | 3.8 |
| 10. Pasta | 2.8 | 3.1 | 2.6 | 2.8 | 2.6 | 2.1 | 2.3 | 2.6 |
| 11. Pizza (no meat) | 2.4 | 1.3 | 2.4 | 2.6 | 3.7 | 2.0 | 2.8 | 4.3 |
| 12. Pasta dishes, italian style | 2.3 | 2.7 | 1.4 | 2.4 | 2.7 | 3.8 | 2.0 | 2.5 |
| 13. Mexican entrees | 2.2 | 2.1 | 2.4 | 2.2 | 2.0 | 1.4 | 2.5 | 1.9 |
| 14. Popcorn | 2.2 | 1.3 u | 1.1 | 2.6 | 3.2 | 3.3 u | 0.5 | 4.1 |
| 15. Pancakes, waffles, french toast | 2.0 | 1.6 | 1.8 | 2.1 | 2.8 | 2.2 | 1.9 | 3.3 |
| 16. Macaroni & cheese | 1.9 | 3.7 | 1.7 | 1.8 | 2.7 | 3.4 | 1.9 | 2.9 |
| 17. Flour tortillas | 1.8 | 1.6 | 2.7 | 1.6 | 1.1 | 1.1 | 1.6 | 0.9 |
| 18. Bagels | 1.7 | 0.6 | 0.7 | 2.0 | 1.4 | 0.9 | 0.8 u | 1.6 |
| 19. Corn tortillas | 1.3 | 0.9 | 3.1 | 0.9 | 0.8 | 0.6 | 1.7 | 0.5 |
| All other food groups | 25.4 | 27.3 | 25.7 | 25.1 | 21.2 | 21.7 | 23.2 | 20.6 |

| | Adults (age 19-59) | | | | Older Adults (age 60+) | | | |
|---|---|---|---|---|---|---|---|---|
| | Total Persons | Food Stamp Program Partic. | Income-eligible Nonpartic. | Higher-income Nonpartic. | Total Persons | Food Stamp Program Partic. | Income-eligible Nonpartic. | Higher-income Nonpartic. |
| Sample size | 5,775 | 593 | 1,124 | 3,587 | 3,061 | 215 | 652 | 1,825 |
| 1. Sandwiches (excl. burgers) | 15.8 | 15.3 | 14.2 | 16.5 | 15.8 | 15.6 | 15.4 | 15.9 |
| 2. Bread | 7.8 | 7.6 | 8.6 | 7.4 | 14.7 | 12.6 | 15.6 | 14.4 |
| 3. Cold cereal | 4.4 | 3.4 | 3.4 | 4.8 | 7.9 | 5.8 | 7.6 | 8.2 |
| 4. Pizza w/ meat | 5.7 | 6.1 | 4.6 | 5.9 | 1.7 | 1.7 u | 0.9 | 2.0 |
| 5. Hamburgers/cheeseburgers | 5.3 | 5.4 | 4.9 | 5.3 | 2.5 | 2.3 u | 2.2 | 2.5 |
| 6. Rice | 4.4 | 5.4 | 6.3 | 3.9 | 3.8 | 7.9 | 5.6 | 2.6 |
| 7. Cookies | 3.4 | 4.0 | 3.5 | 3.4 | 4.1 | 3.0 | 3.7 | 4.2 |
| 8. Corn-based salty snacks | 3.6 | 3.1 | 3.3 | 3.7 | 1.0 | 0.7 u | 0.6 u | 1.1 |
| 9. Crackers | 2.6 | 2.1 | 3.4 | 2.5 | 3.9 | 3.5 | 3.3 | 4.2 |
| 10. Pasta | 3.0 | 3.7 | 3.0 | 3.0 | 2.4 | 2.4 | 1.8 u | 2.5 |
| 11. Pizza (no meat) | 2.3 | 1.3 | 2.8 | 2.4 | 0.7 | 0.1 u | 0.4 u | 0.7 u |
| 12. Pasta dishes, italian style | 2.2 | 2.2 | 0.8 | 2.4 | 2.1 | 2.5 u | 2.6 | 1.9 |
| 13. Mexican entrees | 2.7 | 3.0 | 2.8 | 2.8 | 0.7 | 0.2 u | 0.7 | 0.7 |
| 14. Popcorn | 1.9 | 0.6 u | 1.7 | 2.3 | 1.3 | 0.7 u | 0.3 u | 1.5 |
| 15. Pancakes, waffles, french toast | 1.7 | 1.4 | 1.8 | 1.6 | 1.8 | 1.2 u | 1.8 | 1.9 |
| 16. Macaroni & cheese | 1.6 | 3.4 | 1.5 | 1.4 | 1.9 | 5.1 u | 2.3 u | 1.5 |
| 17. Flour tortillas | 2.3 | 1.9 | 3.6 | 2.1 | 1.0 | 1.2 u | 1.3 u | 0.9 |
| 18. Bagels | 1.9 | 0.6 u | 0.9 | 2.3 | 1.4 | 0.4 u | 0.2 u | 1.8 |
| 19. Corn tortillas | 1.8 | 1.1 | 4.3 | 1.2 | 0.5 | 0.4 u | 1.2 | 0.2 |
| All other food groups | 25.6 | 28.2 | 24.7 | 25.3 | 31.1 | 32.6 | 32.5 | 31.3 |

See notes on Table 6-3.

## Total Grains and Whole Grains

FSP participants and nonparticipants in all age groups had the maximum score of 5.0 for the HEI2005 Total Grains component (Figure 6-2). Scores for Whole Grains were substantially lower, ranging from 0.6 to 1.7 (out of 5).

The top contributors to grain intakes of FSP participants and nonparticipants, by age group, were (Table 6-4):

- Children—sandwiches other than hamburgers and cheeseburgers; ready-to-eat breakfast cereals; pizza with meat; bread (not part of a sandwich)
- Adults— sandwiches other than hamburgers and cheeseburgers; bread (not part of a sandwich)
- Older adults— sandwiches other than hamburgers and cheeseburgers; bread (not part of a sandwich); ready-to-eat breakfast cereals

There was variability across groups of adults and older adults in the leading sources of grains. Ready to-eat breakfast cereals were the third or fourth most important source of grains among older adults, but were a less important source of grains in the diets of other adults.

Differences between FSP participants and nonparticipants in the relative importance of leading sources of grain were generally not statistically significant. Among older adults, however, rice provided 7.9 percent of the grain equivalents consumed by FSP participants (3rd leading source), compared with only 2.6 percent of the grain equivalents consumed by higher-income nonparticipants (6th leading source).

There were scattered differences between FSP participants and one or both groups of nonparticipants in the relative importance of other grain foods. The only differences that were observed for all three age groups were a smaller contribution from meatless pizza for FSP participants, relative to higher-income nonparticipants, and a smaller contribution from corn tortillas among FSP participants, relative to income-eligible nonparticipants.

## Milk and Milk Products

There were no significant differences between FSP participants and income-eligible nonparticipants in scores for the HEI-2005 Milk component (Figure 6-3). However, for all three age groups, FSP participants had significantly lower scores than higher- income nonparticipants.

Unflavored whole milk was the leading contributor to milk intakes of FSP participants in all age groups (Table 6-5). Moreover, among children and adults, FSP participants obtained a significantly larger share of their total milk intakes from unflavored whole milk than either income-eligible or higher-income nonparticipants. This pattern was also observed for older adult FSP participants and higher-income older adults.

Compared with higher-income nonparticipant children, FSP children obtained significantly less of their total milk intakes from unflavored 2 percent, 1 percent, and skim milks and cheese. Similarly, unflavored skim milk and cheese made significantly smaller contributions to intakes of FSP adults than higher-income nonparticipant adults and unflavored one percent milk made a significantly smaller contribution to intakes of FSP older adults than either income-eligible or higher-income older adults. None of the other scattered differences between FSP participants and one or both groups of nonparticipants was observed for all three age groups.

### Table 6-5. Food Sources of MyPyramid Intakes: Milk and Milk Products

| | All Persons | | | | Children (age 2-18) | | | |
|---|---|---|---|---|---|---|---|---|
| | Total Persons | Food Stamp Program Partic. | Income-eligible Nonpartic. | Higher-income Nonpartic. | Total Persons | Food Stamp Program Partic. | Income-eligible Nonpartic. | Higher-income Nonpartic. |
| Sample size | 16,419 | 2,303 | 3,577 | 9,094 | 7,583 | 1,495 | 1,801 | 3,682 |
| 1. Unflavored 2% milk | 15.5 | 12.4 | 14.4 | *16.1 | 19.6 | 14.4 | 18.9 | *21.5 |
| 2. Unflavored whole milk | 13.2 | 27.8 | **19.4 | ***10.3 | 18.5 | 32.2 | *23.6 | ***13.4 |
| 3. Unflavored skim milk | 9.6 | 4.6 | 6.6 | ***11.0 | 5.6 | 1.7 u | 1.3 | ***7.7 |
| 4. Cheese | 9.1 | 6.5 | 8.4 | *9.5 | 6.3 | 5.0 | 5.4 | 6.9 |
| 5. Sandwiches (excl. burgers) | 8.6 | 9.0 | 8.1 | 8.7 | 5.8 | 7.1 | 5.6 | 5.5 |
| 6. Unflavored 1% milk | 5.5 | 1.4 | **4.4 | **6.4 | 5.9 | 1.8 | 3.2 | **7.6 |
| 7. Pizza w/ meat | 4.9 | 5.5 | 4.8 | 4.9 | 5.2 | 4.3 | 6.4 | 5.0 |
| 8. Ice cream | 4.1 | 4.2 | 3.4 | 4.3 | 3.3 | 2.2 | 2.5 | ***3.8 |
| 9. Hamburgers/cheeseburgers | 2.4 | 2.7 | 2.8 | 2.3 | 2.0 | 2.4 | 2.5 | 1.8 |
| 10. Mexican entrees | 2.4 | 2.3 | 2.4 | 2.4 | 2.0 | 1.7 | 2.4 | 2.0 |
| 11. Pizza (no meat) | 2.3 | 1.5 | 2.5 | *2.4 | 2.9 | 1.6 | 2.3 | **3.4 |
| 12. Macaroni & cheese | 2.2 | 3.7 | 2.2 | *2.0 | 2.4 | 2.8 | 2.0 | 2.5 |
| 13. Yogurt | 2.1 | 0.8 | 1.0 | ***2.4 | 1.5 | 0.5 | 0.6 | ***2.0 |
| 14. Flavored whole milk | 1.8 | 2.7 | 3.2 | 1.4 | 3.4 | 4.6 | 4.4 | 2.9 |
| 15. Flavored milk-%fat nfs | 1.4 | 2.6 | 1.6 | *1.2 | 4.4 | 5.9 | 5.6 | 3.8 |
| All other food groups | 14.8 | 12.4 | 14.8 | 14.6 | 11.1 | 12.0 | 13.2 | 10.2 |

| | Adults (age 19-59) | | | | Older Adults (age 60+) | | | |
|---|---|---|---|---|---|---|---|---|
| | Total Persons | Food Stamp Program Partic. | Income-eligible Nonpartic. | Higher-income Nonpartic. | Total Persons | Food Stamp Program Partic. | Income-eligible Nonpartic. | Higher-income Nonpartic. |
| Sample size | 5,775 | 593 | 1,124 | 3,587 | 3,061 | 215 | 652 | 1,825 |
| 1. Unflavored 2% milk | 13.2 | 10.2 | 11.8 | 13.3 | 17.5 | 16.8 | 16.3 | 17.9 |
| 2. Unflavored whole milk | 11.7 | 26.2 | *17.3 | ***9.5 | 10.5 | 26.1 | 20.1 | *8.2 |
| 3. Unflavored skim milk | 9.7 | 3.7 u | 7.6 | **10.8 | 15.2 | 11.9 | 11.6 | 16.7 |
| 4. Cheese | 10.8 | 7.1 | 10.4 | *11.2 | 7.2 | 6.3 | 5.6 | 7.4 |
| 5. Sandwiches (excl. burgers) | 10.2 | 9.9 | 9.9 | 10.3 | 7.7 | 9.0 | 5.8 | 8.1 |
| 6. Unflavored 1% milk | 4.5 | 0.9 u | 3.7 | ***5.1 | 8.7 | 2.5 u | 8.4 | ***9.3 |
| 7. Pizza w/ meat | 5.7 | 7.3 | 5.2 | 5.6 | 1.7 | 1.5 u | 1.2 | 2.0 |
| 8. Ice cream | 3.9 | 4.7 | 3.2 | 4.0 | 5.8 | 5.4 | 5.5 | 6.0 |
| 9. Hamburgers/cheeseburgers | 3.1 | 3.2 | 3.5 | 2.9 | 0.8 | 1.4 u | 0.6 | 0.9 |
| 10. Mexican entrees | 3.0 | 3.1 | 3.1 | 3.1 | 0.6 | 0.2 u | 0.2 u | *0.8 |
| 11. Pizza (no meat) | 2.4 | 1.9 | 3.2 | 2.3 | 0.8 | 0.0 u | 0.4 u | *0.8 u |
| 12. Macaroni & cheese | 2.0 | 4.0 | 2.0 | *1.7 | 2.8 | 4.0 u | 3.6 u | 2.4 |
| 13. Yogurt | 2.4 | 1.0 u | 1.2 | ***2.6 | 2.1 | 1.0 u | 0.8 u | **2.4 |
| 14. Flavored whole milk | 1.4 | 2.6 u | 3.0 | 1.0 | 0.9 | 0.0 | ***1.9 u | **0.7 u |
| 15. Flavored milk-%fat nfs | 0.5 | 1.7 u | 0.3 | 0.5 | 0.2 u | 0.6 u | 0.3 u | 0.0 u |
| All other food groups | 15.6 | 12.5 | 14.7 | *16.0 | 17.4 | 13.2 | 17.8 | 16.4 |

See notes on Table 6-3.

## Meats and Beans

Adults and older adults in all participant/nonparticipant groups had the maximum score of 10 on the Meat and Beans component. FSP children and income-eligible nonparticipant children had comparable scores on this component (about 8.5); and FSP children scored significantly higher than higher- income nonparticipant children on the Meat and Beans component (8.5 vs. 7.6).

With the exception of older adult FSP participants, the top three sources of meat and bean intakes were, in somewhat varying order, sandwiches other than hamburgers and cheeseburgers, chicken, and beef (Table 6-6).[3] Other leading sources of meat among children and adults were hamburgers and cheeseburgers and eggs.

### Table 6-6. Food Sources of MyPyramid Intakes: Meat and Beans

| | All Persons | | | | Children (age 2-18) | | | |
|---|---|---|---|---|---|---|---|---|
| | Total Persons | Food Stamp Program Partic. | Income-eligible Nonpartic. | Higher-income Nonpartic. | Total Persons | Food Stamp Program Partic. | Income-eligible Nonpartic. | Higher-income Nonpartic. |
| Sample size | 16,419 | 2,303 | 3,577 | 9,094 | 7,583 | 1,495 | 1,801 | 3,682 |
| 1. Sandwiches (excl. burgers) | 19.1 | 16.0 | 17.8 | ***20.5 | 21.2 | 20.4 | 19.8 | 22.8 |
| 2. Chicken | 14.7 | 17.1 | 13.9 | 14.6 | 16.4 | 17.7 | 15.8 | 16.8 |
| 3. Beef | 8.3 | 7.1 | 8.0 | 8.3 | 7.7 | 7.4 | 7.9 | 7.1 |
| 4. Hamburgers/cheeseburgers | 6.6 | 6.4 | 6.3 | 6.6 | 8.1 | 8.4 | 7.5 | 8.1 |
| 5. Eggs | 5.5 | 6.5 | 6.4 | * 5.2 | 5.3 | 4.5 | 5.8 | 5.0 |
| 6. Pork | 4.5 | 6.0 | 4.7 | * 4.1 | 3.8 | 4.2 | 3.9 | 3.6 |
| 7. Fish | 4.3 | 4.1 | 4.6 | 4.2 | 2.8 | 2.8 | 2.5 | 3.2 |
| 8. Nuts | 4.0 | 1.1 | ***4.3 | ***4.2 | 1.9 | 0.8 | 1.7 | 2.4 |
| 9. Meat mixtures w/ red meat | 3.4 | 4.5 | 3.4 | 3.3 | 2.7 | 2.8 | 3.1 | 2.5 |
| 10. Meat mixtures w/ chicken/turkey | 2.4 | 3.3 | 2.7 | 2.2 | 2.6 | 4.1 | 2.8 | 1.8 |
| 11. Bacon/sausage | 2.2 | 2.5 | 2.1 | 2.1 | 2.2 | 2.6 | 1.9 | 2.2 |
| 12. Shellfish | 2.0 | 1.7 | 1.3 | 2.0 | 0.8 | 1.4 | 0.8 | 0.8 |
| 13. Ground beef | 2.0 | 2.0 | 2.9 | 1.8 | 2.0 | 1.7 | 2.8 | 1.8 |
| 14. Mexican entrees | 1.9 | 1.7 | 2.0 | 1.9 | 2.1 | 1.3 | ***2.7 | * 2.2 |
| All other food groups | 19.3 | 20.0 | 19.6 | 19.0 | 20.3 | 20.0 | 21.0 | 19.6 |

| | Adults (age 19-59) | | | | Older Adults (age 60+) | | | |
|---|---|---|---|---|---|---|---|---|
| | Total Persons | Food Stamp Program Partic. | Income-eligible Nonpartic. | Higher-income Nonpartic. | Total Persons | Food Stamp Program Partic. | Income-eligible Nonpartic. | Higher-income Nonpartic. |
| Sample size | 5,775 | 593 | 1,124 | 3,587 | 3,061 | 215 | 652 | 1,825 |
| 1. Sandwiches (excl. burgers) | 18.9 | 14.8 | 18.0 | ** 20.3 | 16.7 | 13.5 | 14.4 | 17.8 |
| 2. Chicken | 14.7 | 17.3 | 13.6 | 14.4 | 12.2 | 15.4 | 12.1 | 11.6 |
| 3. Beef | 8.4 | 8.1 | 7.9 | 8.6 | 8.7 | 3.0 | ** 8.0 | ***9.0 |
| 4. Hamburgers/cheeseburgers | 6.8 | 6.1 | 6.8 | 6.8 | 3.6 | 4.0 u | 3.2 | 3.6 |
| 5. Eggs | 5.2 | 6.2 | 6.5 | 4.9 | 6.9 | 10.4 | 7.2 | * 6.7 |
| 6. Pork | 4.9 | 6.8 | 5.3 | 4.5 | 3.9 | 6.2 | 3.9 | 3.7 |
| 7. Fish | 4.3 | 4.2 | 4.8 | 4.0 | 6.4 | 6.0 | 7.5 | 6.1 |
| 8. Nuts | 4.3 | 0.9 | ** 4.4 | ***4.5 | 5.9 | 2.7 u | 7.8 u | 5.8 |
| 9. Meat mixtures w/ red meat | 3.4 | 4.3 | 3.2 | 3.1 | 4.8 | 7.9 | 4.1 | 4.9 |
| 10. Meat mixtures w/ chicken/turkey | 2.3 | 2.4 | 2.6 | 2.2 | 2.6 | 5.3 u | 2.9 | 2.5 |
| 11. Bacon/sausage | 2.1 | 2.3 | 2.2 | 2.0 | 2.5 | 3.1 | 2.1 | 2.4 |
| 12. Shellfish | 2.4 | 2.3 u | 1.4 | 2.5 | 2.2 | 0.0 u | 2.0 u | ***2.3 |
| 13. Ground beef | 2.1 | 2.5 u | 2.9 | 1.8 | 1.8 | 0.8 u | 3.0 u | 1.7 |
| 14. Mexican entrees | 2.2 | 2.3 u | 2.1 | 2.2 | 0.6 | 0.2 u | 0.5 | ** 0.6 |
| All other food groups | 18.2 | 19.6 | 18.3 | 18.1 | 21.3 | 21.6 | 21.4 | 21.4 |

See notes on Table 6-3.

---

[3] The chicken and beef categories do not include those meats consumed as part of sandwiches or other mixed dishes.

There were few significant differences between FSP participants and nonparticipants in the relative contribution of leading sources of meat and bean intakes. Among adults, FSP participants obtained a significantly smaller share of their intakes from sandwiches other than hamburgers and cheeseburgers, relative to higher-income nonparticipants (15 vs. 20 percent). Among older adults, FSP participants obtained a significantly smaller share of their intakes from beef (not part of a sandwich or mixed dish) than either group of nonparticipants (3 vs. 8 and 9 percent).

## Oils

*MyPyramid* encourages use of oils high in polyunsaturated fat and monounsaturated fat as the main sources of fat in the diet. These oils provide essential fatty acids, do not raise levels of LDL ("bad") cholesterol in the blood, and are the major source of vitamin E in the typical American diet (USDA, CNPP, 2008). In the MPED, fat in cooking oils, some salad dressings, and soft tub or squeeze margarines were counted as oils (rather than discretionary solid fats). In addition, fats from fish, nuts, and seeds were classified as oils.

There were no significant differences between FSP children and either group of nonparticipant children in scores for the HEI-2005 Oils component (Figure 6-3). However, among adults and older adults, FSP participants had significantly lower scores for this component than both income-eligible and higher- income nonparticipants (4.5 vs. 5.7 and 6.8 for adults; 3.8 vs. 6.1 and 6.9 for older adults).

There was considerable variation in the leading sources of oil in the diets of FSP participants and nonparticipants and by age group (Table 6-7). Foods that were top contributors to the oil intakes of both FSP participants and nonparticipants were:

- Children— sandwiches,[4] corn-based salty snacks, and potato chips
- Adults—salads and sandwiches
- Older adults—salads, sandwiches, and margarine

Significant differences between FSP participants and nonparticipants, with regard to leading contributors to oil intakes included the following:

- FSP children obtained significantly more of their oil intakes from potato chips (16 vs. 10 percent) and significantly less from chicken (8 vs. 11 percent) and salads (9 vs. 18 percent), than higher-income nonparticipant children.
- FSP adults obtained significantly less of their total oil intakes from salads and nuts (which includes seeds and nut butters) than either group of nonparticipant adults.
- Older adult FSP participants obtained significantly less of their total oil intakes from salads than higher-income nonparticipant adults (6 vs. 21 percent). In addition, FSP participants appear to obtain much larger contributions of oil from potato chips and fats and oils other than margarine or salad dressing. These differences were not

---

[4] Sandwiches do not include hamburgers and cheeseburgers. Oil intake from sandwiches is likely from condiments.

statistically significant, however, probably because of the small sample of FSP participants.

**Table 6-7. Food Sources of MyPyramid Intakes: Oils**

| | All Persons | | | | Children (age 2-18) | | | |
|---|---|---|---|---|---|---|---|---|
| | Total Persons | Food Stamp Program Partic. | Income-eligible Nonpartic. | Higher-income Nonpartic. | Total Persons | Food Stamp Program Partic. | Income-eligible Nonpartic. | Higher-income Nonpartic. |
| Sample size ........................... | 16,419 | 2,303 | 3,577 | 9,094 | 7,583 | 1,495 | 1,801 | 3,682 |
| 1. Salads & salad dressing .............. | 16.5 | 9.2 | 11.6 | ***17.6 | 10.1 | 9.0 | 8.3 | 10.6 |
| 2. Sandwiches (excl. burgers) ......... | 14.0 | 15.0 | 13.7 | 14.5 | 15.1 | 16.1 | 12.2 | 16.3 |
| 3. Corn-based salty snacks ............. | 8.4 | 10.0 | 8.8 | *8.0 | 14.4 | 16.4 | 14.2 | 13.9 |
| 4. Potato chips ............................. | 8.1 | 11.4 | 9.1 | *7.3 | 12.2 | 15.6 | 16.6 | *9.8 |
| 5. Nuts ...................................... | 6.1 | 2.2 | ***6.9 | 6.2 | 2.4 | 1.1 u | 2.1 | *3.0 |
| 6. Chicken ................................. | 5.1 | 5.7 | 4.2 | 5.2 | 10.0 | 7.9 | 8.4 | *10.9 |
| 7. Margarine ............................... | 4.5 | 5.0 | 5.7 | 4.3 | 4.1 | 2.4 | 8.0 | 3.3 |
| 8. Candy .................................... | 3.4 | 2.8 | 3.1 | 3.5 | 3.6 | 2.8 | 4.0 | 3.7 |
| 9. Hamburgers/cheeseburgers ......... | 3.3 | 4.6 | 3.4 | *3.0 | 2.7 | 3.8 | 2.6 | 2.5 |
| 10. Cooked potatoes-fried ............... | 1.8 | 1.0 | **3.0 | 1.7 | 1.2 | 1.4 u | 1.1 | 0.9 |
| 11. Other added fats/oil ................... | 1.8 | 3.2 | 1.6 | 1.7 | 0.8 | 1.2 u | 0.1 u | 1.0 |
| 12. Cake/cupcakes ......................... | 1.5 | 2.2 | 0.8 | 1.7 | 1.3 | 3.0 u | 0.7 | 1.4 |
| All other food groups ......................... | 25.6 | 27.6 | 28.0 | 25.2 | 22.2 | 19.4 | 21.7 | 22.8 |

| | Adults (age 19-59) | | | | Older Adults (age 60+) | | | |
|---|---|---|---|---|---|---|---|---|
| | Total Persons | Food Stamp Program Partic. | Income-eligible Nonpartic. | Higher-income Nonpartic. | Total Persons | Food Stamp Program Partic. | Income-eligible Nonpartic. | Higher-income Nonpartic. |
| Sample size ........................... | 5,775 | 593 | 1,124 | 3,587 | 3,061 | 215 | 652 | 1,825 |
| 1. Salads & salad dressing .............. | 18.0 | 10.5 | 12.7 | *19.6 | 20.9 | 5.5 u | **13.1 | ***21.2 |
| 2. Sandwiches (excl. burgers) ......... | 14.0 | 13.7 | 15.2 | 14.2 | 12.2 | 18.3 | 11.2 | 12.6 |
| 3. Corn-based salty snacks ............. | 7.6 | 9.3 | 8.6 | 7.1 | 2.1 | 3.0 u | 2.0 u | 2.2 |
| 4. Potato chips ............................. | 7.5 | 8.4 | 7.1 | 7.4 | 3.9 | 14.8 u | 4.7 | 3.2 |
| 5. Nuts ...................................... | 6.8 | 1.8 | **7.8 | ***6.9 | 9.0 | 4.9 u | 11.1 u | 8.8 |
| 6. Chicken ................................. | 4.0 | 6.5 | 2.9 | 3.8 | 1.8 | 0.1 u | *2.2 u | **1.8 |
| 7. Margarine ............................... | 3.6 | 5.4 | 3.9 | 3.6 | 8.0 | 8.1 | 9.0 | 8.3 |
| 8. Candy .................................... | 3.5 | 3.1 | 3.1 | 3.7 | 2.7 | 1.8 u | 1.8 | 2.8 |
| 9. Hamburgers/cheeseburgers ......... | 4.0 | 5.9 | 4.6 | *3.6 | 1.7 | 1.4 u | 1.1 | 1.8 |
| 10. Cooked potatoes-fried ............... | 1.9 | 0.9 u | *3.5 | 1.8 | 2.7 | 0.6 u | 4.1 u | *2.4 |
| 11. Other added fats/oil ................... | 1.8 | 1.5 u | 1.5 | 1.8 | 3.2 | 11.1 u | 4.6 | 2.3 |
| 12. Cake/cupcakes ......................... | 1.4 | 2.1 | 0.9 | 1.5 | 2.1 | 1.6 u | 0.4 u | 2.7 |
| All other food groups ......................... | 25.9 | 30.9 | 28.5 | *24.9 | 29.6 | 28.9 | 34.9 | 29.8 |

See notes on Table 6-3.

## Saturated Fat

FSP participants and nonparticipants in all age groups had average scores of 3.0 to 4.3 (out of a possible 10) on the HEI-2005 Saturated Fat component (Figure 6-3). There were no significant differences in scores of FSP participants and nonparticipants, among adults and older adults. FSP children scored significantly below higher- income children (3.6 vs. 4.3). Higher scores on the Saturated Fat component indicate lower consumption of saturated fat.

Sandwiches other than hamburgers and cheeseburgers were the leading contributor to saturated fat intakes of all groups (sandwiches may have included cheese and/or mayonnaise)

(Table 6-8). After this, there was considerable variation by age group and across participant groups in the leading sources of saturated fat.

## Table 6-8. Food Sources of MyPyramid Intakes: Saturated Fat

| | All Persons | | | | Children (age 2-18) | | | |
|---|---|---|---|---|---|---|---|---|
| | Total Persons | Food Stamp Program Partic. | Income-eligible Nonpartic. | Higher-income Nonpartic. | Total Persons | Food Stamp Program Partic. | Income-eligible Nonpartic. | Higher-income Nonpartic. |
| Sample size ........................... | 16,419 | 2,303 | 3,577 | 9,094 | 7,583 | 1,495 | 1,801 | 3,682 |
| 1. Sandwiches (excl. burgers) ......... | 12.6 | 12.3 | 12.1 | 12.7 | 11.8 | 12.7 | 12.4 | 11.5 |
| 2. Hamburgers/cheeseburgers ......... | 5.2 | 5.1 | 5.2 | 5.1 | 5.1 | 5.7 | 5.1 | 4.9 |
| 3. Ice cream ........................... | 5.0 | 4.7 | 4.0 | 5.4 | 5.4 | 3.4 | 3.8 | 6.5 |
| 4. Cheese ............................. | 4.3 | 3.0 | 3.8 | 4.7 | 3.9 | 3.0 | 3.0 | 4.4 |
| 5. Unflavored whole milk ............... | 4.4 | 8.0 | 5.8 | 3.5 | 7.6 | 12.1 | 8.6 | 5.9 |
| 6. Pizza w/ meat ...................... | 3.4 | 3.2 | 3.1 | 3.5 | 4.4 | 3.6 | 4.6 | 4.6 |
| 7. Chicken ............................ | 3.2 | 4.2 | 3.1 | 3.1 | 3.4 | 3.9 | 3.4 | 3.4 |
| 8. Unflavored 2% milk ................. | 3.1 | 2.2 | 2.7 | 3.4 | 4.9 | 3.2 | 4.3 | 5.8 |
| 9. Candy ............................. | 2.6 | 1.8 | 2.4 | 2.7 | 2.6 | 2.1 | 2.9 | 2.7 |
| 10. Mexican entrees .................... | 2.6 | 2.1 | 2.7 | 2.6 | 2.5 | 2.0 | 3.1 | 2.5 |
| 11. Cooked potatoes-fried ............. | 2.6 | 2.8 | 2.5 | 2.5 | 3.0 | 3.2 | 2.9 | 3.0 |
| 12. Eggs ............................. | 2.5 | 2.9 | 3.0 | 2.3 | 1.8 | 1.6 | 2.0 | 1.7 |
| 13. Salad (greens) .................... | 2.4 | 0.9 | 1.5 | 2.7 | 1.0 | 0.8 | 0.8 | 0.9 |
| 14. Beef ............................. | 2.3 | 2.1 | 2.5 | 2.2 | 1.5 | 1.7 | 1.6 | 1.3 |
| 15. Cream /sour cream ................. | 2.1 | 1.9 | 1.6 | 2.2 | 0.7 | 0.5 | 0.6 | 0.8 |
| 16. Cookies .......................... | 2.0 | 2.1 | 2.1 | 2.0 | 2.4 | 2.8 | 2.5 | 2.3 |
| 17. Pork ............................. | 1.6 | 2.5 | 1.8 | 1.5 | 0.9 | 1.1 | 1.0 | 0.8 |
| 18. Macaroni & cheese ................. | 1.6 | 2.6 | 1.5 | 1.5 | 2.2 | 2.5 | 1.6 | 2.5 |
| All other food groups ................. | 36.5 | 35.6 | 38.4 | 36.1 | 34.7 | 34.2 | 35.8 | 34.6 |

| | Adults (age 19-59) | | | | Older Adults (age 60+) | | | |
|---|---|---|---|---|---|---|---|---|
| | Total Persons | Food Stamp Program Partic. | Income-eligible Nonpartic. | Higher-income Nonpartic. | Total Persons | Food Stamp Program Partic. | Income-eligible Nonpartic. | Higher-income Nonpartic. |
| Sample size ........................... | 5,775 | 593 | 1,124 | 3,587 | 3,061 | 215 | 652 | 1,825 |
| 1. Sandwiches (excl. burgers) ......... | 13.1 | 12.3 | 12.2 | 13.5 | 11.6 | 11.6 | 11.1 | 11.9 |
| 2. Hamburgers/cheeseburgers ......... | 6.0 | 5.4 | 6.3 | 5.9 | 2.7 | 3.4 u | 2.2 | 2.7 |
| 3. Ice cream ........................... | 4.4 | 5.1 | 3.1 | 4.5 | 6.9 | 5.2 | 7.6 | 6.9 |
| 4. Cheese ............................. | 4.8 | 3.0 | 4.5 | 5.1 | 3.3 | 3.0 | 2.6 | 3.5 |
| 5. Unflavored whole milk ............... | 3.3 | 6.5 | 4.6 | 2.8 | 3.2 | 7.2 | 5.8 | 2.5 |
| 6. Pizza w/ meat ...................... | 3.6 | 3.6 | 3.1 | 3.7 | 1.2 | 1.0 u | 0.8 | 1.4 |
| 7. Chicken ............................ | 3.3 | 4.2 | 3.2 | 3.2 | 2.5 | 4.4 u | 2.6 | 2.3 |
| 8. Unflavored 2% milk ................. | 2.3 | 1.7 | 2.0 | 2.4 | 3.3 | 2.8 | 3.0 | 3.4 |
| 9. Candy ............................. | 2.7 | 2.0 | 2.6 | 2.8 | 2.5 | 1.0 u | 1.3 | 2.6 |
| 10. Mexican entrees .................... | 3.1 | 2.7 | 3.1 | 3.2 | 0.8 | 0.2 u | 0.7 | 0.8 |
| 11. Cooked potatoes-fried ............. | 2.7 | 2.9 | 2.6 | 2.7 | 1.2 | 1.6 u | 1.3 | 1.2 |
| 12. Eggs ............................. | 2.6 | 3.0 | 3.3 | 2.4 | 3.1 | 4.8 | 3.4 | 3.0 |
| 13. Salad (greens) .................... | 2.8 | 1.1 | 1.7 | 3.2 | 3.1 | 0.5 u | 1.8 | 3.4 |
| 14. Beef ............................. | 2.5 | 2.6 | 2.8 | 2.5 | 2.6 | 0.9 | 2.8 | 2.6 |
| 15. Cream /sour cream ................. | 2.6 | 2.6 | 2.0 | 2.7 | 2.3 | 1.8 | 1.9 | 2.4 |
| 16. Cookies .......................... | 1.9 | 1.7 | 2.1 | 1.9 | 2.1 | 2.4 | 1.8 | 2.2 |
| 17. Pork ............................. | 2.0 | 3.0 | 2.1 | 1.8 | 1.6 | 2.8 | 2.2 u | 1.4 |
| 18. Macaroni & cheese ................. | 1.4 | 2.6 | 1.3 | 1.2 | 1.6 | 3.0 u | 2.0 | 1.4 |
| All other food groups ................. | 35.0 | 34.2 | 37.6 | 34.5 | 44.4 | 42.5 | 45.0 | 44.5 |

See notes on Table 6-3.

Significant differences between FSP participants and nonparticipants included:

- FSP children obtained significantly more of their total saturated fat intake from unflavored whole milk than either income-eligible or higher-income nonparticipant children (12 vs. 9 and 6 percent). In addition, FSP children obtained significantly less of their total saturated fat intake from ice cream and unflavored 2 percent milk (3 vs. 7 percent and 3 vs. 6 percent, respectively).
- FSP adults obtained significantly more of their saturated fat from unflavored whole milk than higher-income nonparticipants (7 vs. 3 percent) and significantly less from cheese (3 vs. 5 percent). In addition, FSP participants obtained significantly more of their saturated fat intake from chicken than either group of nonparticipants, but the magnitude of the differences were small.
- Older adult FSP participants obtained more of their saturated fat intake from unflavored whole milk and eggs than higher-income older adults (7 vs. 3 percent and 5 vs. 3 percent, respectively).

In addition to these differences among the leading sources of saturated fat, results showed that FSP participants consistently obtained smaller shares of their saturated fat intake from candy than higher- income nonparticipants.

## Sodium

There were no significant differences between FSP participants and nonparticipants on scores for the HEI-2005 Sodium component (Figure 6-3). Scores ranged from 5.0 to 7.5 out of a possible 10 across participant/nonparticipant and age groups.

The leading source of sodium in the diets of all groups of FSP participant and nonparticipants was sandwiches other than hamburgers and cheeseburgers (Table 6-9). Other leading sources varied by age group and across participant groups.

Significant differences between FSP participants and nonparticipants included:

- FSP children obtained significantly less of their total sodium intakes from pizza with meat and ready-to-eat breakfast cereals than higher- income nonparticipant children, but the differences were small in magnitude.
- FSP adults obtained a significantly smaller share of their sodium intakes from salads/ greens than higher-income nonparticipant adults, and a significantly larger share from macaroni and cheese (1 vs. 4 percent and 3 vs. 1 percent, respectively). Much of the sodium in salads/greens likely comes from salad dressings.
- Older adult FSP participants obtained a significantly smaller share of their total sodium intake from salads/greens than either income- eligible or higher-income nonparticipant older adults. In addition, FSP older adults obtained a significantly larger share of their sodium from rice than higher-income nonparticipant older adults. The difference in the relative contribution of rice to sodium intakes was also noted for children and adults.

In addition, in all three age groups, FSP participants obtained a significantly smaller share of their sodium intake from cheese than higher-income nonparticipants.

### Table 6-9. Food Sources of MyPyramid Intakes: Sodium

| | All Persons | | | | Children (age 2-18) | | | |
|---|---|---|---|---|---|---|---|---|
| | Total Persons | Food Stamp Program Partic. | Income-eligible Nonpartic. | Higher-income Nonpartic. | Total Persons | Food Stamp Program Partic. | Income-eligible Nonpartic. | Higher-income Nonpartic. |
| Sample size ......................... | 16,419 | 2,303 | 3,577 | 9,094 | 7,583 | 1,495 | 1,801 | 3,682 |
| 1. Sandwiches (excl. burgers) ......... | 15.5 | 15.0 | 14.6 | 15.9 | 15.1 | 16.0 | 16.0 | 14.8 |
| 2. Hamburgers/cheeseburgers ........ | 4.0 | 3.9 | 3.9 | 3.9 | 4.1 | 4.3 | 4.2 | 4.0 |
| 3. Pizza w/ meat ..................... | 3.6 | 3.4 | 3.3 | 3.7 | 4.9 | 3.8 | 5.2 | *5.0 |
| 4. Chicken ........................... | 3.2 | 3.5 | 3.0 | 3.2 | 3.4 | 3.2 | 3.3 | 3.5 |
| 5. Salad (greens) ................... | 2.9 | 1.1 | *1.7 | ***3.2 | 1.3 | 1.0 | 1.1 | 1.2 |
| 6. Cold cereal ...................... | 2.8 | 2.5 | 2.5 | 3.0 | 4.5 | 4.2 | 3.8 | *4.9 |
| 7. Bread ............................ | 2.5 | 2.3 | 2.9 | 2.4 | 2.1 | 1.9 | 2.8 | 2.0 |
| 8. Pasta dishes, italian style ......... | 2.4 | 3.0 | 1.6 | 2.4 | 3.3 | 4.7 | 2.4 | 3.2 |
| 9. Cheese .......................... | 2.1 | 1.5 | 1.8 | ***2.3 | 2.1 | 1.5 | 1.6 | ***2.3 |
| 10. Eggs ............................ | 1.8 | 2.2 | 2.1 | 1.7 | 1.4 | 1.2 | 1.6 | 1.3 |
| 11. Rice ............................ | 1.6 | 2.9 | 2.2 | ***1.3 | 1.6 | 3.2 | 1.9 | *1.2 |
| 12. Grain soups ..................... | 1.5 | 2.0 | 2.4 | 1.3 | 2.3 | 3.5 | 3.0 | *1.9 |
| 13. Macaroni & cheese .............. | 1.5 | 2.6 | *1.3 | *1.4 | 2.2 | 2.4 | 1.5 | 2.4 |
| All other food groups .............. | 54.6 | 54.3 | 56.7 | 54.4 | 51.7 | 49.1 | 51.6 | 52.2 |

| | Adults (age 19-59) | | | | Older Adults (age 60+) | | | |
|---|---|---|---|---|---|---|---|---|
| | Total Persons | Food Stamp Program Partic. | Income-eligible Nonpartic. | Higher-income Nonpartic. | Total Persons | Food Stamp Program Partic. | Income-eligible Nonpartic. | Higher-income Nonpartic. |
| Sample size ......................... | 5,775 | 593 | 1,124 | 3,587 | 3,061 | 215 | 652 | 1,825 |
| 1. Sandwiches (excl. burgers) ......... | 16.0 | 14.7 | 14.6 | 16.7 | 14.4 | 14.3 | 12.7 | 14.8 |
| 2. Hamburgers/cheeseburgers ........ | 4.5 | 4.2 | 4.6 | 4.4 | 1.9 | 2.0 u | 1.6 | 2.0 |
| 3. Pizza w/ meat ..................... | 3.7 | 4.0 | 3.2 | 3.8 | 1.1 | 1.0 u | 0.7 | 1.3 |
| 4. Chicken ........................... | 3.4 | 3.8 | 3.0 | 3.4 | 2.3 | 2.7 u | 2.4 | 2.2 |
| 5. Salad (greens) ................... | 3.4 | 1.2 | 1.8 | ***3.9 | 3.7 | 0.8 u | *2.4 | ***3.9 |
| 6. Cold cereal ...................... | 2.0 | 1.6 | 1.7 | 2.1 | 3.3 | 3.1 u | 3.1 | 3.4 |
| 7. Bread ............................ | 2.2 | 2.1 | 2.5 | 2.1 | 4.2 | 3.9 | 4.5 | 4.1 |
| 8. Pasta dishes, italian style ......... | 2.1 | 2.3 | 0.8 | 2.2 | 2.0 | 2.8 u | 2.8 | 1.8 |
| 9. Cheese .......................... | 2.2 | 1.5 | 1.9 | *2.3 | 1.8 | 1.2 | 1.8 | *1.9 |
| 10. Eggs ............................ | 1.8 | 2.2 | 2.4 | 1.7 | 2.2 | 3.4 | 2.3 | 2.1 |
| 11. Rice ............................ | 1.6 | 2.3 | 2.3 | *1.4 | 1.6 | 4.3 | 2.3 | *1.0 |
| 12. Grain soups ..................... | 1.3 | 1.7 | 2.5 | 1.0 | 1.3 | 0.5 u | 1.2 | 1.3 |
| 13. Macaroni & cheese .............. | 1.2 | 2.5 | 1.2 | *1.0 | 1.4 | 3.5 u | 1.6 u | 1.1 |
| All other food groups .............. | 54.8 | 56.0 | 57.6 | 54.1 | 58.7 | 56.3 | 60.6 | 59.0 |

See notes on Table 6-3.

## Solid Fats, Alcoholic Beverages, and Added Sugars

All age groups and participant groups had low average scores on the Calories from SoFAAS component of the HEI-2005 (which assesses the percentage of total calorie intake contributed by solid fats, alcoholic beverages, and added sugars) (Figure 6-4). Scores ranged from 5.2 to 11.2, out of a possible 20, indicating that, on average, all groups obtained considerably more of their total energy intakes from solid fats, alcoholic beverages, and added sugars than the 20 percent used as the reference for the maximum HEI-2005 score (Table 6-1).

For children and older adults, there were no significant differences between FSP participants and either group of nonparticipants in HEI scores for the SoFAAS component. Among adults, FSP participants had a significantly lower mean score than higher-income nonparticipants (5.2 vs. 7.5, out of a possible 20).

## Food Sources of Solid Fats

Sandwiches other than hamburgers and cheeseburgers were the leading contributor to solid fat intakes of all groups (sandwiches may have included cheese and/or mayonnaise) (Table 6-10).

**Table 6-10. Food Sources of MyPyramid Intakes: Discretionary Solid Fats**

| | All Persons | | | | Children (age 2-18) | | | |
|---|---|---|---|---|---|---|---|---|
| | Total Persons | Food Stamp Program Partic. | Income-eligible Nonpartic. | Higher-income Nonpartic. | Total Persons | Food Stamp Program Partic. | Income-eligible Nonpartic. | Higher-income Nonpartic. |
| Sample size | 16,419 | 2,303 | 3,577 | 9,094 | 7,583 | 1,495 | 1,801 | 3,682 |
| 1. Sandwiches (excl. burgers) | 10.8 | 10.7 | 10.3 | 10.8 | 10.3 | 11.0 | 11.8 | 9.6 |
| 2. Cooked potatoes-fried | 5.0 | 5.0 | 4.6 | 5.0 | 6.0 | 6.2 | 6.0 | 6.0 |
| 3. Hamburgers/cheeseburgers | 4.4 | 4.1 | 4.2 | 4.3 | 4.3 | 4.6 | 4.3 | 4.2 |
| 4. Ice cream | 4.5 | 4.0 | 3.5 | 4.9 | 4.7 | 3.0 | 3.3 | 5.7 |
| 5. Pizza w/ meat | 4.2 | 3.8 | 3.7 | 4.4 | 5.5 | 4.4 | 5.7 | 5.7 |
| 6. Cookies | 4.0 | 4.1 | 4.1 | 4.0 | 4.7 | 5.2 | 4.7 | 4.6 |
| 7. Unflavored whole milk | 4.0 | 6.9 | 5.2 | 3.3 | 6.9 | 10.7 | 7.8 | 5.4 |
| 8. Cheese | 3.8 | 2.5 | 3.3 | 4.2 | 3.5 | 2.6 | 2.6 | 4.0 |
| 9. Mexican entrees | 2.7 | 2.3 | 2.9 | 2.8 | 2.6 | 1.9 | 3.2 | 2.5 |
| 10. Eggs | 2.8 | 3.2 | 3.3 | 2.6 | 2.0 | 1.8 | 2.2 | 1.9 |
| 11. Unflavored 2% milk | 2.6 | 1.8 | 2.3 | 2.9 | 4.1 | 2.7 | 3.6 | 4.9 |
| 12. Cake/cupcakes | 2.6 | 2.1 | 2.4 | 2.7 | 2.2 | 2.2 | 1.9 | 2.3 |
| 13. Chicken | 2.5 | 3.9 | 2.5 | 2.4 | 2.1 | 3.2 | 2.1 | 1.9 |
| 14. Macaroni & cheese | 2.3 | 3.8 | 2.1 | 2.2 | 3.3 | 3.8 | 2.2 | 3.7 |
| 15. Bacon/sausage | 2.3 | 2.5 | 2.1 | 2.3 | 1.6 | 1.9 | 1.5 | 1.6 |
| 16. Cream /sour cream | 1.9 | 1.4 | 1.4 | 2.0 | 0.6 | 0.4 | 0.5 | 0.7 |
| 17. Doughnuts | 1.6 | 1.6 | 2.1 | 1.5 | 1.4 | 1.2 | 1.6 | 1.4 |
| All other food groups | 38.0 | 36.3 | 40.1 | 37.7 | 34.1 | 33.1 | 35.1 | 34.0 |

| | Adults (age 19-59) | | | | Older Adults (age 60+) | | | |
|---|---|---|---|---|---|---|---|---|
| | Total Persons | Food Stamp Program Partic. | Income-eligible Nonpartic. | Higher-income Nonpartic. | Total Persons | Food Stamp Program Partic. | Income-eligible Nonpartic. | Higher-income Nonpartic. |
| Sample size | 5,775 | 593 | 1,124 | 3,587 | 3,061 | 215 | 652 | 1,825 |
| 1. Sandwiches (excl. burgers) | 11.2 | 11.1 | 10.0 | 11.4 | 10.1 | 9.0 | 9.4 | 10.3 |
| 2. Cooked potatoes-fried | 5.4 | 5.1 | 4.8 | 5.5 | 2.0 | 2.5 u | 1.9 | 2.0 |
| 3. Hamburgers/cheeseburgers | 5.1 | 4.3 | 5.0 | 5.0 | 2.2 | 2.7 u | 1.7 | 2.2 |
| 4. Ice cream | 3.9 | 4.4 | 2.7 | 4.1 | 6.0 | 4.0 | 6.3 | 6.2 |
| 5. Pizza w/ meat | 4.4 | 4.3 | 3.7 | 4.6 | 1.5 | 1.1 u | 0.9 | 1.8 |
| 6. Cookies | 3.6 | 3.7 | 4.0 | 3.6 | 4.2 | 3.8 | 3.8 | 4.3 |
| 7. Unflavored whole milk | 3.0 | 5.7 | 4.1 | 2.6 | 2.9 | 5.5 | 5.2 | 2.3 |
| 8. Cheese | 4.2 | 2.5 | 3.9 | 4.6 | 2.9 | 2.3 | 2.2 | 3.1 |
| 9. Mexican entrees | 3.3 | 3.1 u | 3.3 | 3.5 | 0.8 | 0.2 u | 0.8 | 0.9 |
| 10. Eggs | 2.9 | 3.2 | 3.6 | 2.7 | 3.7 | 5.3 | 3.8 | 3.5 |
| 11. Unflavored 2% milk | 2.0 | 1.4 | 1.6 | 2.1 | 2.8 | 2.1 | 2.5 | 3.0 |
| 12. Cake/cupcakes | 2.7 | 2.1 | 2.7 | 2.7 | 3.0 | 2.4 u | 2.4 | 3.3 |
| 13. Chicken | 2.8 | 3.7 | 2.7 | 2.7 | 2.2 | 5.4 u | 2.1 | 1.9 |
| 14. Macaroni & cheese | 1.9 | 3.2 | 1.8 | 1.6 | 2.5 | 6.4 u | 3.0 u | 2.0 |
| 15. Bacon/sausage | 2.3 | 2.2 | 2.2 | 2.3 | 3.2 | 4.1 | 2.7 | 3.2 |
| 16. Cream /sour cream | 2.4 | 1.9 | 1.6 | 2.5 | 2.2 | 1.2 | 1.7 | 2.4 |
| 17. Doughnuts | 1.7 | 1.7 | 2.4 | 1.5 | 1.3 | 1.7 u | 2.0 u | 1.4 |
| All other food groups | 37.2 | 36.6 | 40.1 | 36.9 | 46.6 | 40.2 | 47.8 | 46.2 |

See notes on Table 6-3.

Other "top five" contributors of solid fat for both participants and nonparticipants were:

- Children—fried potatoes and unflavored whole milk
- Adults—fried potatoes and hamburgers and cheeseburgers
- Older adults—eggs

Significant differences between FSP participants and nonparticipants included:

- FSP children obtained more of their solid fat intake from unflavored whole milk than either group of nonparticipant children (11 vs. 8 and 5 percent), and less from ice cream and unflavored 2 percent milk compared with higher-income nonparticipant children (3 vs. 6 percent and 3 vs. 5 percent, respectively).
- FSP adults obtained significantly more of their solid fat intake from unflavored whole milk and chicken than higher-income nonparticipant adults (6 vs. 3 percent and 4 vs. 3 percent, respectively) and significantly less from cheese (3 vs. 5 percent).
- Older adult FSP participants obtained more of their solid fat from unflavored whole milk and less from ice cream than higher-income nonparticipant older adults (6 vs. 2 percent and 4 vs. 6 percent, respectively).

## Food Sources of Added Sugars

The leading source of added sugars for all age groups and all participant groups was regular (not sugar-free) sodas. Overall, sodas contributed about 35 percent of all added sugars (Table 6-11). Other "top five" contributors of added sugars for both participants and nonparticipants were:

- Children—noncarbonated sweetened drinks, candy, and ready-to-eat breakfast cereals
- Adults—noncarbonated sweetened drinks and cake/cupcakes
- Older adults—noncarbonated sweetened drinks, cakes/cupcakes, and ice cream

Significant differences between FSP participants and nonparticipants included:

- FSP children obtained significantly more of their added sugar intakes from regular soda than higher-income nonparticipant children, and significantly less from ice cream (33 vs. 29 percent and 3 vs. 5 percent, respectively).
- FSP adults obtained significantly more of their added sugar intakes from sodas and sugar (46 vs. 39 percent and 7 vs. 4 percent, respectively) and significantly less from candy (3 vs. 6 percent), compared with higher-income nonparticipant adults. FSP adults also obtained significantly more of their added sugar intakes from ice cream than income-eligible nonparticipant adults (4 vs. 2 percent).
- FSP older adults obtained more of their added sugar intakes from sodas than either group of nonparticipant older adults (38 vs. 23 and 17 percent) and less from candy

(2 vs. 5 and 7 percent).[5] In addition, FSP older adults obtained significantly less of their added sugar intakes from ice cream than higher-income nonparticipant older adults (5 vs. 8 percent).

### Table 6-11. Food Sources of MyPyramid Intakes: Added Sugars

| | All Persons | | | | Children (age 2-18) | | | |
|---|---|---|---|---|---|---|---|---|
| | Total Persons | Food Stamp Program Partic. | Income-eligible Nonpartic. | Higher-income Nonpartic. | Total Persons | Food Stamp Program Partic. | Income-eligible Nonpartic. | Higher-income Nonpartic. |
| Sample size | 16,419 | 2,303 | 3,577 | 9,094 | 7,583 | 1,495 | 1,801 | 3,682 |
| 1. Regular soda | 35.1 | 41.4 | 40.8 | 33.2 | 30.8 | 32.6 | 33.8 | 29.4 |
| 2. Noncarbonated sweetened drink | 10.8 | 12.5 | 11.3 | 10.3 | 15.4 | 16.1 | 16.3 | 14.8 |
| 3. Candy | 6.0 | 4.4 | 5.2 | 6.3 | 7.3 | 8.3 | 7.3 | 7.1 |
| 4. Cake/cupcakes | 5.0 | 4.6 | 4.0 | 5.3 | 3.8 | 4.6 | 3.2 | 3.9 |
| 5. Ice cream | 4.6 | 3.7 | 3.3 | 5.1 | 4.1 | 3.1 | 3.1 | 4.8 |
| 6. Cold cereal | 4.2 | 3.1 | 3.3 | 4.5 | 6.9 | 6.7 | 5.5 | 7.3 |
| 7. Cookies | 4.0 | 3.8 | 3.6 | 4.1 | 4.3 | 4.9 | 4.2 | 4.2 |
| 8. Sugar | 3.8 | 6.1 | 4.7 | 3.5 | 0.9 | 1.0 | 0.7 | 1.0 |
| 9. Tea | 3.1 | 2.9 | 3.8 | 3.0 | 1.9 | 2.4 | 3.1 | 1.4 |
| 10. Syrups/sweet toppings | 3.0 | 1.9 | 2.5 | 3.4 | 3.8 | 2.4 | 3.2 | 4.3 |
| 11. Sandwiches (excl. burgers) | 2.0 | 1.8 | 1.7 | 2.1 | 2.1 | 1.8 | 2.2 | 2.1 |
| All other food groups | 18.3 | 13.8 | 16.0 | 19.2 | 18.7 | 16.0 | 17.3 | 19.7 |

| | Adults (age 19-59) | | | | Older Adults (age 60+) | | | |
|---|---|---|---|---|---|---|---|---|
| | Total Persons | Food Stamp Program Partic. | Income-eligible Nonpartic. | Higher-income Nonpartic. | Total Persons | Food Stamp Program Partic. | Income-eligible Nonpartic. | Higher-income Nonpartic. |
| Sample size | 5,775 | 593 | 1,124 | 3,587 | 3,061 | 215 | 652 | 1,825 |
| 1. Regular soda | 41.2 | 46.2 | 48.7 | 39.3 | 19.8 | 37.8 | 22.8 | 17.2 |
| 2. Noncarbonated sweetened drink | 10.0 | 13.0 | 10.2 | 9.4 | 7.0 | 5.4 | 7.7 | 6.3 |
| 3. Candy | 5.4 | 3.4 | 4.4 | 5.9 | 6.5 | 2.2 u | 4.5 | 6.8 |
| 4. Cake/cupcakes | 4.8 | 4.0 | 3.8 | 5.1 | 7.3 | 6.7 u | 5.8 u | 8.1 |
| 5. Ice cream | 3.9 | 3.6 | 2.2 | 4.3 | 7.9 | 5.1 | 8.0 | 8.4 |
| 6. Cold cereal | 2.9 | 1.7 | 2.2 | 3.2 | 4.4 | 2.6 | 3.8 | 5.0 |
| 7. Cookies | 3.4 | 3.1 | 2.8 | 3.7 | 5.4 | 4.3 | 5.2 | 5.7 |
| 8. Sugar | 4.7 | 7.0 | 5.7 | 4.2 | 5.3 | 10.9 | 7.1 | 4.9 |
| 9. Tea | 3.6 | 3.4 | 3.6 | 3.7 | 3.2 | 2.0 u | 5.6 | 2.9 |
| 10. Syrups/sweet toppings | 2.5 | 1.5 | 2.2 | 2.7 | 3.8 | 2.5 u | 2.1 | 4.3 |
| 11. Sandwiches (excl. burgers) | 1.8 | 1.8 | 1.4 | 1.9 | 2.3 | 1.8 | 2.2 | 2.5 |
| All other food groups | 15.7 | 11.4 | 12.8 | 16.6 | 27.0 | 18.7 | 25.3 | 28.0 |

See notes on Table 6-3.

## SUMMARY

The HEI-2005 consists of 12 component scores designed to measure compliance with the Dietary Guidelines for Americans and *MyPyramid* food guidance system. The sum of the component scores yields the Total HEI score. Children ages 2- 18 and adults scored a total of 55 and 58, respectively, out of a possible 100 points on the Total HEI-2005 Score. Older adults scored 68 out of 100 points. These results indicate that the diets of all age groups and participant/nonparticipant groups fell considerably short of the diet recommended in the DGA and *MyPyramid*.

FSP participants, overall and among adults, had lower Total HEI scores than both income-eligible and higher-income nonparticipants. FSP children scored significantly below only higher-income nonparticipant children. There were no statistically significant differences between participants and nonparticipants among older adults.

---

[5] The point estimate for FSP older adults is statistically unreliable, but the differences between groups are statistically significant.

Among all age groups combined, analysis of component scores revealed only two differences between FSP participants and income-eligible nonparticipants: lower scores on the Whole Fruit and Oils components for FSP participants. On the other hand, FSP participants scored significantly below higher-income nonparticipants on 7 of 12 HEI-2005 components. These results indicate that, compared with higher-income groups, lower- income populations have greater difficulty complying with DGA and MyPyramid recommendations, regardless of FSP participation.

Results of the HEI-2005 component scores point to the following key concerns in the diets of *all* age groups and *all* participant/nonparticipant groups:

- Low intakes of fruit, vegetables, whole grains, and oils, relative to the concentrations needed to meet nutrient requirements without exceeding calorie requirements.
- Very low intakes of the most nutritious vegetables—dark green and orange vegetables and legumes.
- High intakes of sodium and of discretionary calories from solid fats, alcoholic beverages, and added sugars (SoFAAS).

All age groups had high intakes of potatoes from high-fat sources: French fries and potato chips accounted for 14 percent of vegetable intakes overall. High potato consumption may help explain low intakes of dark green and orange vegetables and legumes if potatoes substitute for other vegetables. Intakes of potatoes from high fat sources also contribute to SoFAAS intakes.

There were several significant differences in HEI2005 component scores for FSP participants and higher-income nonparticipants. Differences were observed for:

- Total Fruit—FSP adults had significantly lower mean scores than higher-income adults (2.5 vs. 3.1). (The total fruit component includes 100% fruit juices).
- Whole Fruit—FSP children and adults had significantly lower scores on the HEI-2005 component for Whole Fruit than higher-income nonparticipants (2.7 vs. 3.5 out of a possible 5 for children, and 2.5 vs. 3.8 for adults).
- Total Vegetables—FSP adults and older adults scored below higher-income nonparticipants on the Total Vegetables component (3.1 vs. 3.6 for adults; 3.6 vs. 4.2 for older adults). FSP children scored higher than higher-income nonparticipants (2.4 vs. 2.2).
- Milk and milk products—FSP participants in all three age groups had significantly lower scores than higher-income nonparticipants (7.8 vs. 8.8 for children; 4.9 vs. 5.8 for adults; and 4.9 vs. 5.9 for older adults).
- Oils—Among adults and older adults, FSP participants had significantly lower scores than both groups of nonparticipants.

Most of the differences were noted in the diets of FSP participants relative to higher-income (rather than income-eligible) nonparticipants. Key differences between FSP participants and nonparticipants in the relative importance of specific foods to the intakes assessed in HEI-2005 are summarized below.

## Differences between FSP Children and Nonparticipant Children

Unflavored whole milk accounted for significantly larger shares of FSP children's intakes of: milk/milk products, saturated fat, and solid fat. This is consistent with findings from Chapter 5, which showed that FSP children were more likely to consume unflavored whole milk than higher- income nonparticipant children and less likely to consume reduced fat milks.

FSP children obtained a significantly smaller share of their total vegetable intake from salads/greens than higher-income nonparticipant children.

FSP children obtained significantly more of their added sugar intakes from regular soda than higher- income nonparticipant children, and significantly less from ice cream.

## Differences between Adult FSP Participants (age 19-59) and Adult Nonparticipants

There were some significant differences between FSP adults and nonparticipant adults in the relative nutritional quality of foods that were major contributors to fruit and vegetable intakes:

- FSP adults obtained significantly larger shares of their total fruit intake from non-citrus juices and non-carbonated sweetened drinks than either income-eligible or higher-income nonparticipants and significantly smaller shares from fresh apples, melons, and berries.
- FSP adults obtained a significantly smaller share of their total vegetable intake from salads/salad greens, compared with higher- income nonparticipant adults, and a significantly larger share from cooked potatoes that were not fried.

FSP adults obtained significantly less of their total oil intakes from nuts (which includes seeds and nut butters) than either group of nonparticipant adults.

FSP adults had a significantly lower score for the SoFAAS component than higher-income nonparticipants (5.2 vs. 7.5, out of a possible 20). Factors that contributed to this difference were:

- FSP adults obtained significantly more of their solid fat from unflavored whole milk and chicken (likely due to use of solid fats during cooking) and more of their added sugar from regular (not sugar-free) sodas, table sugar, and ice cream.
- On the other hand, FSP adults obtained significantly less of their added sugar intakes from candy, relative to higher-income nonparticipant adults.

## Differences between Older Adult FSP Participants (Age60+) and Nonparticipant Older Adults

FSP older adults obtained a significantly smaller share of their total fruit intakes from fresh apples and fresh berries, relative to higher-income nonparticipant older adults, and a significantly smaller share of their vegetable intake from salads/salad greens.

Similar to children and adults, FSP older adults obtained a significantly larger share of total milk intakes from unflavored whole milk, compared with higher-income nonparticipants. However, in this age group, the difference was not statistically significant, probably because of the small sample size of older adult FSP participants. Nonetheless, FSP older adults obtained a significantly larger share of saturated fat and solid fat intakes from unflavored whole milk, compared with higher- income nonparticipants.

FSP older adults obtained more of their added sugar intakes from sodas than either group of nonparticipant older adults and less from candy. In addition, FSP older adults obtained significantly less of their added sugar intakes from ice cream than higher-income nonparticipant older adults (5 vs. 8 percent).

# Chapter 7

# CONCLUSION

This chapter uses the most recently available data from the National Health and Nutrition Examination Survey (NHANES 1999-2004) to provide an up-to-date and comprehensive picture of the diets of FSP participants in three age groups—children 1-18 years old, adults 19-59 years old, and older adults 60 years and older.[1] The report examines the nutrient intakes, food choices, and diet quality of FSP participants and two groups of nonpartici-pants—those who were income-eligible for the FSP but did not participate in the program, and higher- income individuals who were not eligible for the FSP. This research was not designed to assess the impact of the FSP or in any way attribute differences observed between FSP participants and nonparticipants to an effect of the program. Data on nonparticipants are presented strictly to provide context for data on FSP participants.

Key findings from the preceding chapters are presented here by topic.

## KEY FINDINGS

### Intakes of Vitamins and Minerals

- Over 90 percent of the U.S. population had adequate usual daily intakes of seven essential vitamins and minerals examined in this analysis (folate, vitamin $B_{12}$, thiamin, riboflavin, niacin, phosphorus, and iron). Somewhat smaller proportions had adequate usual daily intakes of zinc (89 percent) and vitamin $B_6$ (87 percent).
- Usual daily intakes of vitamins A, C, and E, and magnesium need improvement—30 percent or more of the U.S. population had inadequate usual daily intakes of these essential vitamins and minerals.[2]
- It is not possible to assess fully the adequacy of calcium, potassium, and fiber because the necessary reference standards have not been defined. Mean usual

---

[1] For some analyses, the sample of children is limited to those 2 years and older because the reference standards used do not apply to younger children.

[2] The prevalence of adequate usual daily intakes of vitamin E was especially low (7.5 percent), consistent with most recent studies of vitamin E intake. Devaney and colleagues have pointed out that vitamin E deficiency is rare in the U.S., despite low measured intakes, and that the Estimated Average Requirements (EARs) for vitamin E may need to be reassessed (Devaney et al., 2007).

daily intakes of calcium were 100, 88, and 62 percent of the defined Adequate Intake level (AI) for children, adults, and older adults, respectively. Mean usual intakes of potassium were 50 to 60 percent of AI. These data indicate that the prevalence of adequate intakes of calcium is likely to be high for children. No firm conclusions can be drawn about the adequacy of calcium intakes of adults and older adults or about the adequacy of potassium or fiber intakes of any age group.[3]

- Sodium intakes were of concern for all age groups. Nearly 90 percent of the population had usual daily intakes that exceeded the Tolerable Upper Intake Level (UL).
- For all nutrients examined, the prevalence of adequate usual daily intakes or mean usual daily intakes relative to AIs were consistently higher for children than for adults and older adults.
- There were no significant differences between FSP participants and income-eligible nonparticipants in the prevalence of adequate usual intakes of vitamins and minerals, or in mean usual intakes of calcium, potassium, fiber, or sodium.
- Compared with higher-income nonparticipants, the prevalence of adequate usual intakes was significantly lower among FSP participants for each of the 13 vitamins and minerals examined, and FSP participants had significantly lower mean usual intakes of calcium, potassium, and fiber. However, FSP participants were less likely than higher-income nonparticipants to have a usual daily sodium intake that exceeded the UL. These general patterns were noted for both adults and older adults, but there were fewer differences between FSP participants and higher-income nonparticipants among children.
- Dietary supplements were used by 47 percent of the population.[4] Supplement use increased with age and FSP participants and income- eligible nonparticipants were about equally likely to use supplements. FSP participants were less likely to use supplements than higher- income nonparticipants.

## Prevalence of Overweight and Obesity

- In all three age groups, female FSP participants were less likely than either group of female nonparticipants to have healthy weights and more likely to be overweight (children) or obese (adults and older adults).
- Among male children, FSP participants were less likely than higher-income nonparticipants to have healthy weights and more likely to be overweight.
- Among adult and older adult males, FSP participants were more likely than higher-income nonparticipants to have healthy weights and less likely to be overweight or obese.

---

[3] Usual daily fiber intakes of all age groups were low, relative to the AIs. Mean usual intakes were equivalent to about half of the 14 grams of fiber per 1,000 calories standard used to establish AIs. Some have suggested that the methods used to establish AIs for fiber may need to be reexamined (Devaney et al., 2007).

[4] Nutrient intake data presented do not include contributions from dietary supplements.

## Sources of Food Energy (Calories)

- Usual daily intakes of protein were within Acceptable Macronutrient Distribution Ranges (AMDRs). However, more than 30 percent of all persons had usual daily intakes of total fat that exceeded the AMDR and a majority had usual daily intakes of saturated fat that exceeded the Dietary Guidelines for Americans recommendation. Specifically:
  - Twenty percent of children consumed too much total fat, as a percentage of total energy intake, and 83 percent consumed too much saturated fat.
  - Close to 40 percent of adults and older adults consumed too much total fat, about 60 percent consumed too much saturated fat, and 20 to 25 percent consumed too few carbohydrates.
- For all persons, an average of 38 percent of calories were consumed from solid fats, alcoholic beverages, and added sugars (SoFAAS). This percentage varied only slightly across age groups and was far in excess of the discretionary calorie allowances included in the MyPyramid food guidance system.
- Among children and older adults, there were no statistically significant differences between FSP participants and nonparticipants in sources of energy.
- Among adults, FSP participants were less likely than higher-income nonparticipants to have fat intakes that exceeded the AMDR and carbohydrate intakes that were less than the AMDR and were more likely to have protein intakes that were less than the AMDR.
- FSP adults consumed more energy from SoFAAS than either group of nonparticipant adults and, relative to higher-income nonparticipant adults, consumed solid foods that had a higher mean energy density.

## Meal and Snack Patterns

- Fewer than half of FSP participants and income-eligible nonparticipants reported all three main meals on the day of the 24-hour recall. In contrast, 63 percent of higher-income nonparticipants reported all three meals.
- About 90 percent of persons in all three age groups reported a dinner.
- Children were most likely to skip breakfast (18 percent), followed by lunch (15 percent). Adults were equally likely to skip breakfast or lunch (23 percent). Older adults were most likely to skip lunch (23 percent).
- Meal and snack patterns were comparable for FSP participants and income-eligible nonparticipants, with two exceptions: smaller percentages of adult and older adult FSP participants reported a lunch.
- FSP participants were less likely than higher- income nonparticipants to eat each meal. Between-group differences were smallest for children and largest for older adults.
- There were no significant differences between FSP participants and nonparticipants in the number of snacks consumed by children and adults. Older adult FSP participants consumed fewer snacks than higher-income older adults.

## Nutrient Density

- Overall diets of FSP participants and income- eligible nonparticipants were comparable in nutrient density, as measured using a modified Nutrient-Rich (NR) score. (Some small offsetting differences were observed for individual meals.)
- Compared with higher-income nonparticipants, FSP participants had overall diets that were lower in nutrient density. Adult FSP participants had significantly lower NR scores for all three meals; FSP children had lower NR scores for breakfast, and older adult FSP participants had lower NR scores for breakfast and lunch. Differences in NR scores for adults and older adults were attributable to differences among females.

## Food Choices

To compare the food choices of FSP participants and nonparticipants, we used two different approaches. The first approach, referred to as the "supermarket aisle approach" looked at the proportions of persons in each group who consumed items within broad food groups. For the second approach, which looked more closely at the nutritional quality of food choices, we classified all foods reported in NHANES 1999-2004 into three categories—foods to consume frequently, selectively, or occasionally—based on *Dietary Guidelines* and *MyPyramid* recommendations.

### Food Choices within Major Food Groups

- FSP participants were less likely than income- eligible nonparticipants to consume vegetables or fruit, but were equally likely to consume foods from all other major food groups (grains, milk/milk products, meat/meat alternates, mixed dishes, beverages other than milk or 100% fruit juice, sweets and desserts, salty snacks, and added fats and oils).
- FSP participants were less likely than higher- income nonparticipants to consume foods from 8 of the 10 major food groups, but were equally likely to consume meat/meat alternates and beverages other than milk and 100% fruit juice.

Findings varied somewhat by age group. Between- group differences for adults reflected the overall differences listed above.

- For children and older adults, there was only one significant difference between FSP participants and income-eligible nonparticipants (older adult FSP participants were less likely than income-eligible older adults to consume vegetables).
- Compared with higher income nonparticipants, FSP children were less likely to consume from 2 of the 10 food groups (grains; added fats and oils). Differences were more widespread for older adults. FSP older adults were less likely to consume from 5 of the 10 food groups, compared with higher-income older adults (grains; vegetables; fruits; milk and milk products; and added fats and oils).

That FSP adults consume from fewer food groups than higher-income adults indicates that FSP adults have less variety in their diets. An alternative explanation would be that FSP adults eat less food and therefore are less likely to consume foods from each food group, however, comparisons of reported energy intakes in Chapter 3 showed no significant differences between FSP adults and higher-income nonparticipant adults. In contrast, FSP older adults had significantly lower energy intakes than higher- income older adults. This suggests that, for older adults, differences in food group consumption may be due to a combination of less variety and a lower overall food intake.

### Food Choices within Food Subgroups

There were no significant differences between FSP participants and income-eligible nonparticipants in the proportions consuming 165 different subgroups.[5] However, compared with higher-income nonparticipants, FSP participants in all three age groups were:

- less likely to consume whole grains
- less likely to consume raw vegetables (including salads), and more likely to consume potatoes
- less likely to consume reduced-fat milk, and more likely to consume whole milk
- less likely to consume sugar-free sodas, and more likely to consume regular sodas.

### Nutritional Quality of Food Choices

Over half of the foods consumed by FSP participants and both groups of nonparticipants were foods that should be consumed only occasionally. Overall, FSP participants were:

- more likely than either income-eligible or higher-income nonparticipants to consume foods recommended for occasional consumption (62% of all food choices vs. 58% and 56%, respectively)
- less likely to consume foods recommended for selective consumption (19% vs. 21% and 21%)
- less likely to consume foods recommended for frequent consumption (19% vs. 21% and 23%).

Differences between FSP participants and income- eligible nonparticipants were largely attributable to differences in the relative nutritional quality of food choices in the milk group. FSP participants were generally more likely to consume milk and milk products from the 'enjoy occasionally' group and less likely to consume milk and milk products from the 'enjoy frequently' and/or 'enjoy selectively' groups. This is consistent with the finding reported above that FSP participants were more likely than income-eligible nonparticipants to consume whole milk and less likely to consume low fat or skim milks.

FSP participants made less nutritious choices than higher-income nonparticipants in the following food groups:

---

[5] These analyses were limited to consumers of each major food group, for example, among those who consumed any grain or grain product, what proportion consumed at least one whole grain food? These conditional proportions allowed us to compare food choices for FSP participants and nonparticipants, while controlling for differences in overall consumption at the level of major food group.

- Milk, cheese, yogurt (all ages) – due to greater consumption of whole milk and less reduced- fat milk
- Beverages other than milk and fruit juice (adults and older adults) – due to greater consumption of regular sodas and less sugar- free sodas
- Salty snacks (all ages) – due to greater consumption of potato chips and less popcorn

## The Healthy Eating Index-2005 (HEI-2005) and Sources of MyPyramid Intakes

The HEI-2005 consists of 12 component scores designed to measure compliance with the Dietary Guidelines for Americans and *MyPyramid* food guidance system. The sum of the component scores yields the Total HEI score. FSP participants, overall and among adults, had lower Total HEI scores than both income-eligible and higher- income nonparticipants. FSP children scored significantly below only higher-income nonparticipant children. There were no statistically significant differences between participants and nonparticipants among older adults.

Analysis of component scores revealed only two differences between FSP participants and income- eligible nonparticipants: lower scores on the Whole Fruit and Oils components for FSP participants. On the other hand, FSP participants scored significantly below higher-income nonparticipants on 7 of 12 HEI-2005 components. These results indicate that, compared with higher-income groups, lower-income populations have greater difficulty complying with DGA and MyPyramid recommendations, regardless of FSP participation.

The HEI component scores point to the following key concerns in the diets of *all* age groups and *all* participant/ nonparticipant groups:

- Low intakes of vegetables and oils, relative to the concentrations needed to meet nutrient requirements without exceeding calorie requirements.
- Very low intakes of the most nutritious vegetables—dark green and orange vegetables and legumes.
- Very low intakes of whole grains.
- High intakes of sodium.

There were several significant differences in HEI2005 component scores for FSP participants and nonparticipants. Differences were observed for:

- Total Fruit—FSP adults had significantly lower mean scores than higher-income adults (2.5 vs. 3.1). (The total fruit component includes 100% fruit juices).
- Whole Fruit—FSP children and adults had significantly lower scores on the HEI-2005 component for Whole Fruit than higher-income nonparticipants (2.7 vs. 3.5 out of a possible 5 for children, and 2.5 vs. 3.8 for adults).
- Total Vegetables—FSP adults and older adults scored below higher-income nonparticipants on the Total Vegetables component (3.1 vs. 3.6 for adults; 3.6 vs. 4.2 for older adults). FSP children scored higher than higher-income nonparticipants (2.4 vs. 2.2).

- Milk and milk products—FSP participants in all three age groups had significantly lower scores than higher-income nonparticipants (7.8 vs. 8.8 for children; 4.9 vs. 5.8 for adults; and 4.9 vs. 5.9 for older adults).
- Oils—Among adults and older adults, FSP participants had significantly lower mean scores than both groups of nonparticipants.

Most of the differences between FSP participants and nonparticipants were noted in the diets of FSP participants relative to higher-income (rather than income-eligible) nonparticipants. Key differences in the relative importance of specific foods to the intakes assessed in HEI-2005 are summarized below.

### Differences between FSP Children and Nonparticipant Children

Unflavored whole milk accounted for significantly larger shares of FSP children's intakes of: milk/milk products, saturated fat, and solid fat. This is consistent with findings from Chapter 5, which showed that FSP children were more likely to consume unflavored whole milk than higher-income nonparticipant children and less likely to consume reduced fat milks.

FSP children obtained a significantly smaller share of their total vegetable intake from salads/greens than higher-income nonparticipant children.

FSP children obtained significantly more of their added sugar intakes from regular soda than higher-income nonparticipant children, and significantly less from ice cream.

### Differences between Adult FSP Participants (Age 19- 59) and Adult Nonparticipants

There were some significant differences between FSP adults and nonparticipant adults in the relative nutritional quality of foods that were major contributors to fruit and vegetable intakes:

- FSP adults obtained significantly larger shares of their total fruit intake from non-citrus juices and non-carbonated sweetened drinks than either income-eligible or higher-income nonparticipants and significantly smaller shares from fresh apples, melons, and berries.
- FSP adults obtained a significantly smaller share of their total vegetable intake from salads/salad greens, compared with higher- income nonparticipant adults, and a significantly larger share from cooked potatoes that were not fried.

FSP adults obtained significantly less of their total oil intakes from nuts (which includes seeds and nut butters) than either group of nonparticipant adults.

FSP adults had a significantly lower mean score for the SoFAAS component than higher-income nonparticipants (5.2 vs. 7.5, out of a possible 20).

Factors that contributed to the difference in SoFAAS scores of FSP participant adults and higher-income nonparticipant adults were:

- FSP adults obtained significantly more of their solid fat from unflavored whole milk and chicken (likely due to use of solid fats during cooking) and more of their added sugar from regular (not sugar-free) sodas, table sugar, and ice cream.

- On the other hand, FSP adults obtained significantly less of their added sugar intakes from candy, relative to higher-income nonparticipant adults.

### *Differences between Older Adult FSP Participants (Age60+) and Nonparticipant Older Adults*

FSP older adults obtained a significantly smaller share of their total fruit intakes from fresh apples and fresh berries, relative to higher-income nonparticipant older adults, and a significantly smaller share of their vegetable intake from salads/salad greens.

Similar to children and adults, FSP older adults obtained a significantly larger share of total milk intakes from unflavored whole milk, compared with higher-income nonparticipants. However, in this age group, the difference was not statistically significant, probably because of the small sample size of older adult FSP participants. Nonetheless, FSP older adults obtained a significantly larger share of saturated fat and solid fat intakes from unflavored whole milk, compared with higher- income nonparticipants.

FSP older adults obtained more of their added sugar intakes from sodas than either group of nonparticipant older adults and less from candy. In addition, FSP older adults obtained significantly less of their added sugar intakes from ice cream than higher-income nonparticipant older adults (5 vs. 8 percent).

## IMPLICATIONS FOR FSP NUTRITION EDUCATION

Primary conclusions from these analyses are that:

- The diets of FSP participants were generally comparable to the diets of income-eligible nonparticipants, but were less adequate and lower in nutritional quality than the diets of higher-income nonparticipants.
- Where differences between FSP participants and income-eligible nonparticipants were observed, diet quality tended to be higher for income-eligible nonparticipants.
- Differences between FSP participants and nonparticipants were more often observed for adults (19 to 59 years) and older adults (60 years and older) than for children (1 to 18 years). Female adult FSP participants emerged as a subgroup of particular concern.

Data from the HEI-2 005 indicate clearly that there is ample room for improvement in the usual diets of all age groups and all participant/nonparticipant groups with respect to the following outcomes:

- Low intakes of vegetables and oils.
- Very low intakes of dark green and orange vegetables and legumes.
- Very low intakes of whole grains.
- High intakes of sodium.

In addition, several factors point to the critical need for improvements in diets of FSP participants:

- FSP participants did not achieve the levels of nutrient adequacy achieved by higher-income nonparticipants.
- FSP children and adult/older adult females exhibited higher levels of overweight and obesity than either group of nonparticipants.
- Foods consumed by adult female FSP participants and older adult FSP participants of both genders were lower in nutrient density than foods consumed by comparable higher- income nonparticipants.
- Foods consumed by adult female FSP participants were higher in energy density than foods consumed by adult female nonparticipants (both income-eligible and higher-income).
- Foods consumed by adult FSP participants of both genders provided, on average, more calories from SoFAAS that foods consumed by adult nonparticipants (both income-eligible and higher-income).

Specific issues that may prove to be useful targets for FSP nutrition education efforts include the following:

- *Use of whole milk.* In all three age groups, FSP participants were more likely than either income-eligible or higher-income nonparticipants to consume whole milk and less likely to consume reduced-fat or skim milks. Whole milk is less nutritionally desirable than reduced-fat/skim versions because it less nutrient dense, contributing more calories from saturated/solid fat.
- •*Low overall consumption of dairy products.* FSP children and adults consumed fewer dairy products, on a cups-per-1,000 calories basis (as measured in the HEI-2005) than higher-income nonparticipants. This pattern is reflected in lower calcium intakes, on average, among FSP participants. In addition to switching from whole milk to reduced-fat and skim milks, FSP participants could benefit from consuming more milk and other low-fat dairy products.(FSP participants in all age groups were less likely than higher-income nonparticipants to consume yogurt).•Low consumption of whole fruit. FSP participants in all three age groups consumed
- *Low consumption of whole fruit.* FSP participants in all three age groups consumed less whole fruit, on a cups-per-1,000 calorie basis, than higher-income nonparticipants. Among adults, this difference extended to 100 percent juices as well.
- *Consumption of regular (not sugar-free) sodas.* In all three age groups, regular sodas accounted for a larger share of the added sugars consumed by FSP participants than higher-income nonparticipants. Among older adults, this was also true for income-eligible nonparticipants.
- *Consumption of potato chips.* FSP adults and children were more likely than higher- income adults and children to consume potato chips. FSP participants were less likely to consume popcorn or pretzels (children only).

Targeting specific food choices, such as those cited above, may be an effective way to affect behavioral change that results in improved diet quality out-comes.

# REFERENCES

Basiotis, P., Guenther, P.M., Lino, M., & Britten, P. (2006). Americans consume too many calories from solid fat, alcohol, and added sugar. *Nutrition Insight, 33*. Alexandria, VA: USDA, Center for Nutrition Policy and Promotion.

Baum, C. (2007). *The effects of food stamps on obesity*. Washington, DC: USDA, Economic Research Service.

Bell, L., Tao, F., Anthony, J., Logan, C., Ledsky, R., Ferreira, M., & Brown, A. (2006). *Food stamp nutrition education systems review: Final report* Cambridge, MA: Abt Associates Inc.

Britten, P., Marcoe, K., Yamini, S., & Davis, C. (2006). Development of food intake patterns for the MyPyramid food guidance system. *Journal of Nutrition Education and Behavior, 38*(6), S78-S92.

Carriquiry A.L. (2003). Estimating usual intake distributions of nutrients and foods. *Journal of Nutrition, 133*, 601S–608S.

Devaney, B., Crepinsek, M.K., Fortson, K., & Quay, L. (2007). *Review of the dietary reference intakes for selected nutrients: Application challenges and implications for food and nutrition assistance programs*. Princeton, NJ: Mathematica Policy Research, Inc.

Devaney, B., Kim, M., Carriquiry, A., & Camaño-Garcia, G. (2005). *Assessing the nutrient intakes of vulnerable subgroups*. Washington, DC: USDA, Economic Research Service.

Drewnowski, A. (2005). Concept of a nutritious food: Toward a nutrient density score. *American Journal of Clinical Nutrition, 82*(4), 72 1–732.

Drewnowski, A., & Specter, S.E. (2004). Poverty and obesity: The role of energy density and energy costs. *American Journal of Clinical Nutrition, 79*(1), 6-16.

Fox, M.K., & Cole, N. (2004). *Nutrition and health characteristics of low-income populations. Volume I: Food stamp participants and nonparticipants* (E-FAN-04-0 14-1). Washington, DC: USDA, Economic Research Service

Guenther, P.M., Reedy, J., & Krebs-Smith, S.M. (in press). Development of the Healthy Eating Index-2005. *Journal of the American Dietetic Association*.

Guthrie, J.F., Frazao, E., Andrews, M., & Smallwood, D. (2007). Improving food choices—Can food stamps do more? *Amber Waves* (April). Washington, DC: USDA, Economic Research Service.

Hamilton, W.L., & Rossi, P.H. (2002). *Effects of Food Assistance and Nutrition Programs on Nutrition and Health: Volume I, Research Design* (Food Assistance and Nutrition Research Report No. 19-1). Washington, DC: USDA, Economic Research Service.

Institute of Medicine [IOM]. (1997). *Dietary reference intakes for calcium, phosphorus, magnesium, vitamin D, and fluoride.* Washington, DC: National Academies Press.

Institute of Medicine [IOM]. (1998). *Dietary reference intakes for thiamin, riboflavin, niacin, vitamin B6, folate, vitamin B12, pantothenic acid, biotin, and choline.* Washington, DC: National Academies Press.

Institute of Medicine [IOM]. (2000a). *Dietary reference intakes for vitamin C, vitamin E, selenium, and carotenoids.* Washington, DC: National Academies Press.

Institute of Medicine [IOM]. (2000b). *Dietary reference intakes: applications in dietary assessment.* Washington, DC: National Academies Press.

Institute of Medicine [IOM]. (2001). *Dietary reference intakes for vitamin A, vitamin K, arsenic, boron, chromium, copper, iodine, iron, manganese, molybdenum, nickel, silicon, vanadium, and zinc.* Washington, DC: National Academies Press.

Institute of Medicine [IOM]. (2005a). *Dietary reference intakes for energy, carbohydrate, fiber, fat, fatty acids, cholesterol, protein and amino acids.* Washington, DC: National Academies Press.

Institute of Medicine [IOM]. (2005b). *Dietary reference intakes for water, potassium, sodium, chloride, and sulfate.* Washington, DC: National Academies Press.

Institute of Medicine [IOM]. (2006). *Dietary reference intakes: The essential guide to nutrient requirements.* Washington, DC: National Academies Press.

Kuczmarski, R.J., & Flegal, K.M. (2000). Criteria for definition of overweight in transition: background and recommendations for the United States. *American Journal of Clinical Nutrition, 72*(5), 1074–1081.

Kuczmarski, R.J., Ogden, C.L., Grummer-Strawn, L.M., Flegal, K.M., Guom, S.S., Wei, R., et al. (2000). CDC growth charts: United States. *Advance Data, 314,* 1–28.

Ledikwe, J., Blanck, H., Khan, L., Serdula, M., Seymour, J., Tohill, B., & Rolls, B. (2005). Dietary energy density determined by eight calculation methods in a nationally representative United States population. *Journal of Nutrition, 135,* 273–278.

Moshfegh, A., Goldman, J., & Cleveland, L. (2005). *What we eat in America, NHANES 2001- 2002: Usual nutrient intakes from food compared to dietary reference intakes.* Washington, DC: USDA, Agricultural Research Service.

Perez-Escamilla, R., & Putnik, P. (2007). The role of acculturation in nutrition, lifestyle, and incidence of type 2 diabetes among Latinos. *Journal of Nutrition, 137,* 860-870.

Shinkle, D. (2006). Food stamp rebates may encourage healthy eating. *National Conference of State Legislatures: State & Federal Issues, 27* (478).

Subar, A.F., Krebs-Smith, S.M., Cook, A., & Kahle, L.L. (1998a). Dietary sources of nutrients among US children, 1989-1991. *Pediatrics, 102*(4), 9 13-923.

Subar, A.F., Krebs-Smith, S.M., Cook, A., & Kahle, L.L. (1 998b). Dietary sources of nutrients among US adults, 1989-1991. *Journal of the American Dietetic Association, 98*(5), 537-547.

U.S. Department of Agriculture [USDA]. (2007). *USDA 2007 farm bill proposals: Title IV, nutrition programs.* Available at: http://www.usda.gov/wps/portal/!ut/p/_s.7_0_A/ 7_0_1UH?navid=FARM_BILL_LEGISLAT&p        arentnav=FARM        _BILL _FORUMS&navtype=R S. Accessed October 2007.

U.S. Department of Agriculture, Center for Nutrition Policy and Promotion [USDA/CNPP]. (2005). *MyPyramid: USDA's new food guidance system.* Available at http://www.mypyramid. gov/downloads/MyPyramid%20Peer%20to%20 Peer.ppt

U.S. Department of Agriculture, Center for Nutrition Policy and Promotion [USDA/CNPP]. (2008). *MyPyramid guidance. Inside the Pyramid: Why is it important to consume oils?* Available at http://www.mypyramid.gov/ pyramid/oils_why.html. Accessed February 24, 2008.

U.S. Department of Agriculture, Food and Nutrition Service [USDA/FNS]. (2005). *Obesity, poverty, and participation in nutrition assistance programs.* Available at http://www. fns.usda.gov/oane/menu/Published/NutritionEdu cation/Files/ObesityPoverty.pdf.

U.S. Department of Agriculture, Food and Nutrition Service [USDA/FNS]. (2007a). *Implications of restricting the use of food stamp benefits.* Available at: www.fns.usda.gov/oane/ menu/Published/FSP/FILES/ProgramOperations /FSPFoodRestrictions.pdf. Published March 2007, accessed October 2007.

U.S. Department of Agriculture, Food and Nutrition Service [USDA/FNS]. (2007b). *Electronic benefits transfer (EBT) status report.* Available at: *www.fns.usda.gov/fsp/ ebt/ebt_status_report.htm.* Accessed October 2007.

U.S. Department of Agriculture, Food and Nutrition Service [USDA/FNS]. (2007c). *Characteristics of food stamp households: Fiscal Year 2006* (FSP-07-CHAR). Available at: *www.fns.usda.gov/oane/menu/Published/FSP/FI LES/Participation/* 2006Characteristics.pdf.

U.S. Department of Agriculture, Food and Nutrition Service [USDA/FNS]. (2008). *Program data: Food stamp program, annual state level data, FY2003-2007.* Available at: http://www.fns.usda.gov/pd/fspmain.htm. Accessed February 2008.

U.S. Department of Health and Human Services & U.S. Department of Agriculture. (2005). *Dietary guidelines for Americans 2005.* Available at: www.healthierus.gov/dietaryguidelines.

U.S. Department of Health and Human Services [U.S. DHHS] (2000). *Tracking healthy people 2010.* Washington, DC: U.S. Government Printing Office.

Ver Ploeg, M., Mancino, L., & Lin, B-H. (2007). *Food and nutrition assistance programs and obesity: 19 76-2002* (ERS Report No. 48). Washington, DC: USDA, Economic Research Service.

Zelman, K., & Kennedy, E. (2005). Naturally nutrient rich... Putting more power on Americans' plates. *Nutrition Today, 40*(2): 60- 68.

# Appendix A: Data and Methods

All tabulations in this chapter are based on NHANES data, analyzed alone or in conjunction with data from the MyPyramid Equivalents Database. In this appendix, we describe the data, variable construction, and statistical methods.

## NHANES Data

The National Health and Nutrition Examination Survey (NHANES) is conducted by the National Center for Health Statistics (NCHS), part of the Centers for Disease Control and Prevention (CDC). NHANES has been conducted on a periodic basis since 1971.[1] Beginning in 1999, NHANES is a continuous annual survey with data released in public data files every two years (e.g., 1999-2000, 200 1-02, 2003-04, etc.).

NCHS recommends combining two or more 2-year cycles of the continuous NHANES to increase sample size and produce estimates with greater statistical reliability. Most of the tabulations in this chapter are based on three 2-year cycles of NHANES data (1999-2004). NHANES 1999-2002 was used in conjunction with the MyPyramid Database (described below).

NHANES includes a 'household interview' conducted in respondents' homes, and a physical examination conducted in Mobile Exam Centers (MEC). Additional interview data were collected at the time of the MEC exam, including a dietary recall interview.

For this study, we used data from the following NHANES data files:

- Body Measures (BMX)
- Demographics (DEMO)
- Diet Behavior and Nutrition (DBQ)
- Dietary Interview Individual Food Files (DRXIFF)
- Dietary Interview, Total Nutrient Intakes (DRXTOT)
- Dietary Supplements (DSQ)
- Food Security (FSQ)
- Reproductive Health (RHQ)

Our sample for all analyses includes persons with complete dietary recalls, excluding pregnant and breastfeeding women, infants, and breastfeeding children. Pregnant and breastfeeding women were excluded due to differences in nutrient requirements and small sample sizes. Infants were excluded because DRI Estimated Average Requirements (EARs) are not defined for infants.

# MYPYRAMID EQUIVALENTS DATABASE FOR USDA FOOD CODES

The *MyPyramid Food Guidance System* (USDA, CNPP 2005), which replaced the Food Guide Pyramid introduced in 1992, provides estimates of the types and quantities of foods individuals should eat from the different food groups, tailored to individuals' age, gender, and activity level.

In contrast to the earlier Food Pyramid, which provided recommended numbers of servings from each food group, MyPyramid recommendations are in cup or ounce 'equivalents.' Recommendations for vegetable, fruit, and milk consumption are measured in cups or 'cup equivalents'; recommendations for grain and meat and bean consumption are measured in ounces or 'ounce equivalents."

The *MyPyramid Equivalents Database* contains records corresponding to NHANES dietary recalls, with NHANES food intakes measured in MyPyramid equivalents (Friday and Bowman, 2006).[2] Measures are provided for major food groups (grains, vegetables, fruits, milk, meat and beans) and subgroups, plus discretionary oils, discretionary solid fats, added sugar, and alcohol.

Each individual food may contain components from multiple MyPyramid food groups.

The MyPyramid database contains files corresponding to the NHANES individual food files (one record per food) and NHANES total nutrient files (one record per person, with total daily intake). We merged MyPyramid data to NHANES data for survey years 1999-2002. All analyses of pyramid intakes are limited to this 4-year period.

## Subgroups for Tabulation

We tabulated NHANES data to provide estimates for the total U.S. population, and for subgroups defined by program participation and income, and by age group.

### *Program Participation and Income*

Food stamp participation is measured at the *household level* based on *reported participation in the last 12 months*. Nonparticipants were further subdivided into those who were income-eligible for the FSP and those whose income exceeded the eligibility standard. These groups were identified by the following NHANES data items:

---

[1] NHANES-I was conducted from 1971-75; NHANES-II from 1976-80; and NHANES-III from 198 8-94.

[2] MyPyramid Equivalents Database version 1.0 contains data corresponding to NHANES 1999-2000 and 200 1-02, and CSFII 1994-96, 1998.

1. FSP participant     *if* FSD170N > 0

   *Nonparticipants:*

2. Income-eligible     *if* $0 \leq$ INDFMPIR $< 1.30$
3. Higher-income      *if* INDFMPIR $> 1.30$

   Where,

FSD170N =   Number of persons in household authorized to receive food stamps in last 12 months

INDFMPIR = Family poverty income ratio


The NHANES survey includes questions about food stamp participation by individuals and household members, currently and in the past 12 months. We used FSD 1 70N to identify FSP participants due to problems with the data item for current participation (FSD200).

The NCHS documentation for the Food Security Questionnaire (FSQ) for 1999-2000 and 200 1-2002 states that, "Computer programming errors resulted in some missing data on how many months each person was authorized to receive food stamps, and whether the person was currently authorized. These data could not be imputed and remain missing." We compared the weighted count of NHANES 1999-2002 respondents reporting "current food stamp participation" with administrative data and found that NHANES identified only 60 percent of current FS participants.

Because of the NHANES data problems, some persons classified as FS participants did not purchase food with food stamps at the time of the dietary recall. However, all persons classified as FS participants received FS benefits (including dollar benefits and nutrition education) in the past year. If FS benefits influence dietary decisions only contemporaneously and impart a positive influence, then this measurement problem results in: a) downward bias on estimates of differences between FS participants and income-eligible nonparticipants (due to misclassification of individuals in these two groups); and b) biased estimates of the differences between FS participants and higher-income nonparticipants (because the FS participant category includes income-eligible nonparticipants).


## Age Groups

Most tabulations for this chapter show data for three age groups:

- Children, age 1 to 18
- Adults, age 19-59
- Older adults, age 60 and above

Age groups were defined by the NHANES data item, RIDAGEYR = age at screening recode (defined as the "best age in years at the time of the household screening"). Infants were excluded from analyses and were identified by the NHANES data item, RIDAGEMN <12, where RIDAGEMN = age in months at screening.

# DIETARY INTAKE DATA, REFERENCE INTAKE STANDARDS, AND ESTIMATION OF USUAL INTAKES

Application of the DRIs requires information about the usual intake distribution for the population of interest. The usual intake distribution can be estimated using two or more days of recall information, or single-day recalls may be adjusted by out of-sample information about the within-person day- to-day variance for each nutrient.

## NHANES Dietary Recalls

Beginning with NHANES 2003-04, NCHS releases two days of dietary recall data for each respondent. The first day (Day 1) is collected in the MEC and the second day (Day 2) is collected by telephone 3 to 10 days later. In 2003-04, 87 percent of respondents completing the first day recall also completed the second day.

For this study, we pooled three 2-year cycles of NHANES (1999-2004). NHANES 1999-2002 public release data contain single-day dietary recalls.[3] Therefore, we estimated usual nutrient intake distributions by first estimating within-person variance components for NHANES 2003-04. These variance components were then used to adjust the single day (first day) intakes of the pooled sample of NHANES 1999-2004.

Usual intakes were estimated using the personal computer version of the *Software for Intake Distribution Estimation* (PC-SIDE). PC-SIDE estimates usual intake distributions from single day intakes when provided with information about variance components and the fourth moments of variance components (fourth moments are measures of skewness).

PC-SIDE was used to estimate means and proportions, standard errors of estimates, and percentiles of dietary intake distributions for gender by age subgroups. Estimates for both sexes were calculated in SAS as the weighted average of the PC- SIDE estimates for males and females.

## Reference Intake Standards

The Dietary Reference Intakes (DRIs) are a group of standards developed by the Food and Nutrition Board of the Institute of Medicine (IOM) to assess the adequacy and quality of nutrient intakes. Four different DRI standards are used to assess the usual nutrient intakes of FSP participants and nonparticipants:

- Estimated Average Requirements (EARs)
- Adequate Intakes (AIs)
- Tolerable Upper Intake Levels (ULs)
- Acceptable Macronutrient Distribution Ranges (AMDRs).

---

[3] Second recalls were collected for the entire sample beginning with NHANES 2002, but the second day recalls from 2002 were not publicly released.

Table A-1 provides the DRI values.

The *Estimated Average Requirement (EAR)* is the level of intake that is estimated to meet the requirements of half of the healthy individuals in a particular life stage and gender group. The EAR is used to assess the prevalence of inadequate intakes using the IOM-recommended "EAR-cut point method" (IOM, 2006).

The EAR cut-point method was used to analyze all nutrients for which EARs have been established. The EAR cut-point method assumes that nutrient requirements are symmetrically distributed. This assumption, however, does not hold for iron requirements among menstruating females. It is not appropriate to use the EAR cut-point method to estimate the prevalence of adequate iron intakes for menstruating females and the full probability approach was used for females aged 9-50 years old (IOM, 2006).

An *Adequate Intake (AI)* was defined when the data available for a particular nutrient were insufficient to estimate requirements and establish an EAR. The AI is the level of intake that is assumed to be adequate, based on observed or experimentally determined estimates of intake. AIs cannot be used to determine the proportion of a population with inadequate intakes. Instead, assessment focuses on comparison of mean usual intakes to the AI. Populations with a mean usual intake equivalent to or greater than the population-specific AI can be assumed to have adequate intakes.

The *Tolerable Upper Intake Level (UL)* is the maximum level of intake that is likely to pose no risks of adverse health effects for all individuals in a population group. As intake increases above the UL, the risk of adverse effects increases. For most nutrients for which ULs have been established, the UL based on intake from food, water, and dietary supplements (e.g., fluoride, phosphorus, and vitamin C) nutrients, the UL applies only to synthetic forms from dietary supplements, fortified foods, or over-the-counter medications (e.g., magnesium, folate, niacin, and vitamin E).

The NHANES nutrient intake files do not include nutrients provided by water, dietary supplements, or over-the-counter medications. Thus, our ability to assess usual intakes relative to ULs is limited. We estimated the prevalence of intakes above the UL for nutrients for which a UL is available, and found prevalence so small that most tables were populated with zeroes. (This is consistent with data presented in Moshfegh et al. (2005) where, with the exception of sodium and a handful of results for other nutrients, every cell in every table is identical ($<3\%$)). For this reason, we included analyses of intake relative to the UL only for sodium.

The DRIs specify *Acceptable Macronutrient Distribution Ranges (AMDRs)* for macronutrients (protein, carbohydrate, and total fat) and fatty acids (linoleic acid and alpha-linolenic acid).[4] AMDRs define ranges of macronutrient intakes that are associated with reduced risk of chronic disease, while providing recommended intakes of other essential nutrients. AMDRs are expressed as percentages of total energy intake because their requirements are *not* independent of each other or of the total energy requirement of the individual (IOM, 2006). A key feature of AMDRs is that each has lower and upper bounds. Intakes that fall below or exceed these levels of intake may increase risk of chronic disease.

---

[4] Usual protein and carbohydrate intakes are also assessed relative to EARs, based on total intake—gm/day for carbohydrate and gm/ day per kg body weight for protein .

## Table A-1. Dietary Reference Intakes for Individuals

| | Estimated Average Requirements (EARs) | | | | | | | |
|---|---|---|---|---|---|---|---|---|
| | Vitamin A (mcg RAE) | Vitamin C (mg) | Vitamin B-6 (mg) | Vitamin B-12 (mcg) | Vitamin E (mg AT) | Folate (mcg DFE) | Niacin (mg) | Riboflavin (mg) |
| Males | | | | | | | | |
| 1-3 years | 210 | 13 | 0.4 | 0.7 | 5 | 120 | 5.0 | 0.4 |
| 4-8 years | 275 | 22 | 0.5 | 1.0 | 6 | 160 | 6.0 | 0.5 |
| 9-13 years | 445 | 39 | 0.8 | 1.5 | 9 | 250 | 9.0 | 0.8 |
| 14-18 years | 630 | 63 | 1.1 | 2.0 | 12 | 330 | 12.0 | 1.1 |
| 19-30 years | 625 | 75 | 1.1 | 2.0 | 12 | 320 | 12.0 | 1.1 |
| 31-50 years | 625 | 75 | 1.1 | 2.0 | 12 | 320 | 12.0 | 1.1 |
| 51-70 years | 625 | 75 | 1.4 | 2.0 | 12 | 320 | 12.0 | 1.1 |
| 71 + years | 625 | 75 | 1.4 | 2.0 | 12 | 320 | 12.0 | 1.1 |
| Females | | | | | | | | |
| 1-3 years | 210 | 13 | 0.4 | 0.7 | 5 | 120 | 5.0 | 0.4 |
| 4-8 years | 275 | 22 | 0.5 | 1.0 | 6 | 160 | 6.0 | 0.5 |
| 9-13 years | 420 | 39 | 0.8 | 1.5 | 12 | 250 | 9.0 | 0.8 |
| 14-18 years | 485 | 56 | 1.0 | 2.0 | 12 | 330 | 11.0 | 0.9 |
| 19-30 years | 500 | 60 | 1.1 | 2.0 | 12 | 320 | 11.0 | 0.9 |
| 31-50 years | 500 | 60 | 1.1 | 2.0 | 12 | 320 | 11.0 | 0.9 |
| 51-70 years | 500 | 60 | 1.3 | 2.0 | 12 | 320 | 11.0 | 0.9 |
| 71 + years | 500 | 60 | 1.3 | 2.0 | 12 | 320 | 11.0 | 0.9 |

| | Estimated Average Requirements (EARs) | | | | | | |
|---|---|---|---|---|---|---|---|
| | Thiamin (mg) | Iron (mg) | Magnesium (mg) | Phosphorus (mg) | Zinc (mg) | Carbohy-drate (g) | Protein (g/kg body wgt) |
| Males | | | | | | | |
| 1-3 years | 0.4 | 3.0 | 65 | 380 | 2.5 | 100 | 0.87 |
| 4-8 years | 0.5 | 4.1 | 110 | 405 | 4.0 | 100 | 0.76 |
| 9-13 years | 0.7 | 5.9 | 200 | 1055 | 7.0 | 100 | 0.76 |
| 14-18 years | 1.0 | 7.7 | 340 | 1055 | 8.5 | 100 | 0.73 |
| 19-30 years | 1.0 | 6.0 | 330 | 580 | 9.4 | 100 | 0.66 |
| 31-50 years | 1.0 | 6.0 | 350 | 580 | 9.4 | 100 | 0.66 |
| 51-70 years | 1.0 | 6.0 | 350 | 580 | 9.4 | 100 | 0.66 |
| 71 + years | 1.0 | 6.0 | 350 | 580 | 9.4 | 100 | 0.66 |
| Females | | | | | | | |
| 1-3 years | 0.4 | 3.0 | 65 | 380 | 2.5 | 100 | 0.87 |
| 4-8 years | 0.5 | 4.1 | 110 | 405 | 4.0 | 100 | 0.76 |
| 9-13 years | 0.7 | 5.7 | 200 | 1055 | 7.0 | 100 | 0.76 |
| 14-18 years | 0.9 | 7.9 | 300 | 1055 | 7.3 | 100 | 0.71 |
| 19-30 years | 0.9 | 8.1 | 255 | 580 | 6.8 | 100 | 0.66 |
| 31-50 years | 0.9 | 8.1 | 265 | 580 | 6.8 | 100 | 0.66 |
| 51-70 years | 0.9 | 5.0 | 265 | 580 | 6.8 | 100 | 0.66 |
| 71 + years | 0.9 | 5.0 | 265 | 580 | 6.8 | 100 | 0.66 |

See note at end of table.

## Table A-1. (Continued)

**Table A-1—Dietary Reference Intakes for Individuals —Continued**

| | Adequate Intakes (AI) | | | | | | Upper Tolerable Intake Level (UL) |
|---|---|---|---|---|---|---|---|
| | Calcium (mg) | Potassium (g) | Sodium (g) | Fiber (g) | Linoleic acid (g) | Linolenic acid (g) | Sodium (g) |
| **Males** | | | | | | | |
| 1-3 years | 500 | 3000 | 1000 | 19 | 7 | 0.7 | 1.5 |
| 4-8 years | 800 | 3800 | 1200 | 25 | 10 | 0.9 | 1.9 |
| 9-13 years | 1300 | 4500 | 1500 | 31 | 12 | 1.2 | 2.2 |
| 14-18 years | 1300 | 4700 | 1500 | 38 | 16 | 1.6 | 2.3 |
| 19-30 years | 1000 | 4700 | 1500 | 38 | 17 | 1.6 | 2.3 |
| 31-50 years | 1000 | 4700 | 1500 | 38 | 17 | 1.6 | 2.3 |
| 51-70 years | 1200 | 4700 | 1300 | 30 | 14 | 1.6 | 2.3 |
| 71 + years | 1200 | 4700 | 1200 | 30 | 14 | 1.6 | 2.3 |
| **Females** | | | | | | | |
| 1-3 years | 500 | 3000 | 1000 | 19 | 7 | 0.7 | 1.5 |
| 4-8 years | 800 | 3800 | 1200 | 25 | 10 | 0.9 | 1.9 |
| 9-13 years | 1300 | 4500 | 1500 | 26 | 10 | 1.0 | 2.2 |
| 14-18 years | 1300 | 4700 | 1500 | 26 | 11 | 1.1 | 2.3 |
| 19-30 years | 1000 | 4700 | 1500 | 25 | 12 | 1.1 | 2.3 |
| 31-50 years | 1000 | 4700 | 1500 | 25 | 12 | 1.1 | 2.3 |
| 51-70 years | 1200 | 4700 | 1300 | 21 | 11 | 1.1 | 2.3 |
| 71 + years | 1200 | 4700 | 1200 | 21 | 11 | 1.1 | 2.3 |

See note at end of table.

## Table A-1. (Continued)

| | Acceptable Macronutrient Distribution Ranges (AMDRs) | | | | |
|---|---|---|---|---|---|
| | Total fat | Linoleic acid | Linolenic acid | Carbohydrate | Protein |
| | Range (% energy) | | | | |
| Children, 1-3 yrs | 30 – 40 | 5 – 10 | 0.6 – 1.2 | 45 – 65 | 5 – 20 |
| Children, 4-18 yrs | 25 – 35 | 5 – 10 | 0.6 – 1.2 | 45 – 65 | 10 – 30 |
| Adults | 20 – 35 | 5 – 10 | 0.6 – 1.2 | 45 – 65 | 10 – 35 |

Source: Institute of Medicine (IOM), Food and Nutrition Board. Dietary Reference Intakes, 1997-2005

# VARIABLE CONSTRUCTION

For several analyses, we constructed new variables from the original NHANES data elements, as described in this section.

## Body Mass Index

NHANES examinations included measurement of body weight and stature (or recumbent length).[5] The NHANES public data files include Body Mass Index (BMI), defined as:

BMI = weight in kilograms / [height in meters]$^2$

We classified adult weight status relative to BMI cutoffs specified by the National Institutes of Health:

- Underweight: BMI < 18.5
- Normal weight: $18.5 \leq$ BMI < 25
- Overweight: $25 \leq$ BMI < 30
- Obese: BMI $\geq$ 30

We classified children's weight status based on comparison of BMI-for-age with the percentiles of the CDC BMI-for-age growth chart using the SAS program provided by the CDC at: http:// www.cdc.gov/nccdphp/dnpa/growthcharts/sas.htm. The CDC SAS program includes LMS parameters of the smoothed growth curve for each age in months, by gender. The LMS parameters are the median (M), the generalized coefficient of variation (S), and the power in the Box-Cox transformation (L) of the growth curve. Documentation of LMS calculations is available at:
http://www.cdc.gov/nchs/about/major/nhanes/growthcharts/datafiles.htm

## Body Weight for Analyzing Usual Intakes of Protein
## Per Kilogram Body Weight

The EAR for protein is specified in terms of protein per kilogram of body weight. We followed the method described in *What We Eat in America* (Moshfegh et al. (2005), Appendix B), which assumes that the EAR refers to the ratio of protein per kg of body weights falling in the healthy range. Thus, if actual body weight is not in the healthy range, a reference body weight is assigned to an individual as follows:

---

[5] Recumbent length was measured for infants and children up to age 3; stature was measured for persons age 2 and over. Both length and height were measured for children age 24 to 36 months.

- Adults—If BMI< 18.5 or BMI>25, the weight closest to actual that yields a BMI, based on height, in the healthy range. For example, since BMI = weight ÷ (height in meters)$^2$, if BMI > 25 then,
  Reference weight = 25 x (height in meters)$^2$
- Children ages 4-18—If BMI-for-age is below the 5$^{th}$ or above the 85$^{th}$ percentile, the reference weight is the weight that places the respondent at the nearest percentile of the healthy range (5$^{th}$ or 85$^{th}$), given their height. Reference weights associated with the 5$^{th}$ and 85$^{th}$ BMI-for-age percentiles (given age and gender) were determined by modifying the CDC SAS program noted above.
- All children ages 1-3—The protein to body weight ratio was computed using a reference weight of 12 kg for all children.

## Meals and Snacks

To analyze meal patterns and nutrient characteristics of meals, we classified all foods in the NHANES food files as part of breakfast lunch, dinner, or snacks. NHANES 1999-2000 and 200 1- 02 contained 16 codes corresponding to English and Spanish meal names, with two additional codes added for NHANES 2003-04. The codes were mapped into four categories as shown in Table A-2.

Foods reported as meals were coded as breakfast, lunch, and dinner without regard to mealtime. Thus persons were observed to consume from zero to three meals. Snack foods were categorized into 'snack periods' according to meal time so that the number of 'snacks' is equal to the number of times a person consumed food and beverages outside of meals, not the number of individual foods consumed as snacks.

## Energy Density

We calculated energy density as the ratio of kilocalories per gram of food. Foods are defined as specified by Ledikwe et al. (2005) as solid and liquid items that are typically consumed as foods. This definition excludes all beverages. Included are soft and liquid foods such as ice cream and soup. Excluded are items typically consumed as beverages, such as milkshakes and liquid meal replacements.[6]

The rationale provided by Ledikwe et al. (2005) for including solid foods and not beverages is that, "Intake of foods, as compared with beverages, is more influenced by hunger and less influenced by fluid balance. Beverages may disproportionately affect energy density values."

---

[6] Liquid meal replacements include instant breakfast, protein supplements and powder, and meal replacement drinks. Meal replacement bars are included in the definition of solid foods.

## Table A-2. NHANES Meal and Snack Codes

| Meal Category / Meal name | NHANES Meal Codes | | |
|---|---|---|---|
| | 1999-00 | 2001-02 | 2003-04 |
| **1. Breakfast** | | | |
| Breakfast | 1 | 1 | 1 |
| Desayuno | 9 | 10 | 10 |
| Almuerzo | 10 | 11 | 11 |
| **2. Lunch** | | | |
| Brunch | 2 | 5 | 5 |
| Lunch | 3 | 2 | 2 |
| Comida | 11 | 12 | 12 |
| **3. Dinner** | | | |
| Dinner | 5 | 3 | 3 |
| Supper | N/A | N/A | 4 |
| Cena | 13 | 14 | 14 |
| **4. Snacks** | | | |
| Snack/ beverage | 4 | 6 | 6/7 |
| Extended consumption | 7 | 9 | 9 |
| Merienda | 12 | 13 | 13 |
| Entre comida, bebida/ tentempie | 14 | 15 | 15/18 |
| Bocadillo | 15 | 17 | 17 |
| Botana | 16 | 16 | 16 |
| Other | 8 | 91 | 91 |
| Don't know | 99 | 99 | 99 |

We implemented this definition by excluding foods at the food group level, after categorizing foods into 3-digit food groups. The following food groups were excluded:

- Milk (white, flavored, soymilk, dry and evaporated milk)
- Protein/meal enhancement drinks
- Non-citrus and citrus juice (juice bars were not excluded)
- Vegetable juice
- Coffee, tea
- Beer, wine, liquor
- Drinking water (identified in NHANES 2003- 04 only)
- Soft drinks; sweetened, low calorie, and sugar- free beverages

In addition, all ingredients of "combination beverages" were excluded. These were identified by the NHANES variable for "combination type."

Total calories and total grams were summed on a per person basis for all foods not excluded, to obtain estimates of the average energy density of daily intake.

## Nutrient Rich (NR) Score

A nutrient rich score is a ratio that measures the nutrient contribution of a food relative to its energy contribution. We calculated NR scores based on the naturally nutrient rich (NNR) score developed by Drewnowski (2005). The NNR score excludes fortified foods; our NR score does not make that exclusion.

We calculated an NR score based on the 16 nutrients shown in Table A-3. For a single food, the NR score is obtained by calculating a score for each nutrient (equation 1 below), and averaging across the 16 nutrients (equation 2):

$$\%DV_x = \frac{amount per 2000kcal_x}{DV_x},\tag{1}$$

where $x = nutrient\ 1\text{-}16$

$$NR = \sum_{x=1}^{16} \%DV_x/16 \tag{2}$$

The NR scores for total daily intakes, meals/snacks, and food groups are obtained by applying equations (1) and (2) to the total nutrients consumed per person at each level of daily intake, meals/snacks, and food groups. Thus, nutrients are summed for each level of analyses; total nutrients are normalized to a "nutrient per 2,000 kcal" measure; the percent DV is calculated for each nutrient; and the NR score is the average of "%DV" across all nutrients. Nutrients are weighted equally. Consistent with Drenowski, the %DV value is truncated at 2000% DV when implementing equation 1, before the average across nutrients is taken, thus limiting the influence of large concentrations of one nutrient.

### Table A-3. Nutrients and Recommended Daily Values (DVs) used to Calculate Nutrient Rich Scores[a]

| Nutrient | Value | Nutrient | Value |
|---|---|---|---|
| Calcium | 1300 mg | Vitamin B12 | 2.4 µg |
| Folate | 400 µg | Vitamin C | 90 mg |
| Iron | 18 mg | Vitamin E | 15 mg |
| Magnesium | 420 mg | Zinc | 11 mg |
| Potassium | 4.7 g | Dietary Fiber | 38 g |
| Riboflavin | 1.3 mg | Linoleic acid | 17 g |
| Thiamin | 1.2 mg | α-Linolenic acid | 1. 6 g |
| Vitamin A (RAE) | 900 mg | Protein | 56 g |

a Daily values are based on maximum RDAs or AIs (calcium, magnesium, potassium, dietary fiber, linoleic acid, and αlinolenic acid), excluding pregnant or lactating women.

The mean NR score must be interpreted with caution. The NR score is not designed to characterize nutrient adequacy or diet quality, but to characterize food choices in terms of nutrient density. The score is normalized to 2,000 kcal, so it does not provide an absolute measure of nutrient intake relative to DVs. Furthermore, the score does not account negatively for "bad nutrients" (saturated fat, cholesterol, and sodium); in contrast, the HEI-2005 accounts for over consumption of "bads." And finally, the score weights all nutrients equally. Thus, a person consuming 2000% DV of one nutrient will have a higher NR score from that single nutrient than a person consuming exactly 100% DV of all nutrients.

The mean NR score for a group of individuals is based on individuals with reported intakes. The score does not weight the contribution of zero intakes (nutrients per 2000 kcal is zero if intake is zero). Thus, the sample size for NR scores per meal varies over meals.

## Percent of Energy from SoFAAS

SoFAAS is an acronym for solid fats, alcoholic beverages, and added sugars. Staff at USDA's Center for Nutrition Policy and Promotion (CNPP) developed the SoFAAS measure to provide insight into discretionary calorie intakes.

We measured SoFAAS calories per food and per NHANES respondent using data from the NHANES individual food file (grams of alcohol) and the MyPyramid Equivalents database (grams of discretionary solid fat and teaspoons of added sugar). Analyses of SoFAAS were limited to NHANES 1999-2002 because MyPyramid data for NHANES 2003-04 had not been released at the time of this study.

The measure of SoFAAS calories was constructed at the level of individual food, and then aggregated for daily intake. The measures from the NHANES and MyPyramid file were converted to measures of calories as follows:

1) Kcal from solid fat = Grams of solid fat × 9
2) Kcal from alcohol[7] = Grams of alcohol × 7 + (Carbohydrates from beer and wine, excluding carbs from added sugar) × 4
3) Kcal from added sugar[8] = Teaspoons of added sugar × 4.2 × 4

Alcoholic beverages have food codes with the first three digits from 931 to 935. Alcohol from cooking wine is not included in SoFAAS (food code 93401300). Carbohydrates from mixed drinks (e.g., orange juice, Bloody Mary mix, soda, etc) are not included in SoFAAS. Note that (2) excludes calories from added sugar to avoid double counting added sugar in steps (2) and (3).

Total calories from SoFAAS were obtained by summing (1) – (3) above, and then expressed as a percentage of total energy:

Percent of total energy from SoFAAS = SoFAAS calories / Total calories × 100

---

[7] The algorithm for computing calories from alcoholic beverages was taken from the HEI-2005 SAS code provided at: www.cnpp.usda.gov/HealthyEatingIndex.htm

[8] Each teaspoon of sugar is equivalent to 4.2 grams of table sugar and each gram of table sugar (carbohydrate) provides 4 calories.

This measure was calculated for total daily intakes, meals/snacks, and food groups by applying steps (1) - (3) to each food record, summing SoFAAS calories and total calories for each level of analysis (daily intake, meals/snacks, and food groups), and calculating the percent SoFAAS based on the summations.

Our analyses of SoFAAS revealed some anomalies with the NHANES data, which we discussed with staff at USDA/ARS. Some food records have grams of discretionary fat in excess of grams of total fat (2,718 records or 1.1 percent), and some food records have calories from added sugar in excess of calories from total sugar.

### Problems with Discretionary Fat

We discussed this problem with ARS staff. They indicated that the problem is due to recipe modifications in the NHANES data that are not accounted for in the MyPyramid data. For example, in the NHANES data, tuna salad might be coded with the same food code but one individual's record was modified to reflect the fact that light mayonnaise rather than regular mayonnaise was used in preparation. In the MyPyramid data, each case of tuna salad coded with the same food code received the same amount of discretionary fat, based on the "original" recipe.[9] ARS staff indicated that this problem will be addressed in future releases of NHANES/MyPyramid data. Our solution was to top code grams of discretionary fat (solids and oils) to sum to grams of total fat, by decreasing both discretionary solid fats and discretionary oils in proportion to their original values.

### Problems with Added Sugar

The MyPyramid Equivalents Database documentation indicates that added sugar was derived by different methods for NHANES 1999-00 and NHANES 2001-02. Methods were improved in the later years and the values of added sugar for 1999-00 were made consistent with 2001-02 for all food codes that appeared in both years with the same total sugar per 100 grams and *same sources of added sugar*. Our examination found that, for some foods, the added sugar values (per 100 grams) for identical food codes in different years varied significantly and calories from added sugar sometimes exceeded calories from total sugar. We chose to use consistent values of added sugar per 100 grams of food across all years of data. The following steps were taken to impose consistency on the added sugar values:

a.  For each food code, added sugar per 100 grams was taken from the MyPyramid equivalents database file for 2001-02 ('Equiv0102').
b.  For each food code, total sugar per 100 grams was calculated as the median in the NHANES 2001-02 food files.
c.  RATIO-1 = ratio of (a) to (b)
d.  1999-2000 NHANES individual food records were merged with 1999-2000 Pyramid data.
e.  RATIO-2 = ratio of added to total sugar per 100 grams on 1999-2000 individual food records
f.  If RATIO-2 did not equal RATIO-1, added sugar on the 1999-2000 food record was set equal to total sugar multiplied by RATIO-1.

---

[9] The data confirm that in the NHANES data there is variation in total fat per 100 grams across records with the same food code, but no variation in discretionary fat for the same records in the MyPyramid data.

g. For all food codes in 1999-2000 and not in 200 1-02, if added sugar (in grams) exceeded total sugar (in grams), added sugar was top coded at the total sugar value.

After "cleaning" the values for discretionary solid fat and added sugar, 2 percent of food records had total SoFAAS calories in excess of total energy. These are mainly the result of rounding error. These records were top coded at SoFAAS percent of calories equal to 100.

## Foods Categorized for Frequent, Selective, and Occasional Consumption

We categorized NHANES foods according to the radiant pyramid/power calories concept, as described by Zelman and Kennedy (2005). This concept recommends that, within food group, the most nutrient-dense choices be consumed most frequently (to obtain recommended levels of nutrients while maintaining energy balance) and choices that are lowest in nutrient density should be consumed only occasionally.

Categorization of foods was implemented through an iterative approach. First, within each of the 10 broad food groups, foods were sorted by Nutrient Rich (NR) score and the percentage of calories from SoFAAS. Decision rules based on the combination of NR score and SoFAAS were applied to each broad food group to provide an initial "break" of foods into 3 categories, thus reducing the need to manually code all foods. Foods were then sorted by 3-digit food subgroup and we reviewed food descriptions, percentage of calories from SoFAAS, and total fat per 100 grams. We divided foods within a food subgroup so that foods with the lowest proportion of calories from SoFAAS/total fat content were included in the "consume frequently" category and foods with the highest proportion of calories from SoFAAS/total fat content were included in the "consume occasionally" category.

The rules used in assigning foods to the three categories were presented in Chapter 5, Table 5-11. These decision rules were informed by general recommendations made in MyPyramid guidance and/or in the Dietary Guidelines for Americans. This categorization was applied only to foods in NHANES 1999-2002 because information about SoFAAS comes from the MyPyramid database, available only for 1999-2002 at the time of this study.

## Healthy Eating Index-2005 (HEI-2005)

HEI-2005 component and total scores were constructed using the following guidance and resources available from USDA/CNPP:[10]

- Healthy Eating Index-2005 Development and Evaluation Technical Report (Guenther, et al. 2007), section on "Using the HEI-2005 to Assess Diets of Groups and Individuals"
- CNPP SAS program for computing HEI -2005 scores for a population or group (HEI2005_NHANES0102_PopulationScore.sas)
- Database for whole fruit

---

[10] The HEI-2005 Technical Report and supporting files are available at
http://www.cnpp.usda.gov/HealthyEatingIndex.htm

The HEI-2005 Technical Report contains the HEI2005 scoring system and guidance for applying the scoring system to population groups.

The SAS program constructs HEI component scores and total score for a population or group. The program reads the NHANES individual food files, MyPyramid Equivalents Database (equiv0102), and the whole fruit database.

The whole fruit database is supplied as a supplement to the Pyramid equivalents database to support the calculation of the HEI component score for whole fruit. The database contains records corresponding to NHANES 2001-02 food records for persons age 2 and above. The file contains two data items—"whole fruit" and "fruit juice"— measured in cup equivalents per 100 grams of food. For each food, the total fruit cup equivalents from the MyPyramid database was assigned to either whole fruit or juice; foods containing both were assigned to one category depending on the majority component.

### Methods for Calculating HEI-2005 Scores

We calculated HEI-2005 scores for groups of program participants and nonparticipants, using the pooled sample of persons in NHANES 1999-2002. These steps were followed:

a)  Merged the whole fruit database to NHANES 1999-2000 food records, by food code and imputed "whole fruit" and "fruit juice" for foods appearing in 1999-2000 and not in the whole fruit database.

b)  Followed the procedures in the CNPP SAS program to apply the HEI scoring system "to the ratio of the population's mean food group (or nutrient) intake to the population's mean energy intake", using the SUDAAN PROC RATIO procedure.

## STATISTICAL METHODS

We produced estimates for this chapter using the following two statistical software packages:

- *PC-SIDE: Software for Intake Distribution Estimation*—used to estimate means, percentiles, and standard errors for nutrient intake tables.

- *SUDAAN (version 9.0)*—used to calculate means, standard errors, and tests of statistical significance for non-nutrient tables, using the DESCRIPT, CROSSTAB, and RATIO procedures.

Sample weights were used to account for sample design and nonresponse. Information about the NHANES survey design (strata and primary sampling units) was used for estimating variances and testing for statistical significance in SUDAAN.

Table A-4 shows the number of foods in the NHANES individual food files (unique food codes) categorized for frequent, selective, or occasional consumption.

**Table A-4. Number and Percent of NHANES Food Codes Categorized as Foods Suggested for Frequent, Selective, or Occasional Consumption**

| | Number of food codes | | | Percent of foods | | |
|---|---|---|---|---|---|---|
| | Foods to enjoy frequently | Foods to enjoy selectively | Foods to enjoy occasionally | Foods to enjoy frequently | Foods to enjoy selectively | Foods to enjoy occasionally |
| **All foods** | 1,244 | 1,426 | 2,021 | 26.5 | 30.4 | 43.1 |
| **Grains** | 147 | 230 | 159 | 27.4 | 42.9 | 29.7 |
| Plain bread, rolls, bagels, Eng muffin | 61 | 68 | 9 | 44.2 | 49.3 | 6.5 |
| Tortillas and taco shells | 2 | 3 | 2 | 28.6 | 42.9 | 28.6 |
| Cereals | 72 | 100 | 67 | 30.1 | 41.8 | 28.0 |
| Rice and pasta | 5 | 29 | 20 | 9.3 | 53.7 | 37.0 |
| Other | 7 | 30 | 61 | 7.1 | 30.6 | 62.2 |
| **Vegetables** | 237 | 382 | 245 | 27.4 | 44.2 | 28.4 |
| Raw | 42 | 6 | 5 | 79.2 | 11.3 | 9.4 |
| Cooked, excl. potatoes | 164 | 238 | 114 | 31.8 | 46.1 | 22.1 |
| Cooked, potatoes | – | 20 | 47 | – | 29.8 | 70.2 |
| Green salads | 1 | 2 | 36 | 2.6 | 5.1 | 92.3 |
| Beans | 24 | 43 | 11 | 30.8 | 55.1 | 14.1 |
| Nuts and seeds | 1 | 58 | 2 | 1.6 | 95.1 | 3.3 |
| Soy products/ meal enhancement | 5 | 15 | 30 | 10.0 | 30.0 | 60.0 |
| **Fruit** | 113 | 86 | 63 | 43.1 | 32.8 | 24.0 |
| Fresh | 39 | 5 | 11 | 70.9 | 9.1 | 20.0 |
| Canned | 35 | 45 | 15 | 36.8 | 47.4 | 15.8 |
| Other fruit | 2 | 12 | 13 | 7.4 | 44.4 | 48.2 |
| Juice (all types) | 37 | 24 | 24 | 43.5 | 28.2 | 28.2 |
| **Milk group** | 20 | 20 | 67 | 18.7 | 18.7 | 62.6 |
| Fluid milk | 8 | 12 | 41 | 13.1 | 19.7 | 67.2 |
| Dry or Evaporated Milk | 7 | 5 | 18 | 23.3 | 16.7 | 60.0 |
| Yogurt | 5 | 3 | 8 | 31.2 | 18.8 | 50.0 |
| **Meat and meat alternates** | 277 | 258 | 325 | 32.2 | 30.0 | 37.8 |
| Red meats (beef, lamb, pork, veal) | 49 | 81 | 76 | 23.8 | 39.3 | 36.9 |
| Other meats | 27 | 20 | 70 | 23.1 | 17.1 | 59.8 |
| Poultry | 84 | 92 | 57 | 36.0 | 39.5 | 24.5 |
| Fish/shellfish | 99 | 27 | 48 | 56.9 | 15.5 | 27.6 |
| Eggs | 2 | 25 | 24 | 3.9 | 49.0 | 47.1 |
| Cheese | 16 | 13 | 50 | 20.2 | 16.5 | 63.3 |
| **Mixed dishes** | 374 | 316 | 294 | 38.0 | 32.1 | 29.9 |
| Mostly meat | 194 | 150 | 76 | 46.2 | 35.7 | 18.1 |
| Mostly grain (incl. pizza) | 106 | 151 | 210 | 22.7 | 32.3 | 45.0 |
| Soup, mostly vegetable | 74 | 15 | 8 | 76.3 | 15.5 | 8.2 |
| **Condiments, Oils, Fats** | 12 | 33 | 99 | 8.3 | 22.9 | 68.8 |
| Added fats | 3 | 31 | 48 | 3.7 | 37.8 | 58.5 |
| Sweet toppings | 9 | 2 | 51 | 14.5 | 3.2 | 82.3 |
| **Sweets** | – | 89 | 562 | – | 13.7 | 86.3 |
| Dairy-based desserts | – | 80 | 48 | – | 62.5 | 37.5 |
| Baked desserts | – | – | 396 | – | – | 100.0 |
| Other | – | 9 | 118 | – | 7.1 | 92.9 |
| **Beverages** | 64 | – | 168 | 27.6 | – | 72.4 |
| Coffee/tea | 35 | – | 35 | 50.0 | – | 50.0 |
| Soft drinks | 16 | – | 13 | 55.2 | – | 44.8 |
| Noncarbonated beverage | 13 | – | 77 | 14.4 | – | 85.6 |
| Alcohol | – | – | 43 | – | – | 100.0 |
| **Salty snacks** | – | 12 | 39 | – | 23.5 | 76.5 |

–No foods in this category.

Source: NHANES 1999–2004 Individual Food Files.

## Sampling Weights

Tables are based on either NHANES 1999-2004 (6 years) or NHANES 1999-2002 (4 years). Accordingly, 6-year weights or 4-year weights were used.

NHANES 1999-2002 public files include two sets of sampling weights: Interview weights and MEC exam weights (MEC weights account for the additional nonresponse to the MEC exam). NHANES 2003-04 also include dietary intake weights. All weights sum to the total US civilian non-institutionalized population in year 2000.

Our sample for analyses includes only persons with complete dietary recalls. We followed the documentation provided in *What We Eat in America (WWEIA)* (Moshfegh et al., 2005, Appendix B) to construct dietary intake sampling weights for NHANES 1999-2002, consistent with the intake weights released with NHANES 2003-04. Dietary intake weights are constructed from the MEC exam weights: a) to account for additional nonresponse to the dietary recall, and b) to provide proportionate weighting of weekday and weekend recalls. The second adjustment is needed because proportionately more dietary recalls occurred on weekends than on weekdays. Since food intake varies by day of week, use of MEC weights would disproportionately represent intakes on weekends. Sample weights for persons with weekday vs. weekend recalls were recalibrated, within demographic group, so that weekday recalls account for 4/7 of the total sample weight.

Dietary intake weights for NHANES 1999-2002 and for NHANES 2003-04 each sum to the US population in year 2000. To construct 6-year weights, we multiplied the 1999-2002 weights by two-thirds and the 2003-04 weights by one-third. Jacknife weights (87 weights) were constructed to account for the NHANES survey design when using PC-SIDE software.

## Age Adjusted Totals

This chapter presents estimates for children, adults, and older adults. In addition, Appendix D presents nutrient intake estimates for age groups consistent with the DRI standards, and for "Total males," "Total females," and "Total both sexes."

We used age-adjustment to produce estimates for children, adults, older adults, total males, total females, and total both sexes. The age-adjusted estimates are calculated as the weighted average of estimates for DRI age groups (or portions of DRI age groups) with the weights equal to year 2000 population. For example, in Appendix D (available online), each DRI-age group estimate is calculated by weighting responses by NHANES dietary intake weights. The "total" rows weight the age group estimates by population weights so that each column in the tables (Total Persons, Food Stamp Participants, Income-eligible Nonparticipants, and Higher-income Nonparticipants) is weighted by the same set of weights. This age adjustment eliminates between-group differences due solely to differences in the age distribution of the groups. Similarly, estimates for Children, Adults, and Older adults are constructed from DRI age group estimates and population weights. Age adjustment is an option within the SUDAAN software.

The HEI-2005 scoring system is shown in Table A5. Population scores were obtained using the SUDAAN PROC RATIO procedure, using dietary recall sampling weights and age adjustment.

### Table A-5. HEI-2005 Scoring System

| Component | Max Score | Criteria for: Zero Score | Criteria for: Max Score | Equation for Score |
|---|---|---|---|---|
| Total fruit | 5 | Zero intake | ≥ 0.8 cup equivalents per 1000 kcal | $\dfrac{5}{0.8} \times \dfrac{f\_total}{energy/1000}$ |
| Whole fruit | 5 | Zero intake | ≥ 0.4 cup equivalents per 1000 kcal | $\dfrac{5}{0.4} \times \dfrac{wholefrt}{energy/1000}$ |
| Total vegetables | 5 | Zero intake | ≥ 1.1 cup equivalents per 1000 kcal | $\dfrac{5}{1.1} \times \dfrac{v\_total}{energy/1000}$ |
| Dark green & orange vegetables & legumes | 5 | Zero intake | ≥ 0.4 cup equivalents per 1000 kcal | $\dfrac{5}{0.4} \times \dfrac{v\_dol}{energy/1000}$ |
| Total grains | 5 | Zero intake | ≥ 3.0 oz equivalents per 1000 kcal | $\dfrac{5}{3.0} \times \dfrac{g\_total}{energy/1000}$ |
| Whole grains | 5 | Zero intake | ≥ 1.5 oz equivalents per 1000 kcal | $\dfrac{5}{1.5} \times \dfrac{g\_whl}{energy/1000}$ |
| Milk | 10 | Zero intake | ≥ 1.3 cup equivalents per 1000 kcal | $\dfrac{10}{1.3} \times \dfrac{d\_total}{energy/1000}$ |
| Meat & beans | 10 | Zero intake | ≥ 2.5 oz equivalents per 1000 kcal | $\dfrac{10}{2.5} \times \dfrac{allmeat}{energy/1000}$ |
| Oils | 10 | Zero intake | ≥ 12 grams per 1000 kcal | $\dfrac{10}{12} \times \dfrac{discfat\_oil}{energy/1000}$ |
| Saturated fat | 10 | ≥ 15% of kcal | ≤ 7% of kcal | For saturated fat between min & max: If >10 then HEI = 8-(8/5 x (%sfat-10)) If ≤10 then HEI =10-(2/3 x (%sfat-7)) |
| Sodium | 10 | ≥ 2.0 grams per 1000 kcal | ≤ 0.7 grams per 1000 kcal | For sodium between min & max: If >1100 then HEI = 8-(8 x (sodium-1100)/900)) If ≤1100 then HEI =10-(2 x (sodium-700)/400)) |
| Calories from SoFAAS | 20 | ≥ 50% of kcal | ≤ 20% of kcal | If % calories from SoFAAS < 50: HEI = Min( (50 - %SoFAAS)/1.5, 20) |

Source: Guenther, et al., 2007.

Table A-6 shows the population distribution used for age-adjustment.

### Table A-6. Census 2000 population for DRI Age Groups

| Age group | Population (1,000's) |
|---|---|
| DRI age groups | |
| 1-3 yrs | 11,444 |
| 4-8 yrs | 20,209 |
| 9-13 yrs | 20,743 |
| 14-18 yrs | 20,144 |
| 19-30 yrs | 46,763 |
| 31-50 yrs | 85,270 |
| 51-70 yrs | 49,460 |
| 71+ | 23,583 |
| Other age groups | |
| 2-3 year | 7,623 |
| 51-59 | 27,246 |
| 60-70 | 22,214 |

Source: Census 2000 Summary File (SF1).

## Tests of Statistical Significance

We tested the statistical significance of differences in means and proportions between FSP participants and each group of nonparticipants using t-tests. When multiple outcome categories were examined simultaneously in Appendix D tables of nutrient intake distributions, we used the Bonferroni adjustment to adjust for multiplicity (Lohr, 1999). The statistical significance of differences in distributions (excluding usual nutrient intake distributions) between FSP participants and each group of nonparticipants was tested using chi-square-tests.

## Indicators of Statistical Reliability

We tested all estimates for statistically reliability according to recommendations in the *NHANES Analytic Guidelines* (NCHS, 1996). Tables include indicators of estimates that are statistically unreliable due to small sample size or large coefficient of variation.

NHANES recommends flagging estimates as unreliable if any of the following conditions are met:

1. *Inadequate sample size for normal approximation.* For means and for proportions based on commonly occurring events (where $0.25 < P < 0.75$), an estimate is flagged if it is based on a cell size of less than 30 times a "broadly calculated average design effect."
2. *Large coefficient of variation.* Estimates are flagged if the coefficient of variation (ratio of the standard error to the mean expressed as a percent) is greater than 30.

3. *Inadequate sample size for uncommon or very common events.* For proportions below 0.25 or above 0.75, the criteria for statistical reliability is that the cell size be sufficiently large that the minimum of nP and n(1-P) be greater than or equal to 8 times a broadly calculated average design effect, where n is the cell size and P is the estimated proportion.

For each data item, the design effect was calculated for each table cell as the ratio of the complex sampling design variance calculated by SUDAAN, to the simple random sample variance. The average design effect for a data item is the average of estimated design effects across age groups (pooled genders) within a program participation/income group (FS participants, income eligible nonparticipants, and higher-income nonparticipants).

## REFERENCES

Drewnowski, A. (2005). "Concept of a nutritious food: toward a nutrient density score," *American Journal of Clinical Nutrition,* 82:721–32.

Friday, J.E., and Bowman, S.A. (2006). *MyPyramid Equivalents Database for USDA Survey Food Codes, 1994-2002 Version 1.0.* [Online]. Beltsville, MD: USDA, Agricultural Research Service, Beltsville Human Nutrition Research Center, Community Nutrition Research Group. Available at: http://www.barc.usda.gov/ bhnrc/cnrg.

Guenther, P.M., Reedy, J., Krebs-Smith, S.M., Reeve, B.B., & Basiotis, P.P. (2007). Development and Evaluation of the Healthy Eating Index-2005: Technical Report. Center for Nutrition Policy and Promotion, U.S. Department of Agriculture. Available at: http://www.cnpp.usda.gov/ HealthyEatingIndex.htm.

IOM (2006). *Dietary Reference Intakes: The Essential Guide to Nutrient Requirements.* Washington, DC: National Academies Press.

Ledikwe, J., Blanck, H., Khan, L., Serdula, M., Seymour, J., Tohill, B., Rolls, B. (2005). "Dietary Energy Density Determined by Eight Calculation Methods in a Nationally Representative United States Population," *Journal of Nutrition*, 135: 273– 278.

Lohr, S. (1999) *Sampling: Design and Analysis.* Pacific Grove, CA: Duxbury Press.

Moshfegh et al. (2005). *What We Eat in America,* NHANES 200 1-2002: Usual Nutrient Intakes from Food Compared to Dietary reference Intakes. USDA, Agricultural Research Service, September 2005.

National Center for Health Statistics (NCHS) (1996). *Analytic and Reporting Guidelines: The Third National Health and Nutrition Examination Survey, NHANES III (1988-94).* Available at: http:// www.cdc.gov/nchs/ about/major/nhanes/ nhanes2003-2004/ analytical _guidelines.htm.

USDA, Center for Nutrition Policy and Promotion (CNPP) (2005). *MyPyramid: USDA's New Food Guidance System.* Available at http:// www.mypyramid.gov/ downloads/ MyPyramid Peer to Peer.ppt.

# APPENDIX B: NUTRIENT INTAKE TABLES

## LIST OF TABLES

# Table B-1. Food Energy (kcal)

| | Total Persons | | | Food Stamp Program Participants | | | Income-eligible Nonparticipants | | | Higher-income Nonparticipants | | |
|---|---|---|---|---|---|---|---|---|---|---|---|---|
| | Sample size | Mean | Standard error | Sample size | Mean | Standard error | Sample size | Mean | Standard error | Sample size | Mean | Standard error |
| **Mean Usual Intake** | | | | | | | | | | | | |
| All persons ......... | 25,170 | 2162 | (12.04) | 4,020 | 2068 | (39.07) | 5,370 | 2095 | (31.57) | 13,934 | ** 2186 | (13.85) |
| Male ......... | 12,747 | 2486 | (19.36) | 1,936 | 2366 | (68.38) | 2,702 | 2464 | (55.53) | 7,201 | 2500 | (21.44) |
| Female ......... | 12,423 | 1834 | (13.94) | 2,084 | 1848 | (45.15) | 2,668 | 1756 | (31.57) | 6,733 | 1842 | (16.50) |
| Children (age 1-18) ...... | 11,878 | 2029 | (18.58) | 2,644 | 1999 | (40.44) | 2,738 | 2057 | (58.29) | 5,727 | 2021 | (20.46) |
| Male ......... | 6,000 | 2215 | (30.88) | 1,343 | 2180 | (61.01) | 1,389 | 2260 | (98.93) | 2,867 | 2211 | (32.26) |
| Female ......... | 5,878 | 1832 | (20.05) | 1,301 | 1841 | (54.25) | 1,349 | 1824 | (46.65) | 2,860 | 1817 | (24.00) |
| Adults (age 19-59) ........ | 8,570 | 2331 | (18.89) | 1,022 | 2261 | (74.34) | 1,629 | 2298 | (48.13) | 5,313 | 2351 | (23.49) |
| Male ......... | 4,424 | 2739 | (30.60) | 441 | 2721 | (140.60) | 854 | 2754 | (78.40) | 2,837 | 2746 | (39.60) |
| Female ......... | 4,146 | 1907 | (21.70) | 581 | 1958 | (81.40) | 775 | 1856 | (56.60) | 2,476 | 1907 | (22.50) |
| Older adults (age 60+) .. | 4,722 | 1765 | (22.17) | 354 | 1583 | (74.06) | 1,003 | 1568 | (53.14) | 2,894 | ** 1814 | (23.57) |
| Male ......... | 2,323 | 2035 | (40.50) | 152 | 1682 | (119.00) | 459 | 1896 | (138.60) | 1,497 | ** 2060 | (33.60) |
| Female ......... | 2,399 | 1555 | (23.70) | 202 | 1522 | (94.60) | 544 | 1402 | (38.50) | 1,397 | 1598 | (33.00) |

Notes: Significant differences in means and proportions are noted by * (.05 level), ** (.01 level), or *** (.001 level). Differences are tested in comparison to FSP participants, identified as persons in households receiving food stamps in the past 12 months.

Source: NHANES 1999-2004 dietary recalls. Excludes pregnant and breastfeeding women and infants. 'Total Persons' includes persons with missing food stamp participation or income. Data reflect nutrient intake from foods and do not include the contribution of vitamin and mineral supplements. Usual intake was estimated using C-SIDE: Software for Intake Distribution Estimation. Estimates are age adjusted.

## Table B-2. Vitamin A (mcg RAE)

| | Total Persons | | | Food Stamp Program Participants | | | Income-eligible Nonparticipants | | | Higher-income Nonparticipants | | |
|---|---|---|---|---|---|---|---|---|---|---|---|---|
| | Sample size | Mean | Standard error | Sample size | Mean | Standard error | Sample size | Mean | Standard error | Sample size | Mean | Standard error |
| **Mean Usual Intake** | | | | | | | | | | | | |
| All persons | 25,170 | 608 | (11.1) | 4,020 | 493 | (20.9) | 5,370 | 563 | (41.6) | 13,934 | ***637 | (14.3) |
| Male | 12,747 | 663 | (18.9) | 1,936 | 545 | (36.7) | 2,702 | 632 | (81.1) | 7,201 | **687 | (23.3) |
| Female | 12,423 | 552 | (11.4) | 2,084 | 456 | (25.3) | 2,668 | 495 | (31.0) | 6,733 | 582 | (15.0) |
| Children (age 1-18) | 11,878 | 571 | (10.1) | 2,644 | 519 | (17.5) | 2,738 | 554 | (31.5) | 5,727 | **593 | (12.9) |
| Male | 6,000 | 610 | (15.5) | 1,343 | 563 | (27.5) | 1,389 | 595 | (46.6) | 2,867 | 637 | (19.3) |
| Female | 5,878 | 529 | (12.8) | 1,301 | 477 | (21.9) | 1,349 | 506 | (39.1) | 2,860 | **548 | (16.6) |
| Adults (age 19-59) | 8,570 | 606 | (18.1) | 1,022 | 458 | (25.3) | 1,629 | 547 | (55.7) | 5,313 | ***640 | (22.3) |
| Male | 4,424 | 668 | (30.4) | 441 | 515 | (38.3) | 854 | 638 | (106.8) | 2,837 | 688 | (36.9) |
| Female | 4,146 | 542 | (19.1) | 581 | 420 | (33.4) | 775 | 459 | (35.8) | 2,476 | ***586 | (22.9) |
| Older adults (age 60+) | 4,722 | 664 | (19.2) | 354 | 551 | (55.5) | 1,003 | 576 | (40.7) | 2,894 | *688 | (26.0) |
| Male | 2,323 | 710 | (29.5) | 152 | 562 | (69.0) | 459 | 558 | (70.0) | 1,497 | 741 | (40.5) |
| Female | 2,399 | 628 | (25.4) | 202 | 544 | (78.9) | 544 | 585 | (50.0) | 1,397 | 642 | (33.6) |
| **Percent of Persons with Usual Intake Greater than Estimated Average Requirement (EAR)[1]** | | | | | | | | | | | | |
| All persons | 25,170 | 55.4 | (1.67) | 4,020 | 41.5 | (3.31) | 5,370 | 48.1 | (3.00) | 13,934 | ***59.8 | (1.69) |
| Male | 12,747 | 52.8 | (2.80) | 1,936 | 39.8 | (5.23) | 2,702 | 47.3 | (4.86) | 7,201 | **56.7 | (2.43) |
| Female | 12,423 | 57.8 | (1.57) | 2,084 | 42.5 | (4.20) | 2,668 | 47.7 | (3.68) | 6,733 | ***63.1 | (2.30) |
| Children (age 1-18) | 11,878 | 75.8 | (1.22) | 2,644 | 69.9 | (2.49) | 2,738 | 70.6 | (2.80) | 5,727 | **78.9 | (1.43) |
| Male | 6,000 | 76.6 | (1.59) | 1,343 | 71.9 | (3.85) | 1,389 | 70.6 | (3.50) | 2,867 | 79.8 | (1.79) |
| Female | 5,878 | 75.0 | (1.86) | 1,301 | 67.8 | (3.09) | 1,349 | 70.3 | (4.43) | 2,860 | **78.1 | (2.21) |
| Adults (age 19-59) | 8,570 | 45.5 | (2.09) | 1,022 | 27.9 | (4.32) | 1,629 | 37.1 | (4.46) | 5,313 | ***50.7 | (2.33) |
| Male | 4,424 | 43.0 | (2.71) | 441 | 26.7 | (6.34) | 854 | 39.8 | (6.98) | 2,837 | 46.4 | (3.24) |
| Female | 4,146 | 48.2 | (3.19) | 581 | 28.6 | (5.82) | 775 | 34.6 | (5.60) | 2,476 | ***55.5 | (3.36) |
| Older adults (age 60+) | 4,722 | 56.1 | (2.06) | 354 | 43.8 | (8.41) | 1,003 | 46.4 | (7.08) | 2,894 | 58.6 | (3.38) |
| Male | 2,323 | 48.0 | (2.50) | 152 | 35.9 | (10.60) | 459 | 30.9 | (8.69) | 1,497 | 51.1 | (4.53) |
| Female | 2,399 | 62.4 | (3.11) | 202 | 48.6 | (11.90) | 544 | 54.3 | (9.72) | 1,397 | 65.1 | (4.94) |

Notes: Significant differences in means and proportions are noted by * (.05 level), ** (.01 level), or *** (.001 level). Differences are tested in comparison to FSP participants, identified as persons in households receiving food stamps in the past 12 months.

[1] The Dietary Reference Intakes (DRI) Estimated Average Requirement (EAR) is used to assess the adequacy of intakes for population groups.

Source: NHANES 1999-2004 dietary recalls. Excludes pregnant and breastfeeding women and infants. 'Total Persons' includes persons with missing food stamp participation or income. Data reflect nutrient intake from foods and do not include the contribution of vitamin and mineral supplements. Usual intake was estimated using C-SIDE: Software for Intake Distribution Estimation. Estimates are age adjusted.

## Table B-3. Vitamin C (mg)

| | Total Persons | | | Food Stamp Program Participants | | | Income-eligible Nonparticipants | | | Higher-income Nonparticipants | | |
|---|---|---|---|---|---|---|---|---|---|---|---|---|
| | Sample size | Mean | Standard error | Sample size | Mean | Standard error | Sample size | Mean | Standard error | Sample size | Mean | Standard error |
| **Mean Usual Intake** | | | | | | | | | | | | |
| All persons | 25,170 | 92.0 | (1.84) | 4,020 | 84.8 | (6.28) | 5,370 | 87.8 | (3.25) | 13,934 | 92.7 | (2.00) |
| Male | 12,747 | 99.5 | (2.74) | 1,936 | 92.6 | (13.76) | 2,702 | 97.4 | (5.60) | 7,201 | 99.4 | (3.03) |
| Female | 12,423 | 84.4 | (2.39) | 2,084 | 78.7 | (4.30) | 2,668 | 79.1 | (3.44) | 6,733 | 85.1 | (2.47) |
| Children (age 1-18) | 11,878 | 89.6 | (2.05) | 2,644 | 95.6 | (3.91) | 2,738 | 94.1 | (4.63) | 5,727 | *85.2 | (2.36) |
| Male | 6,000 | 93.4 | (3.29) | 1,343 | 99.7 | (5.32) | 1,389 | 96.8 | (7.66) | 2,867 | 89.4 | (3.68) |
| Female | 5,878 | 85.5 | (2.39) | 1,301 | 92.0 | (5.85) | 1,349 | 92.0 | (5.20) | 2,860 | 80.6 | (2.95) |
| Adults (age 19-59) | 8,570 | 92.5 | (3.14) | 1,022 | 85.4 | (10.07) | 1,629 | 89.6 | (7.83) | 5,313 | 94.5 | (3.60) |
| Male | 4,424 | 102.5 | (5.05) | 441 | 103.1 | (24.05) | 854 | 103.5 | (14.82) | 2,837 | 103.1 | (5.39) |
| Female | 4,146 | 82.0 | (3.65) | 581 | 73.8 | (5.27) | 775 | 76.1 | (5.58) | 2,476 | 84.9 | (4.65) |
| Older adults (age 60+) | 4,722 | 94.7 | (2.40) | 354 | 72.1 | (6.96) | 1,003 | 76.8 | (4.53) | 2,894 | ***98.2 | (2.90) |
| Male | 2,323 | 99.0 | (3.72) | 152 | 63.8 | (9.17) | 459 | 82.2 | (9.46) | 1,497 | ***102.2 | (4.46) |
| Female | 2,399 | 91.3 | (3.13) | 202 | 77.3 | (9.72) | 544 | 74.1 | (4.87) | 1,397 | 94.8 | (3.77) |
| **Percent of Persons with Usual Intake Greater than Estimated Average Requirement (EAR)[1]** | | | | | | | | | | | | |
| All persons | 25,170 | 68.8 | (1.36) | 4,020 | 60.8 | (3.15) | 5,370 | 64.2 | (2.43) | 13,934 | **70.3 | (1.33) |
| Male | 12,747 | 67.8 | (2.20) | 1,936 | 58.5 | (5.67) | 2,702 | 64.6 | (3.55) | 7,201 | 69.0 | (1.99) |
| Female | 12,423 | 69.6 | (1.59) | 2,084 | 61.8 | (3.55) | 2,668 | 63.7 | (3.26) | 6,733 | *71.7 | (1.72) |
| Children (age 1-18) | 11,878 | 87.6 | (0.98) | 2,644 | 87.3 | (1.61) | 2,738 | 89.2 | (1.79) | 5,727 | 86.5 | (1.12) |
| Male | 6,000 | 88.8 | (1.58) | 1,343 | 89.7 | (2.18) | 1,389 | 89.8 | (2.91) | 2,867 | 87.6 | (1.60) |
| Female | 5,878 | 86.4 | (1.12) | 1,301 | 85.2 | (2.33) | 1,349 | 88.7 | (2.03) | 2,860 | 85.2 | (1.56) |
| Adults (age 19-59) | 8,570 | 61.4 | (3.18) | 1,022 | 53.6 | (5.00) | 1,629 | 57.4 | (4.36) | 5,313 | 63.7 | (2.32) |
| Male | 4,424 | 60.6 | (5.58) | 441 | 54.0 | (10.30) | 854 | 60.3 | (6.99) | 2,837 | 62.0 | (3.32) |
| Female | 4,146 | 62.3 | (2.90) | 581 | 53.4 | (4.78) | 775 | 54.5 | (5.27) | 2,476 | *65.8 | (3.21) |
| Older adults (age 60+) | 4,722 | 64.3 | (1.91) | 354 | 46.5 | (6.07) | 1,003 | 50.8 | (3.57) | 2,894 | **67.6 | (2.24) |
| Male | 2,323 | 59.0 | (2.71) | 152 | 31.4 | (8.89) | 459 | 42.0 | (5.68) | 1,497 | 62.6 | (3.80) |
| Female | 2,399 | 68.4 | (2.67) | 202 | 55.8 | (8.13) | 544 | 55.2 | (4.54) | 1,397 | 72.0 | (2.57) |

Notes: Significant differences in means and proportions are noted by * (.05 level), ** (.01 level), or *** (.001 level). Differences are tested in comparison to FSP participants, identified as persons in households receiving food stamps in the past 12 months.

[1] The Dietary Reference Intakes (DRI) Estimated Average Requirement (EAR) is used to assess the adequacy of intakes for population groups.

Source: NHANES 1999-2004 dietary recalls. Excludes pregnant and breastfeeding women and infants. 'Total Persons' includes persons with missing food stamp participation or income. Data reflect nutrient intake from foods and do not include the contribution of vitamin and mineral supplements. Usual intake was estimated using C-SIDE: Software for Intake Distribution Estimation. Estimates are age adjusted.

## Table B-4. Vitamin $B_6$

| | Total Persons | | | Food Stamp Program Participants | | | Income-eligible Nonparticipants | | | Higher-income Nonparticipants | | |
|---|---|---|---|---|---|---|---|---|---|---|---|---|
| | Sample size | Mean | Standard error | Sample size | Mean | Standard error | Sample size | Mean | Standard error | Sample size | Mean | Standard error |
| **Mean Usual Intake** | | | | | | | | | | | | |
| All persons | 25,170 | 1.81 | (0.016) | 4,020 | 1.61 | (0.038) | 5,370 | 1.67 | (0.034) | 13,934 | ***1.86 | (0.019) |
| Male | 12,747 | 2.09 | (0.023) | 1,936 | 1.85 | (0.067) | 2,702 | 1.99 | (0.051) | 7,201 | 2.13 | (0.027) |
| Female | 12,423 | 1.53 | (0.021) | 2,084 | 1.44 | (0.044) | 2,668 | 1.39 | (0.045) | 6,733 | *1.56 | (0.026) |
| Children (age 1-18) | 11,878 | 1.65 | (0.023) | 2,644 | 1.61 | (0.042) | 2,738 | 1.65 | (0.060) | 5,727 | 1.65 | (0.027) |
| Male | 6,000 | 1.81 | (0.035) | 1,343 | 1.75 | (0.062) | 1,389 | 1.77 | (0.063) | 2,867 | 1.83 | (0.042) |
| Female | 5,878 | 1.48 | (0.030) | 1,301 | 1.48 | (0.059) | 1,349 | 1.52 | (0.101) | 2,860 | 1.45 | (0.031) |
| Adults (age 19-59) | 8,570 | 1.91 | (0.025) | 1,022 | 1.67 | (0.061) | 1,629 | 1.75 | (0.047) | 5,313 | ***1.97 | (0.032) |
| Male | 4,424 | 2.25 | (0.035) | 441 | 2.01 | (0.110) | 854 | 2.15 | (0.072) | 2,837 | 2.30 | (0.043) |
| Female | 4,146 | 1.55 | (0.036) | 581 | 1.45 | (0.070) | 775 | 1.37 | (0.060) | 2,476 | 1.60 | (0.046) |
| Older adults (age 60+) | 4,722 | 1.73 | (0.026) | 354 | 1.43 | (0.090) | 1,003 | 1.46 | (0.048) | 2,894 | ***1.79 | (0.032) |
| Male | 2,323 | 1.99 | (0.037) | 152 | 1.57 | (0.171) | 459 | 1.75 | (0.091) | 1,497 | **2.03 | (0.039) |
| Female | 2,399 | 1.53 | (0.037) | 202 | 1.35 | (0.100) | 544 | 1.31 | (0.055) | 1,397 | 1.58 | (0.050) |
| **Percent of Persons with Usual Intake Greater than Estimated Average Requirement (EAR)[1]** | | | | | | | | | | | | |
| All persons | 25,170 | 87.2 | (0.64) | 4,020 | 77.8 | (2.09) | 5,370 | 79.8 | (1.70) | 13,934 | ***89.3 | (0.67) |
| Male | 12,747 | 93.8 | (0.43) | 1,936 | 85.9 | (2.36) | 2,702 | 89.6 | (1.34) | 7,201 | **94.8 | (0.45) |
| Female | 12,423 | 80.8 | (1.21) | 2,084 | 72.3 | (3.14) | 2,668 | 71.4 | (2.99) | 6,733 | 83.4 | (1.32) |
| Children (age 1-18) | 11,878 | 96.7 | (0.36) | 2,644 | 93.3 | (1.51) | 2,738 | 96.7 | (0.78) | 5,727 | 97.2 | (0.42) |
| Male | 6,000 | 98.4 | (0.37) | 1,343 | 96.8 | (1.34) | 1,389 | 97.9 | (0.82) | 2,867 | 98.8 | (0.36) |
| Female | 5,878 | 94.9 | (0.63) | 1,301 | 90.5 | (2.49) | 1,349 | 95.6 | (1.33) | 2,860 | 95.3 | (0.80) |
| Adults (age 19-59) | 8,570 | 87.5 | (1.06) | 1,022 | 78.3 | (3.04) | 1,629 | 79.6 | (2.65) | 5,313 | ***89.8 | (1.16) |
| Male | 4,424 | 95.5 | (0.50) | 441 | 90.6 | (2.86) | 854 | 92.0 | (1.93) | 2,837 | 96.4 | (0.55) |
| Female | 4,146 | 79.1 | (2.10) | 581 | 70.3 | (4.69) | 775 | 67.5 | (4.87) | 2,476 | 82.6 | (2.40) |
| Older adults (age 60+) | 4,722 | 70.3 | (1.77) | 354 | 52.0 | (6.70) | 1,003 | 52.8 | (3.98) | 2,894 | **73.9 | (2.07) |
| Male | 2,323 | 79.9 | (1.72) | 152 | 54.8 | (10.60) | 459 | 67.1 | (5.01) | 1,497 | 82.3 | (1.65) |
| Female | 2,399 | 62.9 | (2.85) | 202 | 50.2 | (8.64) | 544 | 45.6 | (5.44) | 1,397 | 66.6 | (3.60) |

Notes: Significant differences in means and proportions are noted by * (.05 level), ** (.01 level), or *** (.001 level). Differences are tested in comparison to FSP participants, identified as persons in households receiving food stamps in the past 12 months.

[1] The Dietary Reference Intakes (DRI) Estimated Average Requirement (EAR) is used to assess the adequacy of intakes for population groups.

Source: NHANES 1999-2004 dietary recalls. Excludes pregnant and breastfeeding women and infants. 'Total Persons' includes persons with missing food stamp participation or income. Data reflect nutrient intake from foods and do not include the contribution of vitamin and mineral supplements. Usual intake was estimated using C-SIDE: Software for Intake Distribution Estimation. Estimates are age adjusted.

**Table B-5. Vitamin $B_{12}$**

| | Total Persons | | | Food Stamp Program Participants | | | Income-eligible Nonparticipants | | | Higher-income Nonparticipants | | |
|---|---|---|---|---|---|---|---|---|---|---|---|---|
| | Sample size | Mean | Standard error | Sample size | Mean | Standard error | Sample size | Mean | Standard error | Sample size | Mean | Standard error |
| **Mean Usual Intake** | | | | | | | | | | | | |
| All persons | 25,170 | 5.06 | (0.101) | 4,020 | 4.60 | (0.305) | 5,370 | 4.73 | (0.446) | 13,934 | *5.24 | (0.114) |
| Male | 12,747 | 6.01 | (0.172) | 1,936 | 5.72 | (0.680) | 2,702 | 6.04 | (0.925) | 7,201 | 6.13 | (0.179) |
| Female | 12,423 | 4.11 | (0.100) | 2,084 | 3.79 | (0.195) | 2,668 | 3.54 | (0.172) | 6,733 | *4.28 | (0.136) |
| Children (age 1-18) | 11,878 | 4.77 | (0.090) | 2,644 | 4.66 | (0.177) | 2,738 | 4.87 | (0.279) | 5,727 | 4.81 | (0.101) |
| Male | 6,000 | 5.37 | (0.153) | 1,343 | 5.29 | (0.315) | 1,389 | 5.52 | (0.439) | 2,867 | 5.43 | (0.168) |
| Female | 5,878 | 4.14 | (0.093) | 1,301 | 4.11 | (0.187) | 1,349 | 4.13 | (0.310) | 2,860 | 4.14 | (0.112) |
| Adults (age 19-59) | 8,570 | 5.22 | (0.160) | 1,022 | 4.85 | (0.441) | 1,629 | 4.70 | (0.429) | 5,313 | 5.43 | (0.180) |
| Male | 4,424 | 6.36 | (0.238) | 441 | 6.43 | (1.053) | 854 | 6.15 | (0.851) | 2,837 | 6.46 | (0.261) |
| Female | 4,146 | 4.05 | (0.214) | 581 | 3.81 | (0.234) | 775 | 3.28 | (0.177) | 2,476 | 4.27 | (0.245) |
| Older adults (age 60+) | 4,722 | 4.82 | (0.207) | 354 | 3.53 | (0.350) | 1,003 | 4.00 | (0.292) | 2,894 | ***5.13 | (0.292) |
| Male | 2,323 | 5.69 | (0.344) | 152 | 3.85 | (0.591) | 459 | 5.01 | (0.446) | 1,497 | 5.93 | (0.478) |
| Female | 2,399 | 4.14 | (0.252) | 202 | 3.32 | (0.434) | 544 | 3.48 | (0.377) | 1,397 | 4.43 | (0.352) |
| **Percent of Persons with Usual Intake Greater than Estimated Average Requirement (EAR)[1]** | | | | | | | | | | | | |
| All persons | 25,170 | 96.0 | (0.35) | 4,020 | 92.5 | (1.33) | 5,370 | 92.2 | (1.09) | 13,934 | **97.0 | (0.37) |
| Male | 12,747 | 98.8 | (0.15) | 1,936 | 96.3 | (1.17) | 2,702 | 97.5 | (0.58) | 7,201 | *99.1 | (0.14) |
| Female | 12,423 | 93.4 | (0.68) | 2,084 | 89.9 | (2.11) | 2,668 | 87.6 | (1.96) | 6,733 | 94.6 | (0.78) |
| Children (age 1-18) | 11,878 | 98.6 | (0.22) | 2,644 | 97.3 | (1.25) | 2,738 | 98.0 | (0.57) | 5,727 | 98.9 | (0.25) |
| Male | 6,000 | 99.7 | (0.11) | 1,343 | 99.6 | (0.39) | 1,389 | 99.5 | (0.23) | 2,867 | 99.8 | (0.06) |
| Female | 5,878 | 97.3 | (0.45) | 1,301 | 95.5 | (2.21) | 1,349 | 96.4 | (1.12) | 2,860 | 97.8 | (0.54) |
| Adults (age 19-59) | 8,570 | 95.8 | (0.59) | 1,022 | 92.7 | (1.71) | 1,629 | 91.6 | (1.55) | 5,313 | *96.9 | (0.58) |
| Male | 4,424 | 99.2 | (0.15) | 441 | 98.4 | (0.64) | 854 | 98.2 | (0.60) | 2,837 | 99.4 | (0.13) |
| Female | 4,146 | 92.3 | (1.19) | 581 | 89.0 | (2.81) | 775 | 85.1 | (2.99) | 2,476 | 94.1 | (1.22) |
| Older adults (age 60+) | 4,722 | 92.5 | (0.87) | 354 | 82.5 | (4.16) | 1,003 | 85.7 | (3.28) | 2,894 | **94.2 | (0.94) |
| Male | 2,323 | 97.2 | (0.46) | 152 | 88.5 | (5.91) | 459 | 94.2 | (2.00) | 1,497 | 98.0 | (0.53) |
| Female | 2,399 | 88.9 | (1.50) | 202 | 78.8 | (5.64) | 544 | 81.3 | (4.84) | 1,397 | *91.0 | (1.70) |

Notes: Significant differences in means and proportions are noted by * (.05 level), ** (.01 level), or *** (.001 level). Differences are tested in comparison to FSP participants, identified as persons in households receiving food stamps in the past 12 months.

[1] The Dietary Reference Intakes (DRI) Estimated Average Requirement (EAR) is used to assess the adequacy of intakes for population groups.

Source: NHANES 1999-2004 dietary recalls. Excludes pregnant and breastfeeding women and infants. 'Total Persons' includes persons with missing food stamp participation or income. Data reflect nutrient intake from foods and do not include the contribution of vitamin and mineral supplements. Usual intake was estimated using C-SIDE: Software for Intake Distribution Estimation. Estimates are age adjusted.

## Table B-6. Vitamin E (mg AT)

| | Total Persons | | | Food Stamp Program Participants | | | Income-eligible Nonparticipants | | | Higher-income Nonparticipants | | |
|---|---|---|---|---|---|---|---|---|---|---|---|---|
| | Sample size | Mean | Standard error | Sample size | Mean | Standard error | Sample size | Mean | Standard error | Sample size | Mean | Standard error |
| **Mean Usual Intake** | | | | | | | | | | | | |
| All persons | 25,170 | 6.7 | (0.08) | 4,020 | 5.8 | (0.18) | 5,370 | 6.1 | (0.17) | 13,934 | ***6.9 | (0.10) |
| Male | 12,747 | 7.4 | (0.13) | 1,936 | 6.2 | (0.26) | 2,702 | 7.1 | (0.29) | 7,201 | ***7.6 | (0.16) |
| Female | 12,423 | 6.0 | (0.09) | 2,084 | 5.4 | (0.25) | 2,668 | 5.3 | (0.19) | 6,733 | **6.2 | (0.11) |
| Children (age 1-18) | 11,878 | 5.6 | (0.10) | 2,644 | 5.4 | (0.19) | 2,738 | 5.7 | (0.21) | 5,727 | 5.6 | (0.14) |
| Male | 6,000 | 6.0 | (0.17) | 1,343 | 5.7 | (0.30) | 1,389 | 6.0 | (0.31) | 2,867 | 6.0 | (0.23) |
| Female | 5,878 | 5.2 | (0.11) | 1,301 | 5.2 | (0.25) | 1,349 | 5.3 | (0.28) | 2,860 | 5.1 | (0.14) |
| Adults (age 19-59) | 8,570 | 7.3 | (0.12) | 1,022 | 6.2 | (0.30) | 1,629 | 6.6 | (0.24) | 5,313 | ***7.6 | (0.17) |
| Male | 4,424 | 8.2 | (0.19) | 441 | 6.9 | (0.47) | 854 | 8.0 | (0.40) | 2,837 | * 8.4 | (0.26) |
| Female | 4,146 | 6.4 | (0.15) | 581 | 5.7 | (0.39) | 775 | 5.4 | (0.26) | 2,476 | 6.8 | (0.20) |
| Older adults (age 60+) | 4,722 | 6.5 | (0.16) | 354 | 4.8 | (0.34) | 1,003 | 5.3 | (0.31) | 2,894 | ***6.8 | (0.18) |
| Male | 2,323 | 7.2 | (0.24) | 152 | 4.8 | (0.49) | 459 | 6.0 | (0.59) | 1,497 | ***7.5 | (0.26) |
| Female | 2,399 | 6.0 | (0.20) | 202 | 4.8 | (0.47) | 544 | 5.0 | (0.37) | 1,397 | 6.2 | (0.24) |
| **Percent of Persons with Usual Intake Greater than Estimated Average Requirement (EAR)[1]** | | | | | | | | | | | | |
| All persons | 25,170 | 8.3 | (0.64) | 4,020 | 5.5 | (0.98) | 5,370 | 6.8 | (1.28) | 13,934 | **8.9 | (0.82) |
| Male | 12,747 | 12.1 | (1.10) | 1,936 | 6.3 | (1.42) | 2,702 | 11.2 | (2.34) | 7,201 | ***12.9 | (1.36) |
| Female | 12,423 | 4.4 | (0.64) | 2,084 | 4.9 u | (1.49) | 2,668 | 2.6 u | (1.00) | 6,733 | 4.7 | (0.89) |
| Children (age 1-18) | 11,878 | 11.9 | (1.41) | 2,644 | 13.1 | (2.72) | 2,738 | 12.1 | (3.41) | 5,727 | 11.4 | (1.90) |
| Male | 6,000 | 15.1 | (2.16) | 1,343 | 13.4 | (3.28) | 1,389 | 15.4 u | (5.53) | 2,867 | 15.4 | (3.28) |
| Female | 5,878 | 8.6 | (1.78) | 1,301 | 13.3 u | (4.76) | 1,349 | 8.2 u | (3.34) | 2,860 | 7.4 | (1.93) |
| Adults (age 19-59) | 8,570 | 7.4 | (0.79) | 1,022 | 3.2 u | (1.13) | 1,629 | 5.9 | (1.51) | 5,313 | 8.8 | (1.12) |
| Male | 4,424 | 11.6 | (1.44) | 441 | 5.1 u | (2.15) | 854 | 11.3 | (2.97) | 2,837 | **13.1 | (1.96) |
| Female | 4,146 | 2.9 | (0.57) | 581 | 1.9 u | (1.24) | 775 | 0.7 u | (0.75) | 2,476 | 3.9 | (0.87) |
| Older adults (age 60+) | 4,722 | 5.6 | (0.99) | 354 | 0.5 u | (0.49) | 1,003 | 2.5 u | (1.09) | 2,894 | ***6.0 | (0.90) |
| Male | 2,323 | 8.9 | (1.42) | 152 | 0.8 u | (1.13) | 459 | 5.9 u | (2.92) | 1,497 | ***9.3 | (1.60) |
| Female | 2,399 | 3.0 u | (1.38) | 202 | 0.3 u | (0.38) | 544 | 0.8 u | (0.72) | 1,397 | 3.1 | (0.96) |

Notes: Significant differences in means and proportions are noted by * (.05 level), ** (.01 level), or *** (.001 level). Differences are tested in comparison to FSP participants, identified as persons in households receiving food stamps in the past 12 months.

u Denotes individual estimates not meeting the standards of reliability or precision due to inadequate cell size or large coefficient of variation.

[1] The Dietary Reference Intakes (DRI) Estimated Average Requirement (EAR) is used to assess the adequacy of intakes for population groups.

Source: NHANES 1999-2004 dietary recalls. Excludes pregnant and breastfeeding women and infants. 'Total Persons' includes persons with missing food stamp participation or income. Data reflect nutrient intake from foods and do not include the contribution of vitamin and mineral supplements. Usual intake was estimated using C-SIDE: Software for Intake Distribution Estimation. Estimates are age adjusted.

# Table B-7. Folate (mcg DFE)

| | Total Persons | | | Food Stamp Program Participants | | | Income-eligible Nonparticipants | | | Higher-income Nonparticipants | | |
|---|---|---|---|---|---|---|---|---|---|---|---|---|
| | Sample size | Mean | Standard error | Sample size | Mean | Standard error | Sample size | Mean | Standard error | Sample size | Mean | Standard error |
| **Mean Usual Intake** | | | | | | | | | | | | |
| All persons | 25,170 | 550 | (6.0) | 4,020 | 505 | (14.9) | 5,370 | 511 | (12.3) | 13,934 | ***563 | (7.1) |
| Male | 12,747 | 622 | (8.9) | 1,936 | 584 | (28.1) | 2,702 | 604 | (19.9) | 7,201 | 629 | (9.8) |
| Female | 12,423 | 477 | (7.9) | 2,084 | 446 | (16.0) | 2,668 | 424 | (14.3) | 6,733 | *492 | (10.1) |
| Children (age 1-18) | 11,878 | 550 | (9.4) | 2,644 | 546 | (24.1) | 2,738 | 531 | (18.0) | 5,727 | 554 | (11.0) |
| Male | 6,000 | 608 | (14.6) | 1,343 | 601 | (36.8) | 1,389 | 584 | (28.2) | 2,867 | 613 | (17.2) |
| Female | 5,878 | 489 | (11.6) | 1,301 | 494 | (33.3) | 1,349 | 471 | (20.0) | 2,860 | 492 | (13.8) |
| Adults (age 19-59) | 8,570 | 560 | (10.5) | 1,022 | 506 | (19.9) | 1,629 | 524 | (20.8) | 5,313 | **574 | (11.3) |
| Male | 4,424 | 642 | (16.0) | 441 | 619 | (42.0) | 854 | 640 | (33.0) | 2,837 | 646 | (15.9) |
| Female | 4,146 | 475 | (13.4) | 581 | 431 | (18.1) | 775 | 412 | (25.5) | 2,476 | **494 | (15.9) |
| Older adults (age 60+) | 4,722 | 511 | (9.8) | 354 | 438 | (32.9) | 1,003 | 455 | (25.9) | 2,894 | *529 | (11.0) |
| Male | 2,323 | 570 | (13.9) | 152 | 457 | (67.8) | 459 | 525 | (38.2) | 1,497 | 583 | (14.4) |
| Female | 2,399 | 464 | (13.7) | 202 | 427 | (32.9) | 544 | 420 | (33.9) | 1,397 | 482 | (16.4) |
| **Percent of Persons with Usual Intake Greater than Estimated Average Requirement (EAR)[1]** | | | | | | | | | | | | |
| All persons | 25,170 | 90.3 | (0.53) | 4,020 | 82.4 | (1.88) | 5,370 | 83.8 | (1.66) | 13,934 | ***92.2 | (0.52) |
| Male | 12,747 | 95.5 | (0.33) | 1,936 | 89.4 | (2.10) | 2,702 | 93.2 | (1.07) | 7,201 | **96.1 | (0.36) |
| Female | 12,423 | 85.3 | (1.00) | 2,084 | 77.4 | (2.81) | 2,668 | 75.4 | (2.99) | 6,733 | 88.0 | (1.00) |
| Children (age 1-18) | 11,878 | 96.4 | (0.46) | 2,644 | 93.7 | (1.63) | 2,738 | 95.9 | (1.27) | 5,727 | 97.0 | (0.44) |
| Male | 6,000 | 98.2 | (0.35) | 1,343 | 97.3 | (1.23) | 1,389 | 98.1 | (0.92) | 2,867 | 98.4 | (0.37) |
| Female | 5,878 | 94.5 | (0.87) | 1,301 | 90.8 | (2.75) | 1,349 | 93.7 | (2.34) | 2,860 | 95.2 | (0.86) |
| Adults (age 19-59) | 8,570 | 89.1 | (1.09) | 1,022 | 79.9 | (2.86) | 1,629 | 82.9 | (2.86) | 5,313 | ***91.5 | (1.28) |
| Male | 4,424 | 95.5 | (1.15) | 441 | 90.8 | (2.92) | 854 | 94.7 | (1.62) | 2,837 | 96.2 | (0.69) |
| Female | 4,146 | 82.4 | (1.87) | 581 | 72.7 | (4.33) | 775 | 71.3 | (5.41) | 2,476 | **86.1 | (2.61) |
| Older adults (age 60+) | 4,722 | 83.9 | (1.29) | 354 | 71.8 | (5.33) | 1,003 | 72.3 | (4.00) | 2,894 | *87.0 | (1.31) |
| Male | 2,323 | 89.9 | (1.30) | 152 | 70.2 | (9.70) | 459 | 83.1 | (3.46) | 1,497 | 91.6 | (1.11) |
| Female | 2,399 | 79.3 | (2.05) | 202 | 72.8 | (6.20) | 544 | 66.8 | (5.77) | 1,397 | 82.9 | (2.26) |

Notes: Significant differences in means and proportions are noted by * (.05 level), ** (.01 level), or *** (.001 level). Differences are tested in comparison to FSP participants, identified as persons in households receiving food stamps in the past 12 months.

[1] The Dietary Reference Intakes (DRI) Estimated Average Requirement (EAR) is used to assess the adequacy of intakes for population groups.

Source: NHANES 1999-2004 dietary recalls. Excludes pregnant and breastfeeding women and infants. 'Total Persons' includes persons with missing food stamp participation or income. Data reflect nutrient intake from foods and do not include the contribution of vitamin and mineral supplements. Usual intake was estimated using C-SIDE: Software for Intake Distribution Estimation. Estimates are age adjusted.

# Table B-8. Niacin (mg)

| | Total Persons | | | Food Stamp Program Participants | | | Income-eligible Nonparticipants | | | Higher-income Nonparticipants | | |
|---|---|---|---|---|---|---|---|---|---|---|---|---|
| | Sample size | Mean | Standard error | Sample size | Mean | Standard error | Sample size | Mean | Standard error | Sample size | Mean | Standard error |
| **Mean Usual Intake** | | | | | | | | | | | | |
| All persons | 25,170 | 22.6 | (0.17) | 4,020 | 20.7 | (0.48) | 5,370 | 21.0 | (0.40) | 13,934 | ***23.1 | (0.20) |
| Male | 12,747 | 26.3 | (0.26) | 1,936 | 24.3 | (0.85) | 2,702 | 25.2 | (0.69) | 7,201 | **26.6 | (0.29) |
| Female | 12,423 | 18.9 | (0.21) | 2,084 | 18.1 | (0.54) | 2,668 | 17.2 | (0.45) | 6,733 | ·19.3 | (0.26) |
| Children (age 1-18) | 11,878 | 19.9 | (0.24) | 2,644 | 19.5 | (0.52) | 2,738 | 19.8 | (0.58) | 5,727 | 20.0 | (0.28) |
| Male | 6,000 | 22.0 | (0.39) | 1,343 | 21.5 | (0.85) | 1,389 | 21.4 | (0.84) | 2,867 | 22.2 | (0.45) |
| Female | 5,878 | 17.8 | (0.29) | 1,301 | 17.6 | (0.63) | 1,349 | 17.8 | (0.76) | 2,860 | 17.7 | (0.33) |
| Adults (age 19-59) | 8,570 | 24.5 | (0.29) | 1,022 | 22.4 | (0.83) | 1,629 | 22.8 | (0.65) | 5,313 | **25.0 | (0.35) |
| Male | 4,424 | 29.0 | (0.43) | 441 | 27.8 | (1.68) | 854 | 28.2 | (1.08) | 2,837 | 29.3 | (0.51) |
| Female | 4,146 | 19.7 | (0.40) | 581 | 18.8 | (0.82) | 775 | 17.6 | (0.73) | 2,476 | 20.2 | (0.48) |
| Older adults (age 60+) | 4,722 | 20.4 | (0.28) | 354 | 17.5 | (1.03) | 1,003 | 17.5 | (0.54) | 2,894 | **21.1 | (0.34) |
| Male | 2,323 | 23.6 | (0.41) | 152 | 18.4 | (1.78) | 459 | 21.4 | (1.08) | 1,497 | **24.0 | (0.44) |
| Female | 2,399 | 17.9 | (0.37) | 202 | 16.9 | (1.26) | 544 | 15.5 | (0.61) | 1,397 | 18.5 | (0.50) |
| **Percent of Persons with Usual Intake Greater than Estimated Average Requirement (EAR)[1]** | | | | | | | | | | | | |
| All persons | 25,170 | 98.3 | (0.15) | 4,020 | 94.9 | (0.90) | 5,370 | 95.9 | (0.71) | 13,934 | ***98.8 | (0.14) |
| Male | 12,747 | 99.2 | (0.11) | 1,936 | 96.2 | (1.17) | 2,702 | 98.2 | (0.40) | 7,201 | **99.5 | (0.10) |
| Female | 12,423 | 97.4 | (0.27) | 2,084 | 94.0 | (1.28) | 2,668 | 94.1 | (1.28) | 6,733 | 98.1 | (0.27) |
| Children (age 1-18) | 11,878 | 99.4 | (0.12) | 2,644 | 98.1 | (0.66) | 2,738 | 99.3 | (0.24) | 5,727 | *99.5 | (0.14) |
| Male | 6,000 | 99.6 | (0.09) | 1,343 | 99.1 | (0.58) | 1,389 | 99.4 | (0.31) | 2,867 | 99.8 | (0.07) |
| Female | 5,878 | 99.1 | (0.22) | 1,301 | 97.4 | (1.10) | 1,349 | 99.2 | (0.35) | 2,860 | 99.1 | (0.29) |
| Adults (age 19-59) | 8,570 | 98.6 | (0.23) | 1,022 | 95.9 | (1.35) | 1,629 | 97.0 | (0.95) | 5,313 | *99.1 | (0.21) |
| Male | 4,424 | 99.5 | (0.10) | 441 | 98.4 | (0.84) | 854 | 99.1 | (0.38) | 2,837 | 99.7 | (0.18) |
| Female | 4,146 | 97.7 | (0.46) | 581 | 94.3 | (2.17) | 775 | 94.9 | (1.84) | 2,476 | 98.4 | (0.40) |
| Older adults (age 60+) | 4,722 | 95.4 | (0.56) | 354 | 88.1 | (3.18) | 1,003 | 88.8 | (1.98) | 2,894 | **96.9 | (0.61) |
| Male | 2,323 | 97.9 | (0.35) | 152 | 88.2 | (5.92) | 459 | 93.9 | (1.66) | 1,497 | 98.5 | (0.35) |
| Female | 2,399 | 93.6 | (0.97) | 202 | 88.0 | (3.62) | 544 | 86.2 | (2.86) | 1,397 | 95.5 | (1.11) |

Notes: Significant differences in means and proportions are noted by * (.05 level), ** (.01 level), or *** (.001 level). Differences are tested in comparison to FSP participants, identified as persons in households receiving food stamps in the past 12 months.

[1] The Dietary Reference Intakes (DRI) Estimated Average Requirement (EAR) is used to assess the adequacy of intakes for population groups.

Source: NHANES 1999-2004 dietary recalls. Excludes pregnant and breastfeeding women and infants. 'Total Persons' includes persons with missing food stamp participation or income. Data reflect nutrient intake from foods and do not include the contribution of vitamin and mineral supplements. Usual intake was estimated using C-SIDE: Software for Intake Distribution Estimation. Estimates are age adjusted.

## Table B-9. Riboflavin (mg)

| | Total Persons | | | Food Stamp Program Participants | | | Income-eligible Nonparticipants | | | Higher-income Nonparticipants | | |
|---|---|---|---|---|---|---|---|---|---|---|---|---|
| | Sample size | Mean | Standard error | Sample size | Mean | Standard error | Sample size | Mean | Standard error | Sample size | Mean | Standard error |
| **Mean Usual Intake** | | | | | | | | | | | | |
| All persons | 25,170 | 2.14 | (0.018) | 4,020 | 1.95 | (0.042) | 5,370 | 1.96 | (0.043) | 13,934 | ***2.21 | (0.022) |
| Male | 12,747 | 2.45 | (0.028) | 1,936 | 2.28 | (0.077) | 2,702 | 2.33 | (0.077) | 7,201 | **2.50 | (0.034) |
| Female | 12,423 | 1.83 | (0.021) | 2,084 | 1.71 | (0.048) | 2,668 | 1.63 | (0.042) | 6,733 | 1.89 | (0.028) |
| Children (age 1-18) | 11,878 | 2.14 | (0.026) | 2,644 | 2.07 | (0.052) | 2,738 | 2.06 | (0.057) | 5,727 | 2.18 | (0.030) |
| Male | 6,000 | 2.36 | (0.041) | 1,343 | 2.28 | (0.086) | 1,389 | 2.26 | (0.087) | 2,867 | 2.42 | (0.049) |
| Female | 5,878 | 1.90 | (0.029) | 1,301 | 1.87 | (0.063) | 1,349 | 1.82 | (0.069) | 2,860 | 1.92 | (0.035) |
| Adults (age 19-59) | 8,570 | 2.19 | (0.033) | 1,022 | 1.96 | (0.072) | 1,629 | 2.00 | (0.072) | 5,313 | ***2.26 | (0.040) |
| Male | 4,424 | 2.54 | (0.054) | 441 | 2.41 | (0.151) | 854 | 2.44 | (0.127) | 2,837 | 2.59 | (0.064) |
| Female | 4,146 | 1.82 | (0.037) | 581 | 1.66 | (0.067) | 775 | 1.57 | (0.071) | 2,476 | **1.90 | (0.045) |
| Older adults (age 60+) | 4,722 | 1.97 | (0.030) | 354 | 1.70 | (0.086) | 1,003 | 1.70 | (0.060) | 2,894 | *2.06 | (0.037) |
| Male | 2,323 | 2.25 | (0.051) | 152 | 1.88 | (0.189) | 459 | 2.00 | (0.124) | 1,497 | 2.30 | (0.055) |
| Female | 2,399 | 1.76 | (0.036) | 202 | 1.59 | (0.077) | 544 | 1.54 | (0.064) | 1,397 | ***1.84 | (0.050) |
| **Percent of Persons with Usual Intake Greater than Estimated Average Requirement (EAR)[1]** | | | | | | | | | | | | |
| All persons | 25,170 | 97.5 | (0.17) | 4,020 | 93.4 | (0.94) | 5,370 | 94.6 | (0.78) | 13,934 | ***98.3 | (0.17) |
| Male | 12,747 | 98.2 | (0.18) | 1,936 | 95.1 | (1.26) | 2,702 | 96.2 | (0.74) | 7,201 | **98.7 | (0.18) |
| Female | 12,423 | 96.8 | (0.29) | 2,084 | 92.0 | (1.35) | 2,668 | 92.9 | (1.34) | 6,733 | ***97.9 | (0.31) |
| Children (age 1-18) | 11,878 | 99.0 | (0.15) | 2,644 | 98.2 | (0.57) | 2,738 | 98.3 | (0.50) | 5,727 | 99.4 | (0.14) |
| Male | 6,000 | 99.3 | (0.17) | 1,343 | 98.8 | (0.72) | 1,389 | 99.0 | (0.46) | 2,867 | 99.5 | (0.13) |
| Female | 5,878 | 98.7 | (0.25) | 1,301 | 97.7 | (0.84) | 1,349 | 97.5 | (0.90) | 2,860 | 99.2 | (0.26) |
| Adults (age 19-59) | 8,570 | 97.2 | (0.31) | 1,022 | 92.5 | (1.74) | 1,629 | 93.9 | (1.24) | 5,313 | **98.3 | (0.24) |
| Male | 4,424 | 98.4 | (0.34) | 441 | 96.5 | (1.35) | 854 | 96.7 | (0.93) | 2,837 | 98.9 | (0.24) |
| Female | 4,146 | 96.0 | (0.53) | 581 | 89.9 | (2.75) | 775 | 91.2 | (2.27) | 2,476 | **97.6 | (0.43) |
| Older adults (age 60+) | 4,722 | 96.0 | (0.44) | 354 | 87.8 | (3.25) | 1,003 | 91.8 | (1.60) | 2,894 | 97.3 | (0.45) |
| Male | 2,323 | 96.0 | (0.71) | 152 | 84.3 | (6.61) | 459 | 91.6 | (2.60) | 1,497 | 97.1 | (0.62) |
| Female | 2,399 | 96.0 | (0.56) | 202 | 89.9 | (3.33) | 544 | 91.8 | (2.01) | 1,397 | *97.4 | (0.63) |

Notes: Significant differences in means and proportions are noted by * (.05 level), ** (.01 level), or *** (.001 level). Differences are tested in comparison to FSP participants, identified as persons in households receiving food stamps in the past 12 months.

[1] The Dietary Reference Intakes (DRI) Estimated Average Requirement (EAR) is used to assess the adequacy of intakes for population groups.

Source: NHANES 1999-2004 dietary recalls. Excludes pregnant and breastfeeding women and infants. 'Total Persons' includes persons with missing food stamp participation or income. Data reflect nutrient intake from foods and do not include the contribution of vitamin and mineral supplements. Usual intake was estimated using C-SIDE: Software for Intake Distribution Estimation. Estimates are age adjusted.

## Table B-10. Thiamin (mg)

| | Total Persons | | | Food Stamp Program Participants | | | Income-eligible Nonparticipants | | | Higher-income Nonparticipants | | |
|---|---|---|---|---|---|---|---|---|---|---|---|---|
| | Sample size | Mean | Standard error | Sample size | Mean | Standard error | Sample size | Mean | Standard error | Sample size | Mean | Standard error |
| **Mean Usual Intake** | | | | | | | | | | | | |
| All persons | 25,170 | 1.62 | (0.013) | 4,020 | 1.49 | (0.033) | 5,370 | 1.52 | (0.031) | 13,934 | ***1.66 | (0.015) |
| Male | 12,747 | 1.86 | (0.020) | 1,936 | 1.72 | (0.059) | 2,702 | 1.80 | (0.053) | 7,201 | *1.88 | (0.022) |
| Female | 12,423 | 1.38 | (0.016) | 2,084 | 1.32 | (0.036) | 2,668 | 1.26 | (0.032) | 6,733 | 1.42 | (0.021) |
| Children (age 1-18) | 11,878 | 1.57 | (0.019) | 2,644 | 1.54 | (0.042) | 2,738 | 1.55 | (0.054) | 5,727 | 1.58 | (0.023) |
| Male | 6,000 | 1.73 | (0.032) | 1,343 | 1.71 | (0.072) | 1,389 | 1.72 | (0.091) | 2,867 | 1.74 | (0.039) |
| Female | 5,878 | 1.40 | (0.019) | 1,301 | 1.39 | (0.042) | 1,349 | 1.36 | (0.044) | 2,860 | 1.40 | (0.025) |
| Adults (age 19-59) | 8,570 | 1.69 | (0.022) | 1,022 | 1.52 | (0.058) | 1,629 | 1.59 | (0.048) | 5,313 | **1.72 | (0.026) |
| Male | 4,424 | 1.96 | (0.032) | 441 | 1.84 | (0.109) | 854 | 1.94 | (0.079) | 2,837 | 1.99 | (0.035) |
| Female | 4,146 | 1.39 | (0.032) | 581 | 1.31 | (0.064) | 775 | 1.25 | (0.055) | 2,476 | 1.43 | (0.037) |
| Older adults (age 60+) | 4,722 | 1.49 | (0.022) | 354 | 1.33 | (0.080) | 1,003 | 1.30 | (0.045) | 2,894 | *1.53 | (0.024) |
| Male | 2,323 | 1.71 | (0.038) | 152 | 1.46 | (0.143) | 459 | 1.52 | (0.088) | 1,497 | 1.73 | (0.035) |
| Female | 2,399 | 1.31 | (0.027) | 202 | 1.26 | (0.095) | 544 | 1.18 | (0.051) | 1,397 | 1.36 | (0.034) |
| **Percent of Persons with Usual Intake Greater than Estimated Average Requirement (EAR)[1]** | | | | | | | | | | | | |
| All persons | 25,170 | 94.6 | (0.35) | 4,020 | 89.0 | (1.61) | 5,370 | 89.8 | (1.33) | 13,934 | ***95.9 | (0.35) |
| Male | 12,747 | 97.3 | (0.24) | 1,936 | 93.2 | (1.83) | 2,702 | 94.8 | (0.94) | 7,201 | **97.9 | (0.24) |
| Female | 12,423 | 92.0 | (0.66) | 2,084 | 86.0 | (2.40) | 2,668 | 85.4 | (2.36) | 6,733 | 93.7 | (0.67) |
| Children (age 1-18) | 11,878 | 98.1 | (0.28) | 2,644 | 96.2 | (1.07) | 2,738 | 97.7 | (0.62) | 5,727 | 98.5 | (0.30) |
| Male | 6,000 | 98.8 | (0.28) | 1,343 | 98.2 | (1.06) | 1,389 | 98.4 | (0.85) | 2,867 | 99.2 | (0.24) |
| Female | 5,878 | 97.3 | (0.49) | 1,301 | 94.7 | (1.73) | 1,349 | 97.0 | (0.90) | 2,860 | 97.8 | (0.59) |
| Adults (age 19-59) | 8,570 | 93.9 | (0.80) | 1,022 | 88.0 | (2.72) | 1,629 | 89.8 | (2.19) | 5,313 | **95.3 | (0.65) |
| Male | 4,424 | 97.6 | (0.40) | 441 | 94.4 | (2.63) | 854 | 96.7 | (1.14) | 2,837 | 98.0 | (0.37) |
| Female | 4,146 | 90.0 | (1.58) | 581 | 83.7 | (4.17) | 775 | 83.1 | (4.17) | 2,476 | 92.3 | (1.31) |
| Older adults (age 60+) | 4,722 | 91.1 | (0.91) | 354 | 81.9 | (4.42) | 1,003 | 81.2 | (3.11) | 2,894 | ***93.5 | (0.81) |
| Male | 2,323 | 94.1 | (1.09) | 152 | 82.3 | (6.67) | 459 | 85.6 | (3.70) | 1,497 | 95.5 | (0.79) |
| Female | 2,399 | 88.7 | (1.38) | 202 | 81.6 | (5.84) | 544 | 78.9 | (4.30) | 1,397 | 91.8 | (1.35) |

Notes: Significant differences in means and proportions are noted by * (.05 level), ** (.01 level), or *** (.001 level). Differences are tested in comparison to FSP participants, identified as persons in households receiving food stamps in the past 12 months.

[1] The Dietary Reference Intakes (DRI) Estimated Average Requirement (EAR) is used to assess the adequacy of intakes for population groups.

Source: NHANES 1999-2004 dietary recalls. Excludes pregnant and breastfeeding women and infants. 'Total Persons' includes persons with missing food stamp participation or income. Data reflect nutrient intake from foods and do not include the contribution of vitamin and mineral supplements. Usual intake was estimated using C-SIDE: Software for Intake Distribution Estimation. Estimates are age adjusted.

# Table B-11. Calcium (mg)

| | Total Persons | | | Food Stamp Program Participants | | | Income-eligible Nonparticipants | | | Higher-income Nonparticipants | | |
|---|---|---|---|---|---|---|---|---|---|---|---|---|
| | Sample size | Mean | Standard error | Sample size | Mean | Standard error | Sample size | Mean | Standard error | Sample size | Mean | Standard error |
| **Mean Usual Intake** | | | | | | | | | | | | |
| All persons | 25,170 | 891 | (8.4) | 4,020 | 788 | (20.1) | 5,370 | 815 | (18.9) | 13,934 | ***926 | (10.9) |
| Male | 12,747 | 1003 | (12.7) | 1,936 | 891 | (34.4) | 2,702 | 950 | (32.9) | 7,201 | ***1032 | (15.1) |
| Female | 12,423 | 777 | (10.8) | 2,084 | 709 | (24.0) | 2,668 | 689 | (20.1) | 6,733 | 810 | (15.6) |
| Children (age 1-18) | 11,878 | 975 | (13.5) | 2,644 | 925 | (26.5) | 2,738 | 942 | (28.9) | 5,727 | *1001 | (17.2) |
| Male | 6,000 | 1067 | (21.6) | 1,343 | 1009 | (41.4) | 1,389 | 1028 | (44.5) | 2,867 | *1107 | (27.4) |
| Female | 5,878 | 877 | (16.0) | 1,301 | 849 | (34.9) | 1,349 | 846 | (35.8) | 2,860 | 890 | (20.3) |
| Adults (age 19-59) | 8,570 | 895 | (13.6) | 1,022 | 772 | (32.2) | 1,629 | 817 | (29.3) | 5,313 | *932 | (16.8) |
| Male | 4,424 | 1026 | (18.7) | 441 | 914 | (61.9) | 854 | 987 | (46.3) | 2,837 | *1048 | (22.9) |
| Female | 4,146 | 757 | (19.6) | 581 | 676 | (33.9) | 775 | 652 | (36.3) | 2,476 | 800 | (24.7) |
| Older adults (age 60+) | 4,722 | 744 | (13.6) | 354 | 626 | (39.7) | 1,003 | 643 | (24.4) | 2,894 | *768 | (17.2) |
| Male | 2,323 | 822 | (23.3) | 152 | 661 | (68.1) | 459 | 730 | (52.4) | 1,497 | 840 | (24.8) |
| Female | 2,399 | 683 | (15.9) | 202 | 604 | (48.5) | 544 | 599 | (25.4) | 1,397 | 706 | (23.8) |
| **Mean Usual Intake as a Percent of Adequate Intake (AI)[1]** | | | | | | | | | | | | |
| All persons | 25,170 | 88.1 | (0.82) | 4,020 | 78.2 | (1.95) | 5,370 | 81.1 | (1.83) | 13,934 | ***91.4 | (1.07) |
| Male | 12,747 | 98.8 | (1.24) | 1,936 | 88.3 | (3.33) | 2,702 | 93.9 | (3.16) | 7,201 | ***101.6 | (1.50) |
| Female | 12,423 | 77.1 | (1.07) | 2,084 | 70.4 | (2.34) | 2,668 | 69.2 | (1.98) | 6,733 | ***80.3 | (1.54) |
| Children (age 1-18) | 11,878 | 106.5 | (1.39) | 2,644 | 101.6 | (2.71) | 2,738 | 104.2 | (2.80) | 5,727 | *109.1 | (1.82) |
| Male | 6,000 | 115.2 | (2.15) | 1,343 | 109.6 | (4.03) | 1,389 | 111.4 | (4.05) | 2,867 | *119.3 | (2.84) |
| Female | 5,878 | 97.3 | (1.74) | 1,301 | 94.0 | (3.76) | 1,349 | 95.9 | (3.87) | 2,860 | 98.6 | (2.24) |
| Adults (age 19-59) | 8,570 | 87.2 | (1.34) | 1,022 | 75.1 | (3.18) | 1,629 | 79.7 | (2.86) | 5,313 | ***90.9 | (1.66) |
| Male | 4,424 | 100.1 | (1.85) | 441 | 89.4 | (6.16) | 854 | 96.4 | (4.51) | 2,837 | 102.2 | (2.26) |
| Female | 4,146 | 73.6 | (1.94) | 581 | 65.4 | (3.32) | 775 | 63.4 | (3.54) | 2,476 | *77.9 | (2.44) |
| Older adults (age 60+) | 4,722 | 62.0 | (1.13) | 354 | 52.1 | (3.31) | 1,003 | 53.6 | (2.03) | 2,894 | *64.0 | (1.43) |
| Male | 2,323 | 68.5 | (1.94) | 152 | 55.1 | (5.68) | 459 | 60.9 | (4.36) | 1,497 | 70.0 | (2.07) |
| Female | 2,399 | 56.9 | (1.33) | 202 | 50.4 | (4.04) | 544 | 49.9 | (2.11) | 1,397 | 58.8 | (1.98) |

Notes: Significant differences in means and proportions are noted by * (.05 level), ** (.01 level), or *** (.001 level). Differences are tested in comparison to FSP participants, identified as persons in households receiving food stamps in the past 12 months.

[1] Adequate Intake (AI) is the approximate intake of the nutrient that appears to be adequate for all individuals in the population group. Mean intake at or above the AI implies a low prevalence of inadequate intake.

Source: NHANES 1999-2004 dietary recalls. Excludes pregnant and breastfeeding women and infants. 'Total Persons' includes persons with missing food stamp participation or income. Data reflect nutrient intake from foods and do not include the contribution of vitamin and mineral supplements. Usual intake was estimated using C-SIDE: Software for Intake Distribution Estimation. Estimates are age adjusted.

# Table B-12. Iron (mg)

| | Total Persons | | | Food Stamp Program Participants | | | Income-eligible Nonparticipants | | | Higher-income Nonparticipants | | |
|---|---|---|---|---|---|---|---|---|---|---|---|---|
| | Sample size | Mean | Standard error | Sample size | Mean | Standard error | Sample size | Mean | Standard error | Sample size | Mean | Standard error |
| **Mean Usual Intake** | | | | | | | | | | | | |
| All persons | 25,170 | 15.3 | (0.12) | 4,020 | 14.3 | (0.35) | 5,370 | 14.3 | (0.27) | 13,934 | ***15.6 | (0.15) |
| Male | 12,747 | 17.5 | (0.19) | 1,936 | 16.7 | (0.71) | 2,702 | 16.9 | (0.47) | 7,201 | 17.7 | (0.22) |
| Female | 12,423 | 13.1 | (0.16) | 2,084 | 12.5 | (0.34) | 2,668 | 11.9 | (0.30) | 6,733 | 13.4 | (0.20) |
| Children (age 1-18) | 11,878 | 14.6 | (0.18) | 2,644 | 14.5 | (0.41) | 2,738 | 14.4 | (0.38) | 5,727 | 14.7 | (0.22) |
| Male | 6,000 | 16.2 | (0.29) | 1,343 | 16.0 | (0.67) | 1,389 | 16.0 | (0.60) | 2,867 | 16.3 | (0.36) |
| Female | 5,878 | 13.0 | (0.20) | 1,301 | 13.0 | (0.46) | 1,349 | 12.5 | (0.43) | 2,860 | 13.0 | (0.23) |
| Adults (age 19-59) | 8,570 | 15.9 | (0.18) | 1,022 | 14.7 | (0.48) | 1,629 | 14.8 | (0.43) | 5,313 | 16.3 | (0.22) |
| Male | 4,424 | 18.4 | (0.31) | 441 | 18.2 | (1.11) | 854 | 18.0 | (0.83) | 2,837 | 18.6 | (0.35) |
| Female | 4,146 | 13.3 | (0.25) | 581 | 12.4 | (0.48) | 775 | 11.8 | (0.51) | 2,476 | 13.6 | (0.32) |
| Older adults (age 60+) | 4,722 | 14.5 | (0.23) | 354 | 12.9 | (1.09) | 1,003 | 12.7 | (0.51) | 2,894 | 15.0 | (0.26) |
| Male | 2,323 | 16.6 | (0.37) | 152 | 14.6 | (2.58) | 459 | 15.1 | (0.98) | 1,497 | 16.8 | (0.35) |
| Female | 2,399 | 12.9 | (0.30) | 202 | 11.9 | (0.76) | 544 | 11.5 | (0.58) | 1,397 | 13.4 | (0.39) |
| **Percent of Persons with Usual Intake Greater than Estimated Average Requirement (EAR)[1]** | | | | | | | | | | | | |
| All persons | 25,170 | 95.5 | (0.11) | 4,020 | 92.6 | (0.51) | 5,370 | 93.0 | (0.38) | 13,934 | ***96.4 | (0.12) |
| Male | 12,747 | 99.8 | (0.04) | 1,936 | 98.9 | (0.52) | 2,702 | 99.5 | (0.17) | 7,201 | 99.8 | (0.04) |
| Female | 12,423 | 91.2 | (0.22) | 2,084 | 87.5 | (0.81) | 2,668 | 87.0 | (0.70) | 6,733 | 92.8 | (0.24) |
| Children (age 1-18) | 11,878 | 98.0 | (0.13) | 2,644 | 96.7 | (0.51) | 2,738 | 97.6 | (0.30) | 5,727 | **98.3 | (0.13) |
| Male | 6,000 | 99.8 | (0.07) | 1,343 | 99.4 | (0.41) | 1,389 | 99.7 | (0.22) | 2,867 | 99.9 | (0.07) |
| Female | 5,878 | 96.0 | (0.26) | 1,301 | 93.8 | (0.94) | 1,349 | 95.2 | (0.60) | 2,860 | 96.7 | (0.26) |
| Adults (age 19-59) | 8,570 | 93.8 | (0.21) | 1,022 | 88.7 | (0.92) | 1,629 | 89.5 | (0.62) | 5,313 | ***95.3 | (0.18) |
| Male | 4,424 | 99.8 | (0.04) | 441 | 99.3 | (0.44) | 854 | 99.6 | (0.24) | 2,837 | 99.8 | (0.05) |
| Female | 4,146 | 87.5 | (0.44) | 581 | 81.8 | (1.50) | 775 | 79.6 | (1.20) | 2,476 | 90.1 | (0.38) |
| Older adults (age 60+) | 4,722 | 99.6 | (0.08) | 354 | 98.1 | (1.09) | 1,003 | 98.8 | (0.34) | 2,894 | 99.7 | (0.08) |
| Male | 2,323 | 99.5 | (0.11) | 152 | 96.6 | (2.66) | 459 | 98.6 | (0.54) | 1,497 | 99.6 | (0.14) |
| Female | 2,399 | 99.7 | (0.11) | 202 | 99.1 | (0.66) | 544 | 98.8 | (0.43) | 1,397 | 99.9 | (0.07) |

Notes: Significant differences in means and proportions are noted by * (.05 level), ** (.01 level), or *** (.001 level). Differences are tested in comparison to FSP participants, identified as persons in households receiving food stamps in the past 12 months.

[1] The Dietary Reference Intakes (DRI) Estimated Average Requirement (EAR) is used to assess the adequacy of intakes for population groups. The EAR cut-point method was used for all groups except females age 9-50. The probability approach was used for females of childbearing age because the distribution of nutrient requirements is not symmetrical.

Source: NHANES 1999–2004 dietary recalls. Excludes pregnant and breastfeeding women and infants. 'Total Persons' includes persons with missing food stamp participation or income. Data reflect nutrient intake from foods and do not include the contribution of vitamin and mineral supplements. Usual intake was estimated using C-SIDE: Software for Intake Distribution Estimation. Estimates are age adjusted.

# Table B-13. Magnesium (mg)

| | Total Persons | | | Food Stamp Program Participants | | | Income-eligible Nonparticipants | | | Higher-income Nonparticipants | | |
|---|---|---|---|---|---|---|---|---|---|---|---|---|
| | Sample size | Mean | Standard error | Sample size | Mean | Standard error | Sample size | Mean | Standard error | Sample size | Mean | Standard error |
| **Mean Usual Intake** | | | | | | | | | | | | |
| All persons | 25,170 | 268 | (1.9) | 4,020 | 234 | (5.3) | 5,370 | **253 | (4.3) | 13,934 | ***275 | (2.3) |
| Male | 12,747 | 305 | (2.8) | 1,936 | 271 | (9.0) | 2,702 | *299 | (7.2) | 7,201 | 309 | (3.3) |
| Female | 12,423 | 231 | (2.5) | 2,084 | 207 | (6.3) | 2,668 | 211 | (4.8) | 6,733 | ***238 | (3.2) |
| Children (age 1-18) | 11,878 | 227 | (2.4) | 2,644 | 219 | (4.9) | 2,738 | 228 | (5.7) | 5,727 | 228 | (3.0) |
| Male | 6,000 | 247 | (3.8) | 1,343 | 239 | (7.8) | 1,389 | 248 | (8.7) | 2,867 | 249 | (4.7) |
| Female | 5,878 | 205 | (3.0) | 1,301 | 201 | (6.5) | 1,349 | 206 | (7.0) | 2,860 | 204 | (3.5) |
| Adults (age 19-59) | 8,570 | 289 | (3.1) | 1,022 | 245 | (8.8) | 1,629 | *270 | (7.0) | 5,313 | **299 | (3.7) |
| Male | 4,424 | 334 | (4.4) | 441 | 296 | (15.4) | 854 | 330 | (11.7) | 2,837 | **339 | (5.0) |
| Female | 4,146 | 242 | (4.4) | 581 | 212 | (10.4) | 775 | 214 | (8.0) | 2,476 | ***253 | (5.4) |
| Older adults (age 60+) | 4,722 | 261 | (3.4) | 354 | 218 | (10.8) | 1,003 | 229 | (8.8) | 2,894 | ***269 | (4.2) |
| Male | 2,323 | 296 | (5.4) | 152 | 240 | (18.8) | 459 | 275 | (17.7) | 1,497 | *301 | (5.9) |
| Female | 2,399 | 234 | (4.2) | 202 | 204 | (13.1) | 544 | 206 | (9.8) | 1,397 | 240 | (6.1) |
| **Percent of Persons with Usual Intake Greater than Estimated Average Requirement (EAR)[1]** | | | | | | | | | | | | |
| All persons | 25,170 | 44.1 | (0.84) | 4,020 | 33.6 | (1.96) | 5,370 | 38.2 | (1.73) | 13,934 | ***46.8 | (1.09) |
| Male | 12,747 | 46.9 | (1.13) | 1,936 | 36.1 | (2.98) | 2,702 | 45.4 | (2.48) | 7,201 | 48.6 | (1.52) |
| Female | 12,423 | 41.0 | (1.25) | 2,084 | 31.2 | (2.54) | 2,668 | 31.0 | (2.41) | 6,733 | ***44.8 | (1.59) |
| Children (age 1-18) | 11,878 | 68.0 | (0.98) | 2,644 | 65.5 | (1.80) | 2,738 | 67.3 | (2.40) | 5,727 | 68.4 | (1.16) |
| Male | 6,000 | 73.3 | (1.44) | 1,343 | 70.9 | (2.89) | 1,389 | 72.6 | (3.30) | 2,867 | 74.3 | (1.59) |
| Female | 5,878 | 62.3 | (1.31) | 1,301 | 60.6 | (2.31) | 1,349 | 61.1 | (3.67) | 2,860 | 62.3 | (1.64) |
| Adults (age 19-59) | 8,570 | 38.1 | (1.40) | 1,022 | 24.3 | (3.26) | 1,629 | 30.4 | (3.10) | 5,313 | 41.9 | (1.71) |
| Male | 4,424 | 41.3 | (1.76) | 441 | 27.9 | (5.11) | 854 | 40.5 | (4.19) | 2,837 | 43.1 | (2.21) |
| Female | 4,146 | 34.7 | (2.20) | 581 | 21.9 | (4.22) | 775 | 20.8 | (4.56) | 2,476 | ***40.3 | (2.68) |
| Older adults (age 60+) | 4,722 | 27.1 | (1.40) | 354 | 15.3 u | (4.86) | 1,003 | 17.7 | (3.56) | 2,894 | **29.6 | (1.85) |
| Male | 2,323 | 24.4 | (1.85) | 152 | 11.1 u | (4.90) | 459 | 19.1 | (4.73) | 1,497 | 26.4 | (2.45) |
| Female | 2,399 | 29.2 | (2.04) | 202 | 17.9 u | (7.24) | 544 | 17.0 | (4.79) | 1,397 | 32.5 | (2.74) |

Notes: Significant differences in means and proportions are noted by * (.05 level), ** (.01 level), or *** (.001 level). Differences are tested in comparison to FSP participants, identified as persons in households receiving food stamps in the past 12 months.

u Denotes individual estimates not meeting the standards of reliability or precision due to inadequate cell size or large coefficient of variation.

[1] The Dietary Reference Intakes (DRI) Estimated Average Requirement (EAR) is used to assess the adequacy of intakes for population groups.

Source: NHANES 1999-2004 dietary recalls. Excludes pregnant and breastfeeding women and infants. 'Total Persons' includes persons with missing food stamp participation or income. Data reflect nutrient intake from foods and do not include the contribution of vitamin and mineral supplements. Usual intake was estimated using C-SIDE: Software for Intake Distribution Estimation. Estimates are age adjusted.

# Table B-14. Phosphorus (mg)

| | Total Persons | | | Food Stamp Program Participants | | | Income-eligible Nonparticipants | | | Higher-income Nonparticipants | | |
|---|---|---|---|---|---|---|---|---|---|---|---|---|
| | Sample size | Mean | Standard error | Sample size | Mean | Standard error | Sample size | Mean | Standard error | Sample size | Mean | Standard error |
| **Mean Usual Intake** | | | | | | | | | | | | |
| All persons | 25,170 | 1303 | (8.5) | 4,020 | 1177 | (24.4) | 5,370 | 1230 | (19.4) | 13,934 | ***1337 | (10.6) |
| Male | 12,747 | 1493 | (12.9) | 1,936 | 1356 | (43.5) | 2,702 | 1455 | (33.6) | 7,201 | ***1520 | (15.4) |
| Female | 12,423 | 1109 | (10.8) | 2,084 | 1046 | (27.7) | 2,668 | 1025 | (21.0) | 6,733 | **1138 | (14.4) |
| Children (age 1-18) | 11,878 | 1236 | (13.1) | 2,644 | 1182 | (27.8) | 2,738 | 1214 | (29.2) | 5,727 | *1254 | (16.0) |
| Male | 6,000 | 1356 | (21.4) | 1,343 | 1291 | (43.8) | 1,389 | 1325 | (45.2) | 2,867 | 1390 | (26.5) |
| Female | 5,878 | 1109 | (14.6) | 1,301 | 1085 | (37.3) | 1,349 | 1090 | (36.3) | 2,860 | 1110 | (17.2) |
| Adults (age 19-59) | 8,570 | 1381 | (14.0) | 1,022 | 1238 | (46.6) | 1,629 | 1315 | (30.2) | 5,313 | ***1417 | (18.1) |
| Male | 4,424 | 1612 | (20.9) | 441 | 1508 | (94.6) | 854 | 1597 | (47.0) | 2,837 | 1631 | (28.0) |
| Female | 4,146 | 1141 | (18.4) | 581 | 1060 | (45.7) | 775 | 1041 | (38.1) | 2,476 | 1177 | (22.0) |
| Older adults (age 60+) | 4,722 | 1131 | (14.2) | 354 | 976 | (43.8) | 1,003 | 1005 | (31.5) | 2,894 | ***1166 | (17.3) |
| Male | 2,323 | 1297 | (24.8) | 152 | 1032 | (76.0) | 459 | 1212 | (68.7) | 1,497 | ***1319 | (26.9) |
| Female | 2,399 | 1002 | (16.2) | 202 | 941 | (53.2) | 544 | 900 | (32.2) | 1,397 | 1031 | (22.4) |
| **Percent of Persons with Usual Intake Greater than Estimated Average Requirement (EAR)[1]** | | | | | | | | | | | | |
| All persons | 25,170 | 94.6 | (0.26) | 4,020 | 89.9 | (1.03) | 5,370 | 92.2 | (0.78) | 13,934 | ***95.4 | (0.28) |
| Male | 12,747 | 97.6 | (0.28) | 1,936 | 95.2 | (1.01) | 2,702 | 96.3 | (0.78) | 7,201 | **98.1 | (0.27) |
| Female | 12,423 | 91.5 | (0.44) | 2,084 | 85.9 | (1.60) | 2,668 | 88.3 | (1.33) | 6,733 | ***92.6 | (0.49) |
| Children (age 1-18) | 11,878 | 83.9 | (0.88) | 2,644 | 78.4 | (2.13) | 2,738 | 81.1 | (2.34) | 5,727 | **85.5 | (0.95) |
| Male | 6,000 | 92.0 | (1.05) | 1,343 | 88.7 | (2.69) | 1,389 | 89.7 | (2.76) | 2,867 | 93.7 | (1.02) |
| Female | 5,878 | 75.2 | (1.44) | 1,301 | 69.5 | (3.31) | 1,349 | 71.5 | (3.93) | 2,860 | 76.5 | (1.66) |
| Adults (age 19-59) | 8,570 | 98.9 | (0.17) | 1,022 | 95.5 | (1.27) | 1,629 | 97.6 | (0.61) | 5,313 | 99.4 | (0.11) |
| Male | 4,424 | 99.7 | (0.07) | 441 | 99.0 | (0.56) | 854 | 99.2 | (0.29) | 2,837 | 99.8 | (0.06) |
| Female | 4,146 | 98.0 | (0.33) | 581 | 93.1 | (2.07) | 775 | 96.1 | (1.16) | 2,476 | **98.9 | (0.23) |
| Older adults (age 60+) | 4,722 | 96.7 | (0.39) | 354 | 90.3 | (2.51) | 1,003 | 91.9 | (1.48) | 2,894 | 97.8 | (0.42) |
| Male | 2,323 | 98.9 | (0.19) | 152 | 93.2 | (3.75) | 459 | 97.5 | (0.78) | 1,497 | 99.1 | (0.23) |
| Female | 2,399 | 95.0 | (0.69) | 202 | 88.5 | (3.34) | 544 | 89.1 | (2.19) | 1,397 | *96.6 | (0.76) |

Notes: Significant differences in means and proportions are noted by * (.05 level), ** (.01 level), or *** (.001 level). Differences are tested in comparison to FSP participants, identified as persons in households receiving food stamps in the past 12 months.

[1] The Dietary Reference Intakes (DRI) Estimated Average Requirement (EAR) is used to assess the adequacy of intakes for population groups.

Source: NHANES 1999-2004 dietary recalls. Excludes pregnant and breastfeeding women and infants. 'Total Persons' includes persons with missing food stamp participation or income. Data reflect nutrient intake from foods and do not include the contribution of vitamin and mineral supplements. Usual intake was estimated using C-SIDE: Software for Intake Distribution Estimation. Estimates are age adjusted.

# Table B-15. Potassium (mg)

| | Total Persons | | | Food Stamp Program Participants | | | Income-eligible Nonparticipants | | | Higher-income Nonparticipants | | |
|---|---|---|---|---|---|---|---|---|---|---|---|---|
| | Sample size | Mean | Standard error | Sample size | Mean | Standard error | Sample size | Mean | Standard error | Sample size | Mean | Standard error |
| **Mean Usual Intake** | | | | | | | | | | | | |
| All persons | 25,170 | 2621 | (18.1) | 4,020 | 2365 | (54.2) | 5,370 | 2481 | (39.8) | 13,934 | ***2676 | (21.9) |
| Male | 12,747 | 2960 | (28.0) | 1,936 | 2703 | (90.4) | 2,702 | 2878 | (69.3) | 7,201 | **2996 | (32.6) |
| Female | 12,423 | 2279 | (22.5) | 2,084 | 2121 | (66.1) | 2,668 | 2121 | (42.1) | 6,733 | 2329 | (28.8) |
| Children (age 1-18) | 11,878 | 2283 | (26.7) | 2,644 | 2247 | (49.1) | 2,738 | 2333 | (60.2) | 5,727 | 2262 | (32.0) |
| Male | 6,000 | 2471 | (43.1) | 1,343 | 2434 | (73.0) | 1,389 | 2507 | (96.2) | 2,867 | 2466 | (49.6) |
| Female | 5,878 | 2084 | (30.4) | 1,301 | 2083 | (71.4) | 1,349 | 2137 | (68.9) | 2,860 | 2045 | (38.4) |
| Adults (age 19-59) | 8,570 | 2784 | (31.5) | 1,022 | 2448 | (89.6) | 1,629 | 2583 | (60.9) | 5,313 | ***2878 | (38.9) |
| Male | 4,424 | 3194 | (47.3) | 441 | 2930 | (172.5) | 854 | 3079 | (100.7) | 2,837 | 3256 | (59.9) |
| Female | 4,146 | 2356 | (41.3) | 581 | 2131 | (95.8) | 775 | 2102 | (69.5) | 2,476 | **2452 | (47.8) |
| Older adults (age 60+) | 4,722 | 2605 | (29.7) | 354 | 2210 | (103.7) | 1,003 | 2283 | (53.4) | 2,894 | ***2684 | (37.8) |
| Male | 2,323 | 2928 | (46.7) | 152 | 2395 | (169.6) | 459 | 2684 | (127.1) | 1,497 | *2975 | (55.1) |
| Female | 2,399 | 2354 | (38.3) | 202 | 2097 | (131.1) | 544 | 2080 | (48.2) | 1,397 | 2430 | (51.9) |
| **Mean Usual Intake as a Percent of Adequate Intake (AI)[1]** | | | | | | | | | | | | |
| All persons | 25,170 | 57.8 | (0.39) | 4,020 | 52.4 | (1.16) | 5,370 | 54.9 | (0.86) | 13,934 | ***58.9 | (0.48) |
| Male | 12,747 | 65.1 | (0.60) | 1,936 | 59.7 | (1.93) | 2,702 | 63.4 | (1.49) | 7,201 | **65.8 | (0.71) |
| Female | 12,423 | 50.4 | (0.49) | 2,084 | 47.1 | (1.42) | 2,668 | 47.1 | (0.92) | 6,733 | 51.4 | (0.63) |
| Children (age 1-18) | 11,878 | 56.3 | (0.63) | 2,644 | 55.7 | (1.17) | 2,738 | 57.7 | (1.40) | 5,727 | 55.7 | (0.77) |
| Male | 6,000 | 60.7 | (0.99) | 1,343 | 60.0 | (1.69) | 1,389 | 61.6 | (2.19) | 2,867 | 60.5 | (1.17) |
| Female | 5,878 | 51.7 | (0.76) | 1,301 | 51.9 | (1.74) | 1,349 | 53.2 | (1.69) | 2,860 | 50.7 | (0.96) |
| Adults (age 19-59) | 8,570 | 59.2 | (0.67) | 1,022 | 52.1 | (1.91) | 1,629 | 55.0 | (1.30) | 5,313 | ***61.2 | (0.83) |
| Male | 4,424 | 68.0 | (1.01) | 441 | 62.3 | (3.67) | 854 | 65.5 | (2.14) | 2,837 | 69.3 | (1.27) |
| Female | 4,146 | 50.1 | (0.88) | 581 | 45.3 | (2.04) | 775 | 44.7 | (1.48) | 2,476 | **52.2 | (1.02) |
| Older adults (age 60+) | 4,722 | 55.4 | (0.63) | 354 | 47.0 | (2.21) | 1,003 | 48.6 | (1.14) | 2,894 | ***57.1 | (0.80) |
| Male | 2,323 | 62.3 | (0.99) | 152 | 51.0 | (3.61) | 459 | 57.1 | (2.70) | 1,497 | *63.3 | (1.17) |
| Female | 2,399 | 50.1 | (0.81) | 202 | 44.6 | (2.79) | 544 | 44.3 | (1.03) | 1,397 | 51.7 | (1.10) |

Notes: Significant differences in means and proportions are noted by * (.05 level), ** (.01 level), or *** (.001 level). Differences are tested in comparison to FSP participants, identified as persons in households receiving food stamps in the past 12 months.

[1] Adequate Intake (AI) is the approximate intake of the nutrient that appears to be adequate for all individuals in the population group. Mean intake at or above the AI implies a low prevalence of inadequate intake.

Source: NHANES 1999–2004 dietary recalls. Excludes pregnant and breastfeeding women and infants. 'Total Persons' includes persons with missing food stamp participation or income. Data reflect nutrient intake from foods and do not include the contribution of vitamin and mineral supplements. Usual intake was estimated using C-SIDE: Software for Intake Distribution Estimation. Estimates are age adjusted.

# Table B-16. Sodium (mg)

| | Total Persons | | | Food Stamp Program Participants | | | Income-eligible Nonparticipants | | | Higher-income Nonparticipants | | |
|---|---|---|---|---|---|---|---|---|---|---|---|---|
| | Sample size | Mean | Standard error | Sample size | Mean | Standard error | Sample size | Mean | Standard error | Sample size | Mean | Standard error |
| **Mean Usual Intake** | | | | | | | | | | | | |
| All persons .......... | 25,170 | 3361 | (23.9) | 4,020 | 3152 | (73.7) | 5,370 | 3208 | (63.6) | 13,934 | ***3420 | (27.7) |
| Male .......... | 12,747 | 3851 | (38.3) | 1,936 | 3599 | (125.6) | 2,702 | 3773 | (109.6) | 7,201 | *3894 | (41.9) |
| Female .......... | 12,423 | 2864 | (28.4) | 2,084 | 2819 | (88.0) | 2,668 | 2688 | (65.7) | 6,733 | 2903 | (35.7) |
| Children (age 1-18) .......... | 11,878 | 3079 | (37.5) | 2,644 | 3064 | (78.4) | 2,738 | 3123 | (117.4) | 5,727 | 3056 | (39.8) |
| Male .......... | 6,000 | 3378 | (67.2) | 1,343 | 3380 | (133.2) | 1,389 | 3461 | (202.2) | 2,867 | 3338 | (67.3) |
| Female .......... | 5,878 | 2762 | (31.0) | 1,301 | 2774 | (85.1) | 1,349 | 2737 | (83.1) | 2,860 | 2749 | (39.7) |
| Adults (age 19-59) .......... | 8,570 | 3631 | (37.8) | 1,022 | 3353 | (127.9) | 1,629 | 3416 | (88.3) | 5,313 | **3714 | (42.5) |
| Male .......... | 4,424 | 4235 | (57.0) | 441 | 3953 | (232.8) | 854 | 4097 | (142.4) | 2,837 | 4303 | (65.2) |
| Female .......... | 4,146 | 2998 | (49.3) | 581 | 2949 | (145.2) | 775 | 2756 | (106.5) | 2,476 | 3047 | (52.6) |
| Older adults (age 60+) .. | 4,722 | 2873 | (38.6) | 354 | 2590 | (151.5) | 1,003 | 2646 | (90.9) | 2,894 | 2941 | (44.4) |
| Male .......... | 2,323 | 3279 | (70.0) | 152 | 2853 | (267.2) | 459 | 3075 | (188.1) | 1,497 | 3331 | (68.5) |
| Female .......... | 2,399 | 2555 | (40.5) | 202 | 2452 | (185.5) | 544 | 2399 | (86.3) | 1,397 | 2597 | (57.6) |
| **Mean Usual Intake as a Percent of Adequate Intake (AI)[1]** | | | | | | | | | | | | |
| All persons .......... | 25,170 | 240.2 | (1.66) | 4,020 | 225.6 | (5.09) | 5,370 | 229.3 | (4.51) | 13,934 | ***244.2 | (1.92) |
| Male .......... | 12,747 | 274.6 | (2.69) | 1,936 | 256.5 | (8.68) | 2,702 | 268.8 | (7.86) | 7,201 | *277.5 | (2.91) |
| Female .......... | 12,423 | 205.6 | (1.96) | 2,084 | 202.8 | (6.10) | 2,668 | 193.1 | (4.49) | 6,733 | 208.2 | (2.48) |
| Children (age 1-18) .......... | 11,878 | 230.2 | (2.74) | 2,644 | 230.7 | (5.57) | 2,738 | 233.6 | (8.90) | 5,727 | 227.7 | (2.88) |
| Male .......... | 6,000 | 251.1 | (4.89) | 1,343 | 252.6 | (9.28) | 1,389 | 257.7 | (15.40) | 2,867 | 247.2 | (4.75) |
| Female .......... | 5,878 | 208.0 | (2.31) | 1,301 | 210.5 | (6.32) | 1,349 | 205.9 | (5.92) | 2,860 | 206.7 | (3.09) |
| Adults (age 19-59) .......... | 8,570 | 247.9 | (2.57) | 1,022 | 228.5 | (8.63) | 1,629 | 232.9 | (6.05) | 5,313 | **253.6 | (2.89) |
| Male .......... | 4,424 | 289.2 | (3.88) | 441 | 268.7 | (15.62) | 854 | 279.3 | (9.84) | 2,837 | 294.0 | (4.42) |
| Female .......... | 4,146 | 204.7 | (3.34) | 581 | 201.5 | (9.84) | 775 | 188.0 | (7.21) | 2,476 | 208.0 | (3.57) |
| Older adults (age 60+) .. | 4,722 | 229.9 | (3.07) | 354 | 207.5 | (12.09) | 1,003 | 211.6 | (7.16) | 2,894 | *235.3 | (3.56) |
| Male .......... | 2,323 | 262.3 | (5.56) | 152 | 229.5 | (21.55) | 459 | 246.0 | (14.91) | 1,497 | 266.4 | (5.47) |
| Female .......... | 2,399 | 204.6 | (3.24) | 202 | 195.9 | (14.69) | 544 | 192.1 | (6.83) | 1,397 | 208.0 | (4.63) |

See footnotes at end of table.

## Table B-16. (Continued)

| | Total Persons | | | Food Stamp Program Participants | | | Income-eligible Nonparticipants | | | Higher-income Nonparticipants | | |
|---|---|---|---|---|---|---|---|---|---|---|---|---|
| | Sample size | Mean | Standard error | Sample size | Mean | Standard error | Sample size | Mean | Standard error | Sample size | Mean | Standard error |
| **Percent of Persons with Usual Intake Above the Tolerable Upper Intake Level (UL)[2]** | | | | | | | | | | | | |
| All persons ........ | 25,170 | 86.1 | (0.56) | 4,020 | 78.6 | (2.15) | 5,370 | 80.0 | (1.52) | 13,934 | ***87.9 | (0.63) |
| Male ........ | 12,747 | 94.3 | (0.37) | 1,936 | 87.1 | (2.20) | 2,702 | 90.9 | (1.30) | 7,201 | ***95.2 | (0.37) |
| Female ........ | 12,423 | 78.2 | (1.07) | 2,084 | 72.5 | (3.29) | 2,668 | 70.4 | (2.68) | 6,733 | *80.3 | (1.26) |
| Children (age 1-18) ...... | 11,878 | 90.6 | (0.58) | 2,644 | 88.6 | (1.69) | 2,738 | 90.7 | (1.56) | 5,727 | 90.4 | (0.73) |
| Male ........ | 6,000 | 95.2 | (0.55) | 1,343 | 94.8 | (1.60) | 1,389 | 95.0 | (1.40) | 2,867 | 95.0 | (0.71) |
| Female ........ | 5,878 | 85.8 | (1.05) | 1,301 | 83.0 | (2.85) | 1,349 | 85.7 | (2.90) | 2,860 | 85.6 | (1.31) |
| Adults (age 19-59) ........ | 8,570 | 87.7 | (0.82) | 1,022 | 81.1 | (3.58) | 1,629 | 82.1 | (2.39) | 5,313 | *89.7 | (0.88) |
| Male ........ | 4,424 | 96.6 | (0.38) | 441 | 92.1 | (2.93) | 854 | 94.8 | (1.24) | 2,837 | 97.3 | (0.40) |
| Female ........ | 4,146 | 78.5 | (1.62) | 581 | 73.8 | (5.61) | 775 | 69.8 | (4.56) | 2,476 | 81.1 | (1.82) |
| Older adults (age 60+) .. | 4,722 | 72.0 | (1.41) | 354 | 58.6 | (7.18) | 1,003 | 57.9 | (3.66) | 2,894 | *75.7 | (1.73) |
| Male ........ | 2,323 | 86.2 | (1.50) | 152 | 65.2 | (10.80) | 459 | 74.8 | (6.08) | 1,497 | *88.5 | (1.36) |
| Female ........ | 2,399 | 61.0 | (2.22) | 202 | 54.5 | (9.50) | 544 | 49.4 | (4.57) | 1,397 | 64.4 | (3.02) |

Notes: Significant differences in means and proportions are noted by * (.05 level), ** (.01 level), or *** (.001 level). Differences are tested in comparison to FSP participants, identified as persons in households receiving food stamps in the past 12 months.

[1] Adequate Intake (AI) is the approximate intake of the nutrient that appears to be adequate for all individuals in the population group. Mean intake at or above the AI implies a low prevalence of inadequate intake.

[2] The DRI Tolerable Upper Intake Level (UL) is the highest usual daily intake level that is likely to pose no risk of adverse health effects.

Source: NHANES 1999-2004 dietary recalls. Excludes pregnant and breastfeeding women and infants. 'Total Persons' includes persons with missing food stamp participation or income. Data reflect nutrient intake from foods and do not include the contribution of vitamin and mineral supplements. Usual intake was estimated using C-SIDE: Software for Intake Distribution Estimation. Estimates are age adjusted.

## Table B-17. Zinc (mg)

### Mean Usual Intake

| | Total Persons | | | Food Stamp Program Participants | | | Income-eligible Nonparticipants | | | Higher-income Nonparticipants | | |
|---|---|---|---|---|---|---|---|---|---|---|---|---|
| | Sample size | Mean | Standard error | Sample size | Mean | Standard error | Sample size | Mean | Standard error | Sample size | Mean | Standard error |
| All persons | 25,170 | 11.7 | (0.11) | 4,020 | 10.8 | (0.27) | 5,370 | 10.9 | (0.22) | 13,934 | ***11.9 | (0.12) |
| Male | 12,747 | 13.7 | (0.17) | 1,936 | 12.7 | (0.48) | 2,702 | 13.1 | (0.36) | 7,201 | *13.9 | (0.19) |
| Female | 12,423 | 9.7 | (0.13) | 2,084 | 9.4 | (0.31) | 2,668 | 8.8 | (0.26) | 6,733 | 9.8 | (0.15) |
| Children (age 1-18) | 11,878 | 10.9 | (0.14) | 2,644 | 10.7 | (0.31) | 2,738 | 10.9 | (0.34) | 5,727 | 10.9 | (0.16) |
| Male | 6,000 | 12.3 | (0.22) | 1,343 | 12.1 | (0.53) | 1,389 | 12.3 | (0.56) | 2,867 | 12.3 | (0.26) |
| Female | 5,878 | 9.4 | (0.16) | 1,301 | 9.4 | (0.32) | 1,349 | 9.3 | (0.33) | 2,860 | 9.3 | (0.19) |
| Adults (age 19-59) | 8,570 | 12.4 | (0.16) | 1,022 | 11.6 | (0.49) | 1,629 | 11.4 | (0.34) | 5,313 | 12.7 | (0.18) |
| Male | 4,424 | 14.7 | (0.24) | 441 | 14.4 | (0.96) | 854 | 14.1 | (0.52) | 2,837 | 14.9 | (0.27) |
| Female | 4,146 | 10.0 | (0.21) | 581 | 9.8 | (0.52) | 775 | 8.8 | (0.43) | 2,476 | 10.2 | (0.24) |
| Older adults (age 60+) | 4,722 | 10.5 | (0.22) | 354 | 8.4 | (0.42) | 1,003 | 8.9 | (0.32) | 2,894 | ***10.9 | (0.29) |
| Male | 2,323 | 12.3 | (0.34) | 152 | 9.2 | (0.68) | 459 | 11.1 | (0.60) | 1,497 | ***12.6 | (0.43) |
| Female | 2,399 | 9.1 | (0.28) | 202 | 7.9 | (0.53) | 544 | 7.8 | (0.38) | 1,397 | 9.4 | (0.40) |

### Percent of Persons with Usual Intake Greater than Estimated Average Requirement (EAR)[1]

| | Total Persons | | | Food Stamp Program Participants | | | Income-eligible Nonparticipants | | | Higher-income Nonparticipants | | |
|---|---|---|---|---|---|---|---|---|---|---|---|---|
| | Sample size | Mean | Standard error | Sample size | Mean | Standard error | Sample size | Mean | Standard error | Sample size | Mean | Standard error |
| All persons | 25,170 | 88.0 | (0.56) | 4,020 | 80.1 | (2.10) | 5,370 | 80.9 | (1.66) | 13,934 | ***89.8 | (0.61) |
| Male | 12,747 | 89.1 | (0.64) | 1,936 | 79.1 | (2.88) | 2,702 | 83.8 | (1.79) | 7,201 | **90.6 | (0.69) |
| Female | 12,423 | 86.7 | (0.92) | 2,084 | 80.3 | (2.96) | 2,668 | 77.8 | (2.74) | 6,733 | **88.9 | (1.02) |
| Children (age 1-18) | 11,878 | 94.3 | (0.61) | 2,644 | 90.7 | (1.79) | 2,738 | 93.0 | (1.57) | 5,727 | *95.0 | (0.68) |
| Male | 6,000 | 97.6 | (0.44) | 1,343 | 96.3 | (1.45) | 1,389 | 96.3 | (1.44) | 2,867 | 98.1 | (0.42) |
| Female | 5,878 | 90.9 | (1.17) | 1,301 | 86.1 | (3.04) | 1,349 | 89.6 | (2.98) | 2,860 | 91.5 | (1.36) |
| Adults (age 19-59) | 8,570 | 88.5 | (0.88) | 1,022 | 83.0 | (3.15) | 1,629 | 80.5 | (2.63) | 5,313 | *90.5 | (1.11) |
| Male | 4,424 | 89.7 | (0.93) | 441 | 83.9 | (4.28) | 854 | 84.6 | (2.35) | 2,837 | 91.2 | (1.00) |
| Female | 4,146 | 87.3 | (1.52) | 581 | 82.4 | (4.39) | 775 | 76.5 | (4.65) | 2,476 | 89.8 | (2.07) |
| Older adults (age 60+) | 4,722 | 74.9 | (1.74) | 354 | 56.2 | (7.72) | 1,003 | 61.4 | (3.92) | 2,894 | **78.0 | (2.26) |
| Male | 2,323 | 73.0 | (2.37) | 152 | 41.8 | (10.40) | 459 | 62.3 | (5.70) | 1,497 | 75.7 | (3.70) |
| Female | 2,399 | 76.3 | (2.49) | 202 | 65.0 | (10.70) | 544 | 60.9 | (5.15) | 1,397 | 80.0 | (2.72) |

Notes: Significant differences in means and proportions are noted by * (.05 level), ** (.01 level), or *** (.001 level). Differences are tested in comparison to FSP participants, identified as persons in households receiving food stamps in the past 12 months.

[1] The Dietary Reference Intakes (DRI) Estimated Average Requirement (EAR) is used to assess the adequacy of intakes for population groups.

Source: NHANES 1999-2004 dietary recalls. Excludes pregnant and breastfeeding women and infants. 'Total Persons' includes persons with missing food stamp participation or income. Data reflect nutrient intake from foods and do not include the contribution of vitamin and mineral supplements. Usual intake was estimated using C-SIDE: Software for Intake Distribution Estimation. Estimates are age adjusted.

# Table B-18. Dietary Fiber (g)

| | Total Persons | | | Food Stamp Program Participants | | | Income-eligible Nonparticipants | | | Higher-income Nonparticipants | | |
|---|---|---|---|---|---|---|---|---|---|---|---|---|
| | Sample size | Mean | Standard error | Sample size | Mean | Standard error | Sample size | Mean | Standard error | Sample size | Mean | Standard error |
| **Mean Usual Intake** | | | | | | | | | | | | |
| All persons | 25,170 | 14.9 | (0.15) | 4,020 | 12.9 | (0.43) | 5,370 | *14.3 | (0.35) | 13,934 | ***15.2 | (0.17) |
| Male | 12,747 | 16.6 | (0.23) | 1,936 | 14.6 | (0.69) | 2,702 | *16.6 | (0.64) | 7,201 | **16.7 | (0.25) |
| Female | 12,423 | 13.2 | (0.19) | 2,084 | 11.7 | (0.55) | 2,668 | 12.3 | (0.34) | 6,733 | **13.6 | (0.22) |
| Children (age 1-18) | 11,878 | 12.4 | (0.16) | 2,644 | 11.8 | (0.34) | 2,738 | 12.7 | (0.37) | 5,727 | 12.4 | (0.20) |
| Male | 6,000 | 13.3 | (0.26) | 1,343 | 12.7 | (0.52) | 1,389 | 13.5 | (0.59) | 2,867 | 13.4 | (0.32) |
| Female | 5,878 | 11.5 | (0.19) | 1,301 | 11.1 | (0.47) | 1,349 | 11.8 | (0.43) | 2,860 | 11.4 | (0.24) |
| Adults (age 19-59) | 8,570 | 15.8 | (0.24) | 1,022 | 13.4 | (0.65) | 1,629 | 15.1 | (0.56) | 5,313 | ***16.3 | (0.27) |
| Male | 4,424 | 17.8 | (0.35) | 441 | 15.5 | (0.94) | 854 | 18.0 | (0.94) | 2,837 | 18.1 | (0.39) |
| Female | 4,146 | 13.7 | (0.34) | 581 | 12.0 | (0.86) | 775 | 12.2 | (0.62) | 2,476 | 14.3 | (0.36) |
| Older adults (age 60+) | 4,722 | 15.6 | (0.28) | 354 | 12.9 | (1.24) | 1,003 | 14.1 | (0.57) | 2,894 | 16.1 | (0.34) |
| Male | 2,323 | 17.4 | (0.44) | 152 | 15.1 | (2.79) | 459 | 16.7 | (1.21) | 1,497 | 17.5 | (0.48) |
| Female | 2,399 | 14.2 | (0.36) | 202 | 11.6 | (1.02) | 544 | 12.8 | (0.60) | 1,397 | 14.9 | (0.47) |
| **Mean Usual Intake as a Percent of Adequate Intake (AI)[1]** | | | | | | | | | | | | |
| All persons | 25,170 | 52.8 | (0.52) | 4,020 | 47.4 | (1.65) | 5,370 | 51.0 | (1.13) | 13,934 | ***53.8 | (0.58) |
| Male | 12,747 | 49.8 | (0.66) | 1,936 | 43.8 | (2.04) | 2,702 | 49.8 | (1.80) | 7,201 | **50.3 | (0.74) |
| Female | 12,423 | 55.8 | (0.80) | 2,084 | 49.6 | (2.38) | 2,668 | 51.8 | (1.39) | 6,733 | ***57.7 | (0.93) |
| Children (age 1-18) | 11,878 | 46.4 | (0.57) | 2,644 | 44.9 | (1.23) | 2,738 | 47.7 | (1.31) | 5,727 | 46.3 | (0.73) |
| Male | 6,000 | 46.3 | (0.85) | 1,343 | 44.6 | (1.66) | 1,389 | 47.1 | (1.90) | 2,867 | 46.4 | (1.10) |
| Female | 5,878 | 46.6 | (0.75) | 1,301 | 45.0 | (1.87) | 1,349 | 48.3 | (1.74) | 2,860 | 46.4 | (0.98) |
| Adults (age 19-59) | 8,570 | 52.7 | (0.84) | 1,022 | 46.9 | (2.45) | 1,629 | 49.8 | (1.84) | 5,313 | 54.3 | (0.91) |
| Male | 4,424 | 49.0 | (0.98) | 441 | 42.4 | (2.53) | 854 | 49.2 | (2.59) | 2,837 | 49.9 | (1.09) |
| Female | 4,146 | 56.6 | (1.39) | 581 | 49.7 | (3.64) | 775 | 50.4 | (2.59) | 2,476 | *59.2 | (1.49) |
| Older adults (age 60+) | 4,722 | 63.5 | (1.17) | 354 | 53.4 | (4.65) | 1,003 | 59.1 | (2.33) | 2,894 | *65.1 | (1.41) |
| Male | 2,323 | 57.9 | (1.45) | 152 | 50.3 | (9.30) | 459 | 55.6 | (4.03) | 1,497 | 58.4 | (1.58) |
| Female | 2,399 | 67.8 | (1.74) | 202 | 55.3 | (4.87) | 544 | 60.9 | (2.86) | 1,397 | **70.9 | (2.26) |

Notes: Significant differences in means and proportions are noted by * (.05 level), ** (.01 level), or *** (.001 level). Differences are tested in comparison to FSP participants, identified as persons in households receiving food stamps in the past 12 months.

[1] Adequate Intake (AI) is the approximate intake of the nutrient that appears to be adequate for all individuals in the population group. Mean intake at or above the AI implies a low prevalence of inadequate intake.

Source: NHANES 1999-2004 dietary recalls. Excludes pregnant and breastfeeding women and infants. 'Total Persons' includes persons with missing food stamp participation or income. Data reflect nutrient intake from foods and do not include the contribution of vitamin and mineral supplements. Usual intake was estimated using C-SIDE: Software for Intake Distribution Estimation. Estimates are age adjusted.

## Table B-19. Dietary Fiber (g/1,000 kcal)[1]

| | Total Persons | | | Food Stamp Program Participants | | | Income-eligible Nonparticipants | | | Higher-income Nonparticipants | | |
|---|---|---|---|---|---|---|---|---|---|---|---|---|
| | Sample size | Mean | Standard error | Sample size | Mean | Standard error | Sample size | Mean | Standard error | Sample size | Mean | Standard error |
| **Mean Usual Intake** | | | | | | | | | | | | |
| All persons | 25,165 | 7.2 | (0.05) | 4,017 | 6.6 | (0.17) | 5,368 | **7.2 | (0.14) | 13,934 | ***7.3 | (0.06) |
| Male | 12,743 | 6.9 | (0.07) | 1,934 | 6.6 | (0.24) | 2,700 | 7.0 | (0.22) | 7,201 | ***6.9 | (0.08) |
| Female | 12,422 | 7.5 | (0.08) | 2,083 | 6.6 | (0.22) | 2,668 | **7.4 | (0.19) | 6,733 | ***7.7 | (0.10) |
| Children (age 1-18) | 11,875 | 6.2 | (0.06) | 2,643 | 6.0 | (0.14) | 2,736 | 6.4 | (0.13) | 5,727 | 6.2 | (0.08) |
| Male | 5,997 | 6.1 | (0.09) | 1,342 | 6.0 | (0.20) | 1,387 | 6.2 | (0.20) | 2,867 | 6.1 | (0.11) |
| Female | 5,878 | 6.3 | (0.08) | 1,301 | 6.0 | (0.20) | 1,349 | *6.6 | (0.17) | 2,860 | 6.4 | (0.11) |
| Adults (age 19-59) | 8,569 | 7.1 | (0.11) | 1,021 | 6.2 | (0.23) | 1,629 | *6.8 | (0.24) | 5,313 | ***7.2 | (0.12) |
| Male | 4,423 | 6.7 | (0.14) | 440 | 6.0 | (0.21) | 854 | 6.7 | (0.34) | 2,837 | **6.8 | (0.16) |
| Female | 4,146 | 7.5 | (0.17) | 581 | 6.3 | (0.36) | 775 | 7.0 | (0.34) | 2,476 | ***7.8 | (0.18) |
| Older adults (age 60+) | 4,721 | 9.2 | (0.14) | 353 | 8.6 | (0.63) | 1,003 | 9.3 | (0.25) | 2,894 | 9.2 | (0.17) |
| Male | 2,323 | 8.8 | (0.18) | 152 | 9.2 | (1.26) | 459 | 9.1 | (0.36) | 1,497 | 8.7 | (0.19) |
| Female | 2,398 | 9.5 | (0.21) | 201 | 8.1 | (0.65) | 544 | 9.4 | (0.33) | 1,397 | *9.6 | (0.27) |
| **Percent of Persons with Usual Intake Greater than 14g / 1,000 kcal** | | | | | | | | | | | | |
| All persons | 25,165 | 2.0 | (0.18) | 4,017 | 1.7 u | (0.74) | 5,368 | 2.3 | (0.44) | 13,934 | 2.0 | (0.21) |
| Male | 12,743 | 1.4 | (0.20) | 1,934 | 2.1 u | (1.24) | 2,700 | 2.0 | (0.55) | 7,201 | 1.3 | (0.23) |
| Female | 12,422 | 2.6 | (0.30) | 2,083 | 1.5 u | (0.93) | 2,668 | 2.6 | (0.66) | 6,733 | 2.8 | (0.35) |
| Children (age 1-18) | 11,875 | 0.0 u | (0.01) | 2,643 | 0.0 u | (0.15) | 2,736 | 0.1 u | (0.06) | 5,727 | 0.0 u | (0.02) |
| Male | 5,997 | 0.0 u | (0.02) | 1,342 | 0.0 | (0.00) | 1,387 | 0.1 u | (0.06) | 2,867 | 0.0 u | (0.02) |
| Female | 5,878 | 0.0 u | (0.01) | 1,301 | 0.0 u | (0.27) | 1,349 | 0.1 u | (0.11) | 2,860 | 0.0 u | (0.04) |
| Adults (age 19-59) | 8,569 | 1.7 | (0.27) | 1,021 | 1.1 u | (0.86) | 1,629 | 1.6 u | (0.47) | 5,313 | 1.9 | (0.29) |
| Male | 4,423 | 0.8 | (0.12) | 440 | 0.5 u | (0.44) | 854 | 1.0 u | (0.59) | 2,837 | 0.8 | (0.14) |
| Female | 4,146 | 2.7 | (0.54) | 581 | 1.6 u | (1.40) | 775 | 2.1 u | (0.72) | 2,476 | 3.1 | (0.60) |
| Older adults (age 60+) | 4,721 | 6.3 | (0.80) | 353 | 7.1 u | (3.47) | 1,003 | 6.9 | (1.58) | 2,894 | 6.2 | (1.01) |
| Male | 2,323 | 5.4 | (1.06) | 152 | 13.2 u | (8.46) | 459 | 7.9 | (2.07) | 1,497 | 4.5 | (1.10) |
| Female | 2,398 | 7.0 | (1.15) | 201 | 3.4 u | (2.10) | 544 | 6.4 u | (2.13) | 1,397 | 7.6 | (1.64) |

Notes: Significant differences in means and proportions are noted by * (.05 level), ** (.01 level), or *** (.001 level). Differences are tested in comparison to FSP participants, identified as persons in households receiving food stamps in the past 12 months.

[1] The AIs for fiber are based on an intake of 14g of total fiber per 1,000 kcal (IOM, 2006). Intakes of dietary fiber understate total fiber intake.

Source: NHANES 1999–2004 dietary recalls. Excludes pregnant and breastfeeding women and infants. 'Total Persons' includes persons with missing food stamp participation or income. Data reflect nutrient intake from foods and do not include the contribution of vitamin and mineral supplements. Usual intake was estimated using C-SIDE: Software for Intake Distribution Estimation. Estimates are age adjusted.

## Table B-20. Total Fat (g)

| | Total Persons | | | Food Stamp Program Participants | | | Income-eligible Nonparticipants | | | Higher-income Nonparticipants | | |
|---|---|---|---|---|---|---|---|---|---|---|---|---|
| | Sample size | Mean | Standard error | Sample size | Mean | Standard error | Sample size | Mean | Standard error | Sample size | Mean | Standard error |
| **Mean Usual Intake** | | | | | | | | | | | | |
| All persons ......... | 25,170 | 80 | (0.6) | 4,020 | 76 | (1.8) | 5,370 | 77 | (1.6) | 13,934 | ** 81 | (0.7) |
| Male ......... | 12,747 | 92 | (1.0) | 1,936 | 85 | (3.2) | 2,702 | 90 | (2.8) | 7,201 | * 93 | (1.1) |
| Female ......... | 12,423 | 69 | (0.7) | 2,084 | 68 | (2.1) | 2,668 | 65 | (1.5) | 6,733 | 69 | (0.8) |
| Children (age 1-18) ...... | 11,878 | 74 | (0.8) | 2,644 | 74 | (1.9) | 2,738 | 76 | (2.7) | 5,727 | 73 | (0.9) |
| Male ......... | 6,000 | 81 | (1.3) | 1,343 | 81 | (2.7) | 1,389 | 84 | (4.6) | 2,867 | 79 | (1.4) |
| Female ......... | 5,878 | 67 | (0.9) | 1,301 | 69 | (2.6) | 1,349 | 67 | (2.1) | 2,860 | 66 | (1.1) |
| Adults (age 19-59) ...... | 8,570 | 87 | (1.1) | 1,022 | 82 | (3.4) | 1,629 | 83 | (2.3) | 5,313 | 89 | (1.3) |
| Male ......... | 4,424 | 101 | (1.9) | 441 | 97 | (6.4) | 854 | 98 | (3.7) | 2,837 | 103 | (2.2) |
| Female ......... | 4,146 | 72 | (1.0) | 581 | 72 | (3.9) | 775 | 68 | (2.9) | 2,476 | 73 | (1.1) |
| Older adults (age 60+) .. | 4,722 | 67 | (1.0) | 354 | 58 | (3.9) | 1,003 | 60 | (2.7) | 2,894 | ** 69 | (1.1) |
| Male ......... | 2,323 | 78 | (1.7) | 152 | 59 | (5.7) | 459 | 71 | (6.8) | 1,497 | *** 79 | (1.5) |
| Female ......... | 2,399 | 59 | (1.3) | 202 | 58 | (5.2) | 544 | 54 | (2.2) | 1,397 | 60 | (1.7) |

Notes: Significant differences in means and proportions are noted by * (.05 level), ** (.01 level), or *** (.001 level). Differences are tested in comparison to FSP participants, identified as persons in households receiving food stamps in the past 12 months.

Source: NHANES 1999-2004 dietary recalls. Excludes pregnant and breastfeeding women and infants. 'Total Persons' includes persons with missing food stamp participation or income. Data reflect nutrient intake from foods and do not include the contribution of vitamin and mineral supplements. Usual intake was estimated using C-SIDE: Software for Intake Distribution Estimation. Estimates are age adjusted.

## Table B-21. Total Fat (% of energy intake)

### Mean Usual Intake

| | Total Persons | | | Food Stamp Program Participants | | | Income-eligible Nonparticipants | | | Higher-income Nonparticipants | | |
|---|---|---|---|---|---|---|---|---|---|---|---|---|
| | Sample size | Mean | Standard error | Sample size | Mean | Standard error | Sample size | Mean | Standard error | Sample size | Mean | Standard error |
| All persons | 25,165 | 33.0 | (0.13) | 4,017 | 32.4 | (0.38) | 5,368 | 32.5 | (0.31) | 13,934 | 33.1 | (0.16) |
| Male | 12,743 | 32.9 | (0.19) | 1,934 | 32.3 | (0.59) | 2,700 | 32.3 | (0.48) | 7,201 | 33.0 | (0.24) |
| Female | 12,422 | 33.2 | (0.19) | 2,083 | 32.5 | (0.50) | 2,668 | 32.8 | (0.41) | 6,733 | 33.4 | (0.22) |
| Children (age 1-18) | 11,875 | 32.4 | (0.16) | 2,643 | 33.0 | (0.41) | 2,736 | 32.8 | (0.36) | 5,727 | 32.2 | (0.21) |
| Male | 5,997 | 32.3 | (0.21) | 1,342 | 32.8 | (0.62) | 1,387 | 32.8 | (0.49) | 2,867 | 31.9 | (0.27) |
| Female | 5,878 | 32.6 | (0.24) | 1,301 | 33.3 | (0.51) | 1,349 | 32.7 | (0.51) | 2,860 | 32.4 | (0.32) |
| Adults (age 19-59) | 8,569 | 33.2 | (0.23) | 1,021 | 32.0 | (0.58) | 1,629 | 32.1 | (0.50) | 5,313 | 33.6 | (0.26) |
| Male | 4,423 | 33.0 | (0.33) | 440 | 32.3 | (0.66) | 854 | 31.7 | (0.69) | 2,837 | 33.3 | (0.40) |
| Female | 4,146 | 33.5 | (0.33) | 581 | 31.9 | (0.86) | 775 | 32.5 | (0.73) | 2,476 | 34.0 | (0.34) |
| Older adults (age 60+) | 4,721 | 33.5 | (0.25) | 353 | 32.5 | (1.10) | 1,003 | 33.3 | (0.59) | 2,894 | 33.7 | (0.29) |
| Male | 2,323 | 33.8 | (0.28) | 152 | 31.6 | (1.61) | 459 | 33.0 | (0.98) | 1,497 | 34.0 | (0.33) |
| Female | 2,398 | 33.3 | (0.38) | 201 | 33.0 | (1.47) | 544 | 33.4 | (0.74) | 1,397 | 33.4 | (0.45) |

### Percent of Persons with Usual Intake Below the AMDR[1]

| | Total Persons | | | Food Stamp Program Participants | | | Income-eligible Nonparticipants | | | Higher-income Nonparticipants | | |
|---|---|---|---|---|---|---|---|---|---|---|---|---|
| | Sample size | Mean | Standard error | Sample size | Mean | Standard error | Sample size | Mean | Standard error | Sample size | Mean | Standard error |
| All persons | 25,165 | 2.1 | (0.16) | 4,017 | 2.6 | (0.44) | 5,368 | 2.3 | (0.33) | 13,934 | 2.1 | (0.23) |
| Male | 12,743 | 2.0 | (0.22) | 1,934 | 2.5 | (0.69) | 2,700 | 2.3 | (0.39) | 7,201 | 2.0 | (0.30) |
| Female | 12,422 | 2.3 | (0.23) | 2,083 | 2.8 | (0.60) | 2,668 | 2.2 | (0.54) | 6,733 | 2.2 | (0.35) |
| Children (age 1-18) | 11,875 | 6.4 | (0.56) | 2,643 | 5.5 | (0.95) | 2,736 | 6.0 | (0.93) | 5,727 | 6.8 | (0.84) |
| Male | 5,997 | 5.9 | (0.77) | 1,342 | 4.6 | (1.35) | 1,387 | 6.4 | (1.21) | 2,867 | 6.5 | (1.10) |
| Female | 5,878 | 6.8 | (0.81) | 1,301 | 6.5 | (1.32) | 1,349 | 5.5 | (1.43) | 2,860 | 7.2 | (1.28) |
| Adults (age 19-59) | 8,569 | 0.7 | (0.17) | 1,021 | 1.5 u | (0.66) | 1,629 | 1.0 u | (0.34) | 5,313 | 0.6 | (0.13) |
| Male | 4,423 | 0.7 u | (0.21) | 440 | 1.2 u | (0.58) | 854 | 0.9 u | (0.38) | 2,837 | 0.6 u | (0.21) |
| Female | 4,146 | 0.7 u | (0.26) | 581 | 1.8 u | (1.02) | 775 | 1.2 u | (0.56) | 2,476 | 0.4 u | (0.13) |
| Older adults (age 60+) | 4,721 | 0.6 u | (0.13) | 353 | 2.4 u | (1.25) | 1,003 | 0.9 u | (0.39) | 2,894 | 0.5 u | (0.12) |
| Male | 2,323 | 0.6 u | (0.12) | 152 | 4.4 u | (2.62) | 459 | 1.2 u | (0.62) | 1,497 | 0.4 u | (0.14) |
| Female | 2,398 | 0.6 u | (0.22) | 201 | 1.2 u | (1.22) | 544 | 0.8 u | (0.50) | 1,397 | 0.6 u | (0.19) |

See footnotes at end of table.

# Table B-21. (Continued)

| | Total Persons | | | Food Stamp Program Participants | | | Income-eligible Nonparticipants | | | Higher-income Nonparticipants | | |
|---|---|---|---|---|---|---|---|---|---|---|---|---|
| | Sample size | Mean | Standard error | Sample size | Mean | Standard error | Sample size | Mean | Standard error | Sample size | Mean | Standard error |
| **Percent of Persons with Usual Intake Within the AMDR[1]** | | | | | | | | | | | | |
| All persons | 25,165 | 66.0 | (1.00) | 4,017 | 68.0 | (2.72) | 5,368 | 68.6 | (2.21) | 13,934 | 65.3 | (1.21) |
| Male | 12,743 | 67.7 | (1.43) | 1,934 | 69.9 | (4.10) | 2,700 | 70.5 | (3.36) | 7,201 | 67.2 | (1.78) |
| Female | 12,422 | 64.2 | (1.38) | 2,083 | 66.3 | (3.59) | 2,668 | 67.0 | (2.90) | 6,733 | 63.2 | (1.62) |
| Children (age 1-18) | 11,875 | 73.4 | (1.41) | 2,643 | 68.4 | (3.77) | 2,736 | 70.2 | (3.36) | 5,727 | 75.2 | (1.84) |
| Male | 5,997 | 76.4 | (1.88) | 1,342 | 73.2 | (5.62) | 1,387 | 69.3 | (4.80) | 2,867 | 78.3 | (2.37) |
| Female | 5,878 | 70.3 | (2.11) | 1,301 | 62.7 | (4.95) | 1,349 | 70.9 | (4.61) | 2,860 | 72.1 | (2.82) |
| Adults (age 19-59) | 8,569 | 62.7 | (1.81) | 1,021 | 69.1 | (3.74) | 1,629 | 70.2 | (3.32) | 5,313 | 60.0 | (2.16) |
| Male | 4,423 | 64.4 | (2.78) | 440 | 68.7 | (4.21) | 854 | 73.2 | (4.53) | 2,837 | 62.4 | (3.46) |
| Female | 4,146 | 61.0 | (2.30) | 581 | 69.3 | (5.55) | 775 | 67.3 | (4.85) | 2,476 | 57.4 | (2.44) |
| Older adults (age 60+) | 4,721 | 60.4 | (1.77) | 353 | 62.8 | (7.00) | 1,003 | 61.5 | (4.22) | 2,894 | 60.0 | (2.05) |
| Male | 2,323 | 58.4 | (2.06) | 152 | 64.7 | (9.16) | 459 | 62.3 | (6.89) | 1,497 | 57.4 | (2.59) |
| Female | 2,398 | 62.1 | (2.70) | 201 | 61.7 | (9.80) | 544 | 61.0 | (5.31) | 1,397 | 62.3 | (3.11) |
| **Percent of Persons with Usual Intake Above the AMDR[1]** | | | | | | | | | | | | |
| All persons | 25,165 | 31.9 | (0.98) | 4,017 | 29.4 | (2.69) | 5,368 | 29.1 | (2.18) | 13,934 | 32.5 | (1.19) |
| Male | 12,743 | 30.4 | (1.42) | 1,934 | 27.6 | (4.04) | 2,700 | 27.2 | (3.33) | 7,201 | 30.8 | (1.75) |
| Female | 12,422 | 33.6 | (1.36) | 2,083 | 30.9 | (3.54) | 2,668 | 30.8 | (2.85) | 6,733 | 34.6 | (1.58) |
| Children (age 1-18) | 11,875 | 20.2 | (1.29) | 2,643 | 26.1 | (3.65) | 2,736 | 23.8 | (3.23) | 5,727 | 18.0 | (1.64) |
| Male | 5,997 | 17.6 | (1.72) | 1,342 | 22.1 | (5.46) | 1,387 | 24.3 | (4.64) | 2,867 | 15.2 | (2.10) |
| Female | 5,878 | 22.9 | (1.95) | 1,301 | 30.8 | (4.77) | 1,349 | 23.6 | (4.38) | 2,860 | 20.6 | (2.52) |
| Adults (age 19-59) | 8,569 | 36.6 | (1.80) | 1,021 | 29.4 | (3.68) | 1,629 | 28.8 | (3.30) | 5,313 | 39.4 | (2.16) |
| Male | 4,423 | 34.9 | (2.77) | 440 | 30.1 | (4.17) | 854 | 25.9 | (4.51) | 2,837 | 37.0 | (3.45) |
| Female | 4,146 | 38.3 | (2.29) | 581 | 28.9 | (5.46) | 775 | 31.5 | (4.82) | 2,476 | 42.2 | (2.44) |
| Older adults (age 60+) | 4,721 | 38.9 | (1.76) | 353 | 34.8 | (6.89) | 1,003 | 37.6 | (4.20) | 2,894 | 39.5 | (2.05) |
| Male | 2,323 | 41.1 | (2.06) | 152 | 31.0 | (8.78) | 459 | 36.5 | (6.86) | 1,497 | 42.2 | (2.59) |
| Female | 2,398 | 37.3 | (2.69) | 201 | 37.1 | (9.72) | 544 | 38.2 | (5.29) | 1,397 | 37.2 | (3.10) |

Notes: Significant differences in means and proportions are noted by * (.05 level), ** (.01 level), or *** (.001 level). Differences are tested in comparison to FSP participants, identified as persons in households receiving food stamps in the past 12 months.

[u] Denotes individual estimates not meeting the standards of reliability or precision due to inadequate cell size or large coefficient of variation.

[1] Acceptable Macronutrient Distribution Ranges (AMDR) are the ranges of intake for macronutrients, as a percent of total food energy, associated with reduced risk of chronic disease while providing intakes of essential nutrients.

Source: NHANES 1999-2004 dietary recalls. Excludes pregnant and breastfeeding women and infants. 'Total Persons' includes persons with missing food stamp participation or income. Data reflect nutrient intake from foods and do not include the contribution of vitamin and mineral supplements. Usual intake was estimated using C-SIDE: Software for Intake Distribution Estimation. Estimates are age adjusted.

# Table B-22. Saturated Fat (g)

| | Total Persons | | | Food Stamp Program Participants | | | Income-eligible Nonparticipants | | | Higher-income Nonparticipants | | |
|---|---|---|---|---|---|---|---|---|---|---|---|---|
| | Sample size | Mean | Standard error | Sample size | Mean | Standard error | Sample size | Mean | Standard error | Sample size | Mean | Standard error |
| **Mean Usual Intake** | | | | | | | | | | | | |
| All persons ............ | 24,385 | 27 | (0.2) | 3,783 | 26 | (0.7) | 5,174 | 26 | (0.6) | 13,619 | *27 | (0.3) |
| Male .................. | 12,338 | 31 | (0.3) | 1,813 | 29 | (1.2) | 2,601 | 30 | (1.0) | 7,028 | 31 | (0.4) |
| Female ............... | 12,047 | 23 | (0.3) | 1,970 | 23 | (0.7) | 2,573 | 22 | (0.6) | 6,591 | 23 | (0.3) |
| Children (age 2–18)[1] ..... | 11,093 | 27 | (0.3) | 2,407 | 27 | (0.7) | 2,542 | 27 | (0.9) | 5,412 | 26 | (0.4) |
| Male .................. | 5,591 | 29 | (0.5) | 1,220 | 29 | (1.2) | 1,288 | 30 | (1.6) | 2,694 | 29 | (0.6) |
| Female ............... | 5,502 | 24 | (0.4) | 1,187 | 25 | (0.9) | 1,254 | 24 | (0.9) | 2,718 | 24 | (0.5) |
| Adults (age 19–59) ....... | 8,570 | 29 | (0.3) | 1,022 | 27 | (1.3) | 1,629 | 27 | (0.9) | 5,313 | 29 | (0.4) |
| Male .................. | 4,424 | 34 | (0.5) | 441 | 33 | (2.4) | 854 | 32 | (1.3) | 2,837 | 34 | (0.7) |
| Female ............... | 4,146 | 24 | (0.4) | 581 | 24 | (1.4) | 775 | 22 | (1.2) | 2,476 | 24 | (0.4) |
| Older adults (age 60+) .. | 4,722 | 21 | (0.4) | 354 | 19 | (1.3) | 1,003 | 19 | (0.8) | 2,894 | *22 | (0.5) |
| Male .................. | 2,323 | 25 | (0.6) | 152 | 20 | (2.1) | 459 | 23 | (1.9) | 1,497 | 25 | (0.6) |
| Female ............... | 2,399 | 19 | (0.5) | 202 | 19 | (1.7) | 544 | 17 | (0.7) | 1,397 | 19 | (0.6) |

Notes: Significant differences in means and proportions are noted by * (.05 level), ** (.01 level), or *** (.001 level). Differences are tested in comparison to FSP participants, identified as persons in households receiving food stamps in the past 12 months.

[1] Data are not presented for children under age 2 because the Dietary Guidelines recommendations for saturated fat apply to persons age 2 and older.

Source: NHANES 1999–2004 dietary recalls. Excludes pregnant and breastfeeding women and infants. 'Total Persons' includes persons with missing food stamp participation or income. Data reflect nutrient intake from foods and do not include the contribution of vitamin and mineral supplements. Usual intake was estimated using C-SIDE: Software for Intake Distribution Estimation. Estimates are age adjusted.

# Table B-23. Saturated Fat (% of energy intake)

| | Total Persons | | | Food Stamp Program Participants | | | Income-eligible Nonparticipants | | | Higher-income Nonparticipants | | |
|---|---|---|---|---|---|---|---|---|---|---|---|---|
| | Sample size | Mean | Standard error | Sample size | Mean | Standard error | Sample size | Mean | Standard error | Sample size | Mean | Standard error |
| **Mean Usual Intake** | | | | | | | | | | | | |
| All persons | 24,380 | 11.0 | (0.06) | 3,780 | 11.0 | (0.17) | 5,172 | 10.7 | (0.13) | 13,619 | 11.0 | (0.07) |
| Male | 12,334 | 11.0 | (0.08) | 1,811 | 10.9 | (0.25) | 2,599 | 10.6 | (0.18) | 7,028 | 11.1 | (0.09) |
| Female | 12,046 | 11.0 | (0.09) | 1,969 | 11.1 | (0.22) | 2,573 | 10.8 | (0.19) | 6,591 | 11.0 | (0.11) |
| Children (age 2–18)[1] | 11,090 | 11.5 | (0.07) | 2,406 | 11.8 | (0.22) | 2,540 | 11.6 | (0.16) | 5,412 | 11.4 | (0.10) |
| Male | 5,588 | 11.5 | (0.10) | 1,219 | 11.8 | (0.33) | 1,286 | 11.6 | (0.22) | 2,694 | 11.4 | (0.14) |
| Female | 5,502 | 11.5 | (0.11) | 1,187 | 11.8 | (0.27) | 1,254 | 11.6 | (0.23) | 2,718 | 11.4 | (0.14) |
| Adults (age 19–59) | 8,569 | 10.9 | (0.10) | 1,021 | 10.8 | (0.26) | 1,629 | 10.3 | (0.21) | 5,313 | 11.0 | (0.12) |
| Male | 4,423 | 10.9 | (0.13) | 440 | 10.8 | (0.28) | 854 | 10.1 | (0.28) | 2,837 | 11.0 | (0.16) |
| Female | 4,146 | 10.9 | (0.16) | 581 | 10.8 | (0.40) | 775 | 10.6 | (0.32) | 2,476 | 11.1 | (0.18) |
| Older adults (age 60+) | 4,721 | 10.6 | (0.11) | 353 | 10.6 | (0.43) | 1,003 | 10.7 | (0.22) | 2,894 | 10.6 | (0.14) |
| Male | 2,323 | 10.8 | (0.15) | 152 | 10.5 | (0.66) | 459 | 10.7 | (0.36) | 1,497 | 10.8 | (0.18) |
| Female | 2,398 | 10.5 | (0.16) | 201 | 10.7 | (0.57) | 544 | 10.7 | (0.28) | 1,397 | 10.4 | (0.21) |
| **Percent of Persons Meeting Dietary Guidelines Recommendation[2]** | | | | | | | | | | | | |
| All persons | 24,380 | 31.0 | (1.05) | 3,780 | 32.3 | (2.94) | 5,172 | 37.0 | (2.49) | 13,619 | 29.9 | (1.25) |
| Male | 12,334 | 29.9 | (1.43) | 1,811 | 32.8 | (4.54) | 2,599 | 39.2 | (3.72) | 7,028 | 28.6 | (1.73) |
| Female | 12,046 | 32.0 | (1.52) | 1,969 | 32.2 | (3.85) | 2,573 | 35.2 | (3.38) | 6,591 | 31.4 | (1.79) |
| Children (age 2–18)[1] | 11,090 | 16.7 | (1.29) | 2,406 | 14.5 | (3.21) | 2,540 | 15.9 | (2.62) | 5,412 | 18.0 | (1.76) |
| Male | 5,588 | 15.0 | (1.76) | 1,219 | 13.6 u | (5.02) | 1,286 | 13.2 | (3.30) | 2,694 | 16.3 | (2.58) |
| Female | 5,502 | 18.6 | (1.89) | 1,187 | 15.2 | (3.94) | 1,254 | 18.6 | (4.13) | 2,718 | 20.0 | (2.43) |
| Adults (age 19–59) | 8,569 | 34.8 | (1.90) | 1,021 | 38.0 | (4.29) | 1,629 | 45.6 | (4.03) | 5,313 | 32.2 | (2.42) |
| Male | 4,423 | 34.5 | (2.57) | 440 | 36.4 | (5.81) | 854 | 49.6 | (5.55) | 2,837 | 31.7 | (3.73) |
| Female | 4,146 | 35.1 | (2.82) | 581 | 39.1 | (5.99) | 775 | 41.7 | (5.84) | 2,476 | 32.7 | (2.96) |
| Older adults (age 60+) | 4,721 | 40.2 | (2.08) | 353 | 41.0 | (7.32) | 1,003 | 38.8 | (4.12) | 2,894 | 40.7 | (2.57) |
| Male | 2,323 | 38.0 | (2.56) | 152 | 43.8 | (9.98) | 459 | 40.3 | (6.66) | 1,497 | 37.7 | (2.90) |
| Female | 2,398 | 42.0 | (3.12) | 201 | 39.2 | (10.10) | 544 | 38.1 | (5.21) | 1,397 | 43.3 | (4.11) |

Notes: Significant differences in means and proportions are noted by * (.05 level), ** (.01 level), or *** (.001 level). Differences are tested in comparison to FSP participants, identified as persons in households receiving food stamps in the past 12 months.

u Denotes individual estimates not meeting the standards of reliability or precision due to inadequate cell size or large coefficient of variation.

[1] Data are not presented for children under age 2 because the Dietary Guidelines recommendations for saturated fat apply to persons age 2 and older.

[2] Recommended intake of saturated fat is less than 10 percent of total calories.

Source: NHANES 1999–2004 dietary recalls. Excludes pregnant and breastfeeding women and infants. 'Total Persons' includes persons with missing food stamp participation or income. Data reflect nutrient intake from foods and do not include the contribution of vitamin and mineral supplements. Usual intake was estimated using C-SIDE: Software for Intake Distribution Estimation. Estimates are age adjusted.

# Table B-24. Linoleic Acid (g)

| | Total Persons | | | Food Stamp Program Participants | | | Income-eligible Nonparticipants | | | Higher-income Nonparticipants | | |
|---|---|---|---|---|---|---|---|---|---|---|---|---|
| | Sample size | Mean | Standard error | Sample size | Mean | Standard error | Sample size | Mean | Standard error | Sample size | Mean | Standard error |
| **Mean Usual Intake** | | | | | | | | | | | | |
| All persons | 25,170 | 14.4 | (0.14) | 4,020 | 13.0 | (0.39) | 5,370 | 14.0 | (0.34) | 13,934 | ***14.6 | (0.18) |
| Male | 12,747 | 16.2 | (0.23) | 1,936 | 14.4 | (0.70) | 2,702 | 16.2 | (0.62) | 7,201 | *16.2 | (0.29) |
| Female | 12,423 | 12.7 | (0.16) | 2,084 | 12.1 | (0.45) | 2,668 | 11.9 | (0.31) | 6,733 | 12.9 | (0.20) |
| Children (age 1-18) | 11,878 | 12.5 | (0.21) | 2,644 | 12.4 | (0.45) | 2,738 | 13.0 | (0.62) | 5,727 | 12.3 | (0.23) |
| Male | 6,000 | 13.4 | (0.34) | 1,343 | 13.2 | (0.70) | 1,389 | 14.4 | (1.06) | 2,867 | 13.1 | (0.35) |
| Female | 5,878 | 11.5 | (0.23) | 1,301 | 11.8 | (0.62) | 1,349 | 11.4 | (0.45) | 2,860 | 11.4 | (0.29) |
| Adults (age 19-59) | 8,570 | 15.8 | (0.23) | 1,022 | 14.1 | (0.66) | 1,629 | 15.2 | (0.46) | 5,313 | **16.1 | (0.30) |
| Male | 4,424 | 18.0 | (0.35) | 441 | 16.4 | (1.35) | 854 | 17.9 | (0.77) | 2,837 | 18.1 | (0.49) |
| Female | 4,146 | 13.5 | (0.29) | 581 | 12.6 | (0.62) | 775 | 12.6 | (0.52) | 2,476 | 13.9 | (0.34) |
| Older adults (age 60+) | 4,722 | 12.9 | (0.27) | 354 | 10.1 | (0.81) | 1,003 | 11.4 | (0.70) | 2,894 | ***13.4 | (0.31) |
| Male | 2,323 | 14.4 | (0.49) | 152 | 9.4 | (1.02) | 459 | 13.0 | (1.74) | 1,497 | ***14.8 | (0.49) |
| Female | 2,399 | 11.7 | (0.29) | 202 | 10.5 | (1.15) | 544 | 10.5 | (0.60) | 1,397 | 12.2 | (0.38) |
| **Mean Usual Intake as a Percent of Adequate Intake (AI)[1]** | | | | | | | | | | | | |
| All persons | 25,170 | 111.5 | (1.04) | 4,020 | 104.1 | (2.93) | 5,370 | 108.5 | (2.61) | 13,934 | **112.4 | (1.27) |
| Male | 12,747 | 109.5 | (1.53) | 1,936 | 97.6 | (4.35) | 2,702 | 110.1 | (4.45) | 7,201 | **109.8 | (1.82) |
| Female | 12,423 | 113.5 | (1.42) | 2,084 | 108.5 | (3.94) | 2,668 | 106.4 | (2.72) | 6,733 | 115.5 | (1.75) |
| Children (age 1-18) | 11,878 | 115.8 | (1.82) | 2,644 | 117.1 | (3.99) | 2,738 | 119.9 | (5.73) | 5,727 | 113.7 | (2.03) |
| Male | 6,000 | 114.9 | (2.82) | 1,343 | 114.0 | (5.46) | 1,389 | 123.3 | (9.66) | 2,867 | 112.3 | (2.82) |
| Female | 5,878 | 116.8 | (2.28) | 1,301 | 120.5 | (6.09) | 1,349 | 115.3 | (4.40) | 2,860 | 115.6 | (2.93) |
| Adults (age 19-59) | 8,570 | 111.7 | (1.61) | 1,022 | 103.6 | (4.51) | 1,629 | 107.5 | (3.23) | 5,313 | *113.7 | (2.05) |
| Male | 4,424 | 109.4 | (2.14) | 441 | 99.0 | (8.04) | 854 | 109.1 | (4.76) | 2,837 | 110.4 | (2.92) |
| Female | 4,146 | 114.2 | (2.41) | 581 | 106.5 | (5.23) | 775 | 106.0 | (4.39) | 2,476 | 117.5 | (2.84) |
| Older adults (age 60+) | 4,722 | 105.1 | (2.11) | 354 | 84.5 | (7.05) | 1,003 | 94.9 | (5.50) | 2,894 | ***108.4 | (2.48) |
| Male | 2,323 | 102.9 | (3.47) | 152 | 67.3 | (7.29) | 459 | 93.2 | (12.39) | 1,497 | 106.1 | (3.53) |
| Female | 2,399 | 106.8 | (2.61) | 202 | 95.0 | (10.45) | 544 | 95.7 | (5.42) | 1,397 | 110.5 | (3.47) |

Notes: Significant differences in means and proportions are noted by * (.05 level), ** (.01 level), or *** (.001 level). Differences are tested in comparison to FSP participants, identified as persons in households receiving food stamps in the past 12 months.

[1] Adequate Intake (AI) is the approximate intake of the nutrient that appears to be adequate for all individuals in the population group. Mean intake at or above the AI implies a low prevalence of inadequate intake.

Source: NHANES 1999–2004 dietary recalls. Excludes pregnant and breastfeeding women and infants. 'Total Persons' includes persons with missing food stamp participation or income. Data reflect nutrient intake from foods and do not include the contribution of vitamin and mineral supplements. Usual intake was estimated using C-SIDE: Software for Intake Distribution Estimation. Estimates are age adjusted.

# Table B-25. Linoleic Acid (% of energy intake)

| | Total Persons | | | Food Stamp Program Participants | | | Income-eligible Nonparticipants | | | Higher-income Nonparticipants | | |
|---|---|---|---|---|---|---|---|---|---|---|---|---|
| | Sample size | Mean | Standard error | Sample size | Mean | Standard error | Sample size | Mean | Standard error | Sample size | Mean | Standard error |
| **Mean Usual Intake** | | | | | | | | | | | | |
| All persons | 25,165 | 5.95 | (0.042) | 4,017 | 5.60 | (0.114) | 5,368 | *5.96 | (0.097) | 13,934 | **5.98 | (0.051) |
| Male | 12,743 | 5.77 | (0.060) | 1,934 | 5.40 | (0.177) | 2,700 | 5.79 | (0.129) | 7,201 | 5.77 | (0.077) |
| Female | 12,422 | 6.12 | (0.058) | 2,083 | 5.74 | (0.149) | 2,668 | 6.09 | (0.142) | 6,733 | **6.21 | (0.068) |
| Children (age 1-18) | 11,875 | 5.40 | (0.056) | 2,643 | 5.46 | (0.117) | 2,736 | 5.47 | (0.134) | 5,727 | 5.37 | (0.072) |
| Male | 5,997 | 5.27 | (0.080) | 1,342 | 5.26 | (0.157) | 1,387 | 5.49 | (0.203) | 2,867 | 5.19 | (0.101) |
| Female | 5,878 | 5.53 | (0.079) | 1,301 | 5.66 | (0.175) | 1,349 | 5.46 | (0.160) | 2,860 | 5.56 | (0.102) |
| Adults (age 19-59) | 8,569 | 6.07 | (0.063) | 1,021 | 5.59 | (0.142) | 1,629 | *6.05 | (0.134) | 5,313 | ***6.15 | (0.080) |
| Male | 4,423 | 5.87 | (0.082) | 440 | 5.51 | (0.238) | 854 | 5.90 | (0.168) | 2,837 | 5.90 | (0.112) |
| Female | 4,146 | 6.28 | (0.096) | 581 | 5.64 | (0.175) | 775 | *6.20 | (0.209) | 2,476 | ***6.44 | (0.114) |
| Older adults (age 60+) | 4,721 | 6.44 | (0.092) | 353 | 5.63 | (0.263) | 1,003 | *6.29 | (0.203) | 2,894 | *6.54 | (0.118) |
| Male | 2,323 | 6.25 | (0.147) | 152 | 5.02 | (0.393) | 459 | 5.86 | (0.271) | 1,497 | **6.39 | (0.192) |
| Female | 2,398 | 6.58 | (0.117) | 201 | 6.00 | (0.350) | 544 | 6.51 | (0.273) | 1,397 | 6.66 | (0.142) |
| **Percent of Persons with Usual Intake Below the AMDR[1]** | | | | | | | | | | | | |
| All persons | 25,165 | 24.3 | (1.06) | 4,017 | 32.3 | (3.57) | 5,368 | *23.4 | (2.22) | 13,934 | *24.0 | (1.35) |
| Male | 12,743 | 28.3 | (1.72) | 1,934 | 39.0 | (6.14) | 2,700 | 26.0 | (3.35) | 7,201 | 29.1 | (2.29) |
| Female | 12,422 | 20.2 | (1.21) | 2,083 | 27.6 | (4.09) | 2,668 | 22.0 | (2.96) | 6,733 | 18.2 | (1.44) |
| Children (age 1-18) | 11,875 | 34.3 | (2.54) | 2,643 | 32.4 | (6.27) | 2,736 | 30.2 | (4.60) | 5,727 | 36.1 | (3.43) |
| Male | 5,997 | 36.5 | (4.28) | 1,342 | 38.1 | (10.44) | 1,387 | 27.9 | (6.57) | 2,867 | 40.6 | (6.14) |
| Female | 5,878 | 31.9 | (2.70) | 1,301 | 26.8 | (5.37) | 1,349 | 33.3 | (6.06) | 2,860 | 31.2 | (3.65) |
| Adults (age 19-59) | 8,569 | 21.4 | (1.24) | 1,021 | 33.8 | (4.50) | 1,629 | *22.0 | (3.07) | 5,313 | **19.8 | (1.65) |
| Male | 4,423 | 26.5 | (1.79) | 440 | 38.0 | (6.44) | 854 | 24.8 | (4.29) | 2,837 | 25.8 | (2.76) |
| Female | 4,146 | 16.1 | (1.70) | 581 | 31.0 | (6.14) | 775 | 19.2 | (4.38) | 2,476 | **13.1 | (1.61) |
| Older adults (age 60+) | 4,721 | 15.0 | (1.64) | 353 | 32.1 | (7.40) | 1,003 | 17.7 | (3.64) | 2,894 | *13.4 | (1.82) |
| Male | 2,323 | 19.0 | (2.83) | 152 | 51.9 | (12.60) | 459 | 27.7 | (6.95) | 1,497 | **16.3 | (3.27) |
| Female | 2,398 | 11.8 | (1.90) | 201 | 20.0 u | (9.11) | 544 | 12.6 u | (4.20) | 1,397 | 10.9 | (1.87) |

See footnotes at end of table.

**Table B-25. (Continued)**

### Percent of Persons with Usual Intake Within the AMDR[1]

| | Total Persons | | | Food Stamp Program Participants | | | Income-eligible Nonparticipants | | | Higher-income Nonparticipants | | |
|---|---|---|---|---|---|---|---|---|---|---|---|---|
| | Sample size | Mean | Standard error | Sample size | Mean | Standard error | Sample size | Mean | Standard error | Sample size | Mean | Standard error |
| All persons | 25,165 | 75.0 | (1.06) | 4,017 | 67.5 | (3.57) | 5,368 | 75.9 | (2.25) | 13,934 | *75.2 | (1.36) |
| Male | 12,743 | 71.1 | (1.73) | 1,934 | 60.8 | (6.14) | 2,700 | 73.5 | (3.35) | 7,201 | 70.2 | (2.30) |
| Female | 12,422 | 79.0 | (1.22) | 2,083 | 72.2 | (4.09) | 2,668 | 77.1 | (3.03) | 6,733 | *80.8 | (1.46) |
| Children (age 1-18) | 11,875 | 65.6 | (2.54) | 2,643 | 67.5 | (6.27) | 2,736 | 69.6 | (4.60) | 5,727 | 63.8 | (3.44) |
| Male | 5,997 | 63.5 | (4.28) | 1,342 | 61.8 | (10.44) | 1,387 | 71.9 | (6.58) | 2,867 | 59.4 | (6.14) |
| Female | 5,878 | 68.0 | (2.71) | 1,301 | 73.2 | (5.37) | 1,349 | 66.7 | (6.06) | 2,860 | 68.6 | (3.66) |
| Adults (age 19-59) | 8,569 | 78.0 | (1.25) | 1,021 | 66.0 | (4.50) | 1,629 | *77.3 | (3.10) | 5,313 | **79.4 | (1.66) |
| Male | 4,423 | 73.0 | (1.80) | 440 | 61.6 | (6.45) | 854 | 74.7 | (4.30) | 2,837 | 73.7 | (2.78) |
| Female | 4,146 | 83.1 | (1.72) | 581 | 68.8 | (6.14) | 775 | 79.8 | (4.45) | 2,476 | **85.9 | (1.64) |
| Older adults (age 60+) | 4,721 | 83.7 | (1.67) | 353 | 67.9 | (7.41) | 1,003 | 81.5 | (3.68) | 2,894 | *84.9 | (1.89) |
| Male | 2,323 | 79.9 | (2.86) | 152 | 48.1 | (12.60) | 459 | 71.8 | (6.96) | 1,497 | 82.4 | (3.33) |
| Female | 2,398 | 86.6 | (1.96) | 201 | 80.0 | (9.11) | 544 | 86.4 | (4.28) | 1,397 | 87.1 | (2.02) |

### Percent of Persons with Usual Intake Above the AMDR[1]

| | Total Persons | | | Food Stamp Program Participants | | | Income-eligible Nonparticipants | | | Higher-income Nonparticipants | | |
|---|---|---|---|---|---|---|---|---|---|---|---|---|
| | Sample size | Mean | Standard error | Sample size | Mean | Standard error | Sample size | Mean | Standard error | Sample size | Mean | Standard error |
| All persons | 25,165 | 0.7 | (0.12) | 4,017 | 0.2 u | (0.11) | 5,368 | 0.7 u | (0.36) | 13,934 | **0.8 | (0.16) |
| Male | 12,743 | 0.6 | (0.17) | 1,934 | 0.2 u | (0.14) | 2,700 | 0.5 u | (0.22) | 7,201 | 0.6 u | (0.23) |
| Female | 12,422 | 0.8 | (0.17) | 2,083 | 0.2 u | (0.15) | 2,668 | 1.0 u | (0.64) | 6,733 | **1.0 | (0.23) |
| Children (age 1-18) | 11,875 | 0.1 u | (0.05) | 2,643 | 0.1 u | (0.06) | 2,736 | 0.1 u | (0.11) | 5,727 | 0.1 u | (0.12) |
| Male | 5,997 | 0.1 u | (0.03) | 1,342 | 0.1 u | (0.10) | 1,387 | 0.2 u | (0.22) | 2,867 | 0.0 u | (0.04) |
| Female | 5,878 | 0.1 u | (0.11) | 1,301 | 0.0 u | (0.08) | 1,349 | 0.0 u | (0.03) | 2,860 | 0.2 u | (0.26) |
| Adults (age 19-59) | 8,569 | 0.6 | (0.16) | 1,021 | 0.2 u | (0.17) | 1,629 | 0.7 u | (0.42) | 5,313 | 0.7 u | (0.22) |
| Male | 4,423 | 0.5 u | (0.22) | 440 | 0.4 u | (0.39) | 854 | 0.5 u | (0.29) | 2,837 | 0.5 u | (0.31) |
| Female | 4,146 | 0.8 u | (0.25) | 581 | 0.2 u | (0.12) | 775 | 1.0 u | (0.78) | 2,476 | 1.0 | (0.32) |
| Older adults (age 60+) | 4,721 | 1.4 | (0.31) | 353 | 0.1 u | (0.19) | 1,003 | 0.9 u | (0.55) | 2,894 | **1.7 | (0.50) |
| Male | 2,323 | 1.1 u | (0.40) | 152 | 0.0 u | (0.25) | 459 | 0.5 u | (0.30) | 1,497 | *1.3 | (0.63) |
| Female | 2,398 | 1.6 | (0.46) | 201 | 0.1 u | (0.27) | 544 | 1.0 u | (0.81) | 1,397 | 2.0 | (0.76) |

Notes: Significant differences in means and proportions are noted by * (.05 level), ** (.01 level), or *** (.001 level). Differences are tested in comparison to FSP participants, identified as persons in households receiving food stamps in the past 12 months.

[1] Acceptable Macronutrient Distribution Ranges (AMDR) are the ranges of intake for macronutrients, as a percent of total food energy, associated with reduced risk of chronic disease while providing intakes of essential nutrients.

Source: NHANES 1999-2004 dietary recalls. Excludes pregnant and breastfeeding women and infants. 'Total Persons' includes persons with missing food stamp participation or income. Data reflect nutrient intake from foods and do not include the contribution of vitamin and mineral supplements. Usual intake was estimated using C-SIDE: Software for Intake Distribution Estimation. Estimates are age adjusted.

# Table B-26. Linolenic Acid (g)

| | Total Persons | | | Food Stamp Program Participants | | | Income-eligible Nonparticipants | | | Higher-income Nonparticipants | | |
|---|---|---|---|---|---|---|---|---|---|---|---|---|
| | Sample size | Mean | Standard error | Sample size | Mean | Standard error | Sample size | Mean | Standard error | Sample size | Mean | Standard error |
| **Mean Usual Intake** | | | | | | | | | | | | |
| All persons | 25,170 | 1.43 | (0.01) | 4,020 | 1.28 | (0.04) | 5,370 | 1.34 | (0.03) | 13,934 | ***1.46 | (0.02) |
| Male | 12,747 | 1.59 | (0.02) | 1,936 | 1.43 | (0.06) | 2,702 | 1.53 | (0.05) | 7,201 | *1.60 | (0.03) |
| Female | 12,423 | 1.26 | (0.02) | 2,084 | 1.16 | (0.04) | 2,668 | 1.15 | (0.04) | 6,733 | **1.30 | (0.02) |
| Children (age 1-18) | 11,878 | 1.21 | (0.02) | 2,644 | 1.24 | (0.04) | 2,738 | 1.22 | (0.05) | 5,727 | 1.19 | (0.02) |
| Male | 6,000 | 1.28 | (0.03) | 1,343 | 1.34 | (0.06) | 1,389 | 1.33 | (0.08) | 2,867 | 1.25 | (0.03) |
| Female | 5,878 | 1.13 | (0.03) | 1,301 | 1.17 | (0.07) | 1,349 | 1.10 | (0.04) | 2,860 | 1.12 | (0.03) |
| Adults (age 19-59) | 8,570 | 1.56 | (0.02) | 1,022 | 1.38 | (0.06) | 1,629 | 1.46 | (0.05) | 5,313 | ***1.60 | (0.03) |
| Male | 4,424 | 1.76 | (0.03) | 441 | 1.64 | (0.11) | 854 | 1.72 | (0.07) | 2,837 | 1.79 | (0.05) |
| Female | 4,146 | 1.34 | (0.03) | 581 | 1.21 | (0.06) | 775 | 1.21 | (0.07) | 2,476 | *1.39 | (0.04) |
| Older adults (age 60+) | 4,722 | 1.33 | (0.03) | 354 | 0.99 | (0.07) | 1,003 | 1.12 | (0.05) | 2,894 | *1.39 | (0.05) |
| Male | 2,323 | 1.48 | (0.06) | 152 | 0.95 | (0.10) | 459 | *1.23 | (0.09) | 1,497 | *1.53 | (0.07) |
| Female | 2,399 | 1.22 | (0.04) | 202 | 1.02 | (0.10) | 544 | 1.06 | (0.06) | 1,397 | *1.27 | (0.08) |
| **Mean Usual Intake as a Percent of Adequate Intake (AI)[1]** | | | | | | | | | | | | |
| All persons | 25,170 | 113.7 | (1.15) | 4,020 | 105.9 | (2.87) | 5,370 | 107.7 | (2.57) | 13,934 | ***115.2 | (1.41) |
| Male | 12,747 | 108.1 | (1.49) | 1,936 | 98.9 | (4.00) | 2,702 | 105.1 | (3.60) | 7,201 | *108.8 | (1.82) |
| Female | 12,423 | 119.1 | (1.74) | 2,084 | 110.2 | (4.04) | 2,668 | 109.0 | (3.57) | 6,733 | **122.0 | (2.17) |
| Children (age 1-18) | 11,878 | 116.5 | (1.82) | 2,644 | 121.7 | (4.14) | 2,738 | 117.6 | (4.59) | 5,727 | 114.2 | (2.04) |
| Male | 6,000 | 114.5 | (2.54) | 1,343 | 119.9 | (4.67) | 1,389 | 118.4 | (7.43) | 2,867 | 111.8 | (2.94) |
| Female | 5,878 | 118.6 | (2.62) | 1,301 | 123.6 | (7.39) | 1,349 | 116.3 | (4.53) | 2,860 | 117.1 | (2.91) |
| Adults (age 19-59) | 8,570 | 116.0 | (1.74) | 1,022 | 106.8 | (4.33) | 1,629 | 108.9 | (3.98) | 5,313 | 118.8 | (2.27) |
| Male | 4,424 | 110.3 | (2.17) | 441 | 102.4 | (7.07) | 854 | 107.4 | (4.35) | 2,837 | 112.1 | (3.01) |
| Female | 4,146 | 121.9 | (2.74) | 581 | 109.7 | (5.47) | 775 | 110.3 | (6.61) | 2,476 | 126.3 | (3.45) |
| Older adults (age 60+) | 4,722 | 102.9 | (2.73) | 354 | 80.1 | (6.01) | 1,003 | 90.0 | (3.96) | 2,894 | ***106.3 | (4.23) |
| Male | 2,323 | 92.6 | (3.46) | 152 | 59.6 | (6.35) | 459 | *76.8 | (5.92) | 1,497 | 95.7 | (4.29) |
| Female | 2,399 | 111.0 | (4.04) | 202 | 92.6 | (8.88) | 544 | 96.7 | (5.15) | 1,397 | 115.6 | (7.00) |

Notes: Significant differences in means and proportions are noted by * (.05 level), ** (.01 level), or *** (.001 level). Differences are tested in comparison to FSP participants, identified as persons in households receiving food stamps in the past 12 months.

[1] Adequate Intake (AI) is the approximate intake of the nutrient that appears to be adequate for all individuals in the population group. Mean intake at or above the AI implies a low prevalence of inadequate intake.

Source: NHANES 1999-2004 dietary recalls. Excludes pregnant and breastfeeding women and infants. 'Total Persons' includes persons with missing food stamp participation or income. Data reflect nutrient intake from foods and do not include the contribution of vitamin and mineral supplements. Usual intake was estimated using C-SIDE: Software for Intake Distribution Estimation. Estimates are age adjusted.

# Table B-27. Linolenic Acid (% of energy intake)

| | Total Persons | | | Food Stamp Program Participants | | | Income-eligible Nonparticipants | | | Higher-income Nonparticipants | | |
|---|---|---|---|---|---|---|---|---|---|---|---|---|
| | Sample size | Mean | Standard error | Sample size | Mean | Standard error | Sample size | Mean | Standard error | Sample size | Mean | Standard error |
| **Mean Usual Intake** | | | | | | | | | | | | |
| All persons ............. | 25,165 | 0.59 | (0.005) | 4,017 | 0.55 | (0.011) | 5,368 | 0.58 | (0.011) | 13,934 | ***0.60 | (0.006) |
| Male ...................... | 12,743 | 0.57 | (0.007) | 1,934 | 0.54 | (0.015) | 2,700 | 0.56 | (0.014) | 7,201 | 0.57 | (0.008) |
| Female .................. | 12,422 | 0.61 | (0.008) | 2,083 | 0.56 | (0.016) | 2,668 | 0.59 | (0.017) | 6,733 | ***0.63 | (0.009) |
| Children (age 1-18) ...... | 11,875 | 0.53 | (0.006) | 2,643 | 0.55 | (0.012) | 2,736 | 0.53 | (0.011) | 5,727 | 0.53 | (0.007) |
| Male ...................... | 5,997 | 0.51 | (0.008) | 1,342 | 0.54 | (0.015) | 1,387 | 0.52 | (0.016) | 2,867 | 0.50 | (0.010) |
| Female .................. | 5,878 | 0.55 | (0.008) | 1,301 | 0.56 | (0.021) | 1,349 | 0.54 | (0.016) | 2,860 | 0.55 | (0.011) |
| Adults (age 19-59) ....... | 8,569 | 0.60 | (0.007) | 1,021 | 0.55 | (0.015) | 1,629 | 0.58 | (0.020) | 5,313 | **0.61 | (0.009) |
| Male ...................... | 4,423 | 0.57 | (0.008) | 440 | 0.54 | (0.022) | 854 | 0.56 | (0.021) | 2,837 | 0.58 | (0.010) |
| Female .................. | 4,146 | 0.63 | (0.012) | 581 | 0.55 | (0.020) | 775 | 0.60 | (0.034) | 2,476 | ***0.65 | (0.014) |
| Older adults (age 60+) .. | 4,721 | 0.67 | (0.013) | 353 | 0.56 | (0.028) | 1,003 | *0.63 | (0.020) | 2,894 | ***0.69 | (0.018) |
| Male ...................... | 2,323 | 0.65 | (0.020) | 152 | 0.51 | (0.042) | 459 | 0.59 | (0.029) | 1,497 | **0.66 | (0.026) |
| Female .................. | 2,398 | 0.69 | (0.018) | 201 | 0.59 | (0.036) | 544 | 0.66 | (0.026) | 1,397 | **0.71 | (0.026) |
| **Percent of Persons with Usual Intake Below the AMDR[1]** | | | | | | | | | | | | |
| All persons ............. | 25,165 | 59.7 | (1.30) | 4,017 | 70.9 | (9.85) | 5,368 | 63.5 | (3.17) | 13,934 | 57.8 | (1.58) |
| Male ...................... | 12,743 | 65.1 | (1.81) | 1,934 | 73.6 | (4.51) | 2,700 | 69.2 | (3.92) | 7,201 | 64.4 | (2.27) |
| Female .................. | 12,422 | 54.3 | (1.86) | 2,083 | 69.5 | (19.49) | 2,668 | 59.2 | (4.94) | 6,733 | 50.5 | (2.21) |
| Children (age 1-18) ...... | 11,875 | 82.2 | (1.75) | 2,643 | 78.8 u | (35.72) | 2,736 | 82.9 | (3.55) | 5,727 | 82.6 | (2.28) |
| Male ...................... | 5,997 | 83.0 | (2.27) | 1,342 | 77.5 | (5.55) | 1,387 | 81.6 | (4.64) | 2,867 | 85.2 | (3.10) |
| Female .................. | 5,878 | 81.3 | (2.67) | 1,301 | 80.0 u | (72.68) | 1,349 | 84.2 | (5.64) | 2,860 | 79.4 | (3.41) |
| Adults (age 19-59) ....... | 8,569 | 55.5 | (1.89) | 1,021 | 70.9 | (4.54) | 1,629 | 61.5 | (5.63) | 5,313 | ***51.9 | (2.23) |
| Male ...................... | 4,423 | 63.0 | (2.27) | 440 | 72.3 | (6.56) | 854 | 67.7 | (6.36) | 2,837 | 60.9 | (2.88) |
| Female .................. | 4,146 | 47.8 | (3.04) | 581 | 69.9 | (6.17) | 775 | 55.4 | (9.22) | 2,476 | ***41.9 | (3.45) |
| Older adults (age 60+) .. | 4,721 | 37.3 | (3.16) | 353 | 65.1 | (8.26) | 1,003 | *42.8 | (5.88) | 2,894 | ***34.7 | (3.41) |
| Male ...................... | 2,323 | 43.8 | (4.09) | 152 | 78.2 | (10.40) | 459 | 56.8 | (8.55) | 1,497 | **40.7 | (5.14) |
| Female .................. | 2,398 | 32.2 | (4.62) | 201 | 57.1 | (11.70) | 544 | 35.8 | (7.73) | 1,397 | *29.4 | (4.55) |

See footnotes at end of table.

# Table B-27. (Continued)

| | Total Persons | | | Food Stamp Program Participants | | | Income-eligible Nonparticipants | | | Higher-income Nonparticipants | | |
|---|---|---|---|---|---|---|---|---|---|---|---|---|
| | Sample size | Mean | Standard error | Sample size | Mean | Standard error | Sample size | Mean | Standard error | Sample size | Mean | Standard error |
| **Percent of Persons with Usual Intake Within the AMDR[1]** | | | | | | | | | | | | |
| All persons | 25,165 | 40.0 | (1.30) | 4,017 | 29.1 u | (9.85) | 5,368 | 36.4 | (3.17) | 13,934 | 41.9 | (1.58) |
| Male | 12,743 | 34.7 | (1.82) | 1,934 | 26.3 | (4.51) | 2,700 | 30.7 | (3.92) | 7,201 | 35.4 | (2.28) |
| Female | 12,422 | 45.3 | (1.87) | 2,083 | 30.5 u | (19.49) | 2,668 | 40.6 | (4.95) | 6,733 | 49.1 | (2.22) |
| Children (age 1-18) | 11,875 | 17.8 | (1.75) | 2,643 | 21.2 u | (35.72) | 2,736 | 17.1 | (3.55) | 5,727 | 17.4 | (2.28) |
| Male | 5,997 | 17.0 | (2.27) | 1,342 | 22.5 | (5.55) | 1,387 | 18.4 | (4.64) | 2,867 | 14.8 | (3.10) |
| Female | 5,878 | 18.7 | (2.67) | 1,301 | 20.0 u | (72.68) | 1,349 | 15.8 u | (5.64) | 2,860 | 20.6 | (3.41) |
| Adults (age 19-59) | 8,569 | 44.3 | (1.89) | 1,021 | 29.1 | (4.54) | 1,629 | 38.4 | (5.63) | 5,313 | ***47.8 | (2.23) |
| Male | 4,423 | 37.0 | (2.27) | 440 | 27.7 | (6.56) | 854 | 32.3 | (6.36) | 2,837 | 39.1 | (2.88) |
| Female | 4,146 | 51.9 | (3.04) | 581 | 30.1 | (6.17) | 775 | 44.3 | (9.22) | 2,476 | ***57.7 | (3.46) |
| Older adults (age 60+) | 4,721 | 61.9 | (3.21) | 353 | 34.9 | (8.26) | 1,003 | 57.1 | (5.88) | 2,894 | **64.1 | (3.57) |
| Male | 2,323 | 55.3 | (4.11) | 152 | 21.8 u | (10.41) | 459 | 43.1 | (8.55) | 1,497 | **58.3 | (5.18) |
| Female | 2,398 | 67.0 | (4.73) | 201 | 42.9 | (11.70) | 544 | 64.2 | (7.73) | 1,397 | 69.2 | (4.92) |
| **Percent of Persons with Usual Intake Above the AMDR[1]** | | | | | | | | | | | | |
| All persons | 25,165 | 0.3 u | (0.11) | 4,017 | 0.0 u | (0.06) | 5,368 | 0.1 u | (0.12) | 13,934 | *0.3 | (0.12) |
| Male | 12,743 | 0.2 u | (0.08) | 1,934 | 0.0 u | (0.11) | 2,700 | 0.1 u | (0.10) | 7,201 | 0.2 u | (0.15) |
| Female | 12,422 | 0.4 u | (0.20) | 2,083 | 0.0 u | (0.06) | 2,668 | 0.1 u | (0.21) | 6,733 | *0.4 | (0.18) |
| Children (age 1-18) | 11,875 | 0.0 | (0.00) | 2,643 | 0.0 | (0.00) | 2,736 | 0.0 u | (0.03) | 5,727 | 0.0 u | (0.03) |
| Male | 5,997 | 0.0 | (0.00) | 1,342 | 0.0 | (0.00) | 1,387 | 0.0 u | (0.05) | 2,867 | 0.0 | (0.00) |
| Female | 5,878 | 0.0 | (0.00) | 1,301 | 0.0 | (0.00) | 1,349 | 0.0 | (0.00) | 2,860 | 0.0 u | (0.07) |
| Adults (age 19-59) | 8,569 | 0.2 u | (0.09) | 1,021 | 0.0 | (0.00) | 1,629 | 0.1 u | (0.15) | 5,313 | 0.2 u | (0.13) |
| Male | 4,423 | 0.0 u | (0.09) | 440 | 0.0 | (0.00) | 854 | 0.0 u | (0.01) | 2,837 | 0.0 u | (0.14) |
| Female | 4,146 | 0.3 u | (0.17) | 581 | 0.0 | (0.00) | 775 | 0.2 u | (0.29) | 2,476 | 0.4 u | (0.23) |
| Older adults (age 60+) | 4,721 | 0.9 u | (0.60) | 353 | 0.0 u | (0.18) | 1,003 | 0.1 u | (0.12) | 2,894 | 1.2 u | (1.03) |
| Male | 2,323 | 0.8 u | (0.43) | 152 | 0.1 u | (0.47) | 459 | 0.0 u | (0.20) | 1,497 | 1.1 u | (0.64) |
| Female | 2,398 | 0.9 u | (1.01) | 201 | 0.0 | (0.00) | 544 | 0.1 u | (0.15) | 1,397 | 1.3 u | (1.86) |

Notes: Significant differences in means and proportions are noted by * (.05 level), ** (.01 level), or *** (.001 level). Differences are tested in comparison to FSP participants, identified as persons in households receiving food stamps in the past 12 months.

[1] Acceptable Macronutrient Distribution Ranges (AMDR) are the ranges of intake for macronutrients, as a percent of total food energy, associated with reduced risk of chronic disease while providing intakes of essential nutrients.

Source: NHANES 1999-2004 dietary recalls. Excludes pregnant and breastfeeding women and infants. 'Total Persons' includes persons with missing food stamp participation or income. Data reflect nutrient intake from foods and do not include the contribution of vitamin and mineral supplements. Usual intake was estimated using C-SIDE: Software for Intake Distribution Estimation. Estimates are age adjusted.

# Table B-28. Protein (g)

| | Total Persons | | | Food Stamp Program Participants | | | Income-eligible Nonparticipants | | | Higher-income Nonparticipants | | |
|---|---|---|---|---|---|---|---|---|---|---|---|---|
| | Sample size | Mean | Standard error | Sample size | Mean | Standard error | Sample size | Mean | Standard error | Sample size | Mean | Standard error |
| **Mean Usual Intake** | | | | | | | | | | | | |
| All persons ............ | 25,170 | 78.7 | (0.51) | 4,020 | 73.4 | (1.58) | 5,370 | 74.6 | (1.20) | 13,934 | ***80.0 | (0.60) |
| Male ............... | 12,747 | 91.4 | (0.79) | 1,936 | 85.5 | (2.69) | 2,702 | 89.6 | (2.04) | 7,201 | *92.2 | (0.92) |
| Female ............. | 12,423 | 65.8 | (0.63) | 2,084 | 64.5 | (1.88) | 2,668 | 61.0 | (1.37) | 6,733 | 66.7 | (0.74) |
| Children (age 1-18) ...... | 11,878 | 69.1 | (0.74) | 2,644 | 68.2 | (1.63) | 2,738 | 69.8 | (1.90) | 5,727 | 68.7 | (0.85) |
| Male ............... | 6,000 | 76.3 | (1.26) | 1,343 | 75.6 | (2.70) | 1,389 | 76.8 | (3.13) | 2,867 | 76.2 | (1.44) |
| Female ............. | 5,878 | 61.6 | (0.74) | 1,301 | 61.7 | (2.00) | 1,349 | 61.9 | (2.01) | 2,860 | 60.7 | (0.83) |
| Adults (age 19-59) ...... | 8,570 | 85.8 | (0.84) | 1,022 | 79.6 | (2.94) | 1,629 | 80.8 | (1.80) | 5,313 | **87.6 | (0.99) |
| Male ............... | 4,424 | 101.7 | (1.27) | 441 | 98.3 | (5.55) | 854 | 99.5 | (2.74) | 2,837 | 102.6 | (1.52) |
| Female ............. | 4,146 | 69.3 | (1.09) | 581 | 67.2 | (3.23) | 775 | 62.7 | (2.36) | 2,476 | 70.7 | (1.22) |
| Older adults (age 60+) .. | 4,722 | 68.7 | (0.81) | 354 | 61.3 | (3.33) | 1,003 | 61.5 | (1.61) | 2,894 | **70.7 | (1.06) |
| Male ............... | 2,323 | 79.6 | (1.30) | 152 | 63.6 | (5.54) | 459 | 76.0 | (3.87) | 1,497 | **80.7 | (1.66) |
| Female ............. | 2,399 | 60.3 | (1.02) | 202 | 59.8 | (4.16) | 544 | 54.1 | (1.44) | 1,397 | 61.8 | (1.35) |

Notes: Significant differences in means and proportions are noted by * (.05 level), ** (.01 level), or *** (.001 level). Differences are tested in comparison to FSP participants, identified as persons in households receiving food stamps in the past 12 months.

Source: NHANES 1999-2004 dietary recalls. Excludes pregnant and breastfeeding women and infants. 'Total Persons' includes persons with missing food stamp participation or income. Data reflect nutrient intake from foods and do not include the contribution of vitamin and mineral supplements. Usual intake was estimated using C-SIDE: Software for Intake Distribution Estimation. Estimates are age adjusted.

# Table B-29. Protein (g/kg body weight)

**Mean Usual Intake**

| | Total Persons | | | Food Stamp Program Participants | | | Income-eligible Nonparticipants | | | Higher-income Nonparticipants | | |
|---|---|---|---|---|---|---|---|---|---|---|---|---|
| | Sample size | Mean | Standard error | Sample size | Mean | Standard error | Sample size | Mean | Standard error | Sample size | Mean | Standard error |
| All persons | 24,544 | 1.49 | (0.009) | 3,911 | 1.47 | (0.028) | 5,212 | 1.46 | (0.021) | 13,626 | 1.49 | (0.012) |
| Male | 12,443 | 1.61 | (0.013) | 1,888 | 1.59 | (0.044) | 2,621 | 1.62 | (0.032) | 7,050 | 1.60 | (0.017) |
| Female | 12,101 | 1.37 | (0.013) | 2,023 | 1.37 | (0.036) | 2,591 | 1.31 | (0.028) | 6,576 | 1.37 | (0.016) |
| Children (age 1-18) | 11,615 | 2.34 | (0.023) | 2,585 | 2.41 | (0.053) | 2,685 | 2.38 | (0.049) | 5,599 | 2.30 | (0.031) |
| Male | 5,874 | 2.49 | (0.034) | 1,312 | 2.55 | (0.077) | 1,364 | 2.51 | (0.070) | 2,809 | 2.45 | (0.046) |
| Female | 5,741 | 2.19 | (0.032) | 1,273 | 2.28 | (0.074) | 1,321 | 2.22 | (0.074) | 2,790 | 2.13 | (0.041) |
| Adults (age 19-59) | 8,438 | 1.23 | (0.012) | 999 | 1.20 | (0.048) | 1,592 | 1.19 | (0.028) | 5,249 | 1.24 | (0.014) |
| Male | 4,357 | 1.35 | (0.016) | 432 | 1.38 | (0.085) | 832 | 1.38 | (0.039) | 2,805 | 1.35 | (0.020) |
| Female | 4,081 | 1.11 | (0.019) | 567 | 1.08 | (0.057) | 760 | 1.01 | (0.040) | 2,444 | 1.13 | (0.021) |
| Older adults (age 60+) | 4,491 | 1.03 | (0.013) | 327 | 0.96 | (0.049) | 935 | 0.97 | (0.030) | 2,778 | 1.05 | (0.015) |
| Male | 2,212 | 1.09 | (0.018) | 144 | 0.91 | (0.080) | 425 | 1.09 | (0.063) | 1,436 | 1.09 | (0.022) |
| Female | 2,279 | 0.99 | (0.017) | 183 | 0.99 | (0.063) | 510 | 0.91 | (0.032) | 1,342 | 1.01 | (0.020) |

**Percent of Persons with Usual Intake Greater than Estimated Average Requirement (EAR)[1]**

| | Total Persons | | | Food Stamp Program Participants | | | Income-eligible Nonparticipants | | | Higher-income Nonparticipants | | |
|---|---|---|---|---|---|---|---|---|---|---|---|---|
| | Sample size | Mean | Standard error | Sample size | Mean | Standard error | Sample size | Mean | Standard error | Sample size | Mean | Standard error |
| All persons | 24,544 | 96.8 | (0.24) | 3,911 | 93.0 | (1.21) | 5,212 | 93.9 | (0.88) | 13,626 | *** 97.5 | (0.22) |
| Male | 12,443 | 98.6 | (0.15) | 1,888 | 95.7 | (1.57) | 2,621 | 97.5 | (0.53) | 7,050 | ** 98.8 | (0.16) |
| Female | 12,101 | 95.0 | (0.45) | 2,023 | 91.0 | (1.76) | 2,591 | 90.8 | (1.59) | 6,576 | ** 96.0 | (0.43) |
| Children (age 1-18) | 11,615 | 97.9 | (0.22) | 2,585 | 96.4 | (0.84) | 2,685 | 97.4 | (0.63) | 5,599 | * 98.2 | (0.25) |
| Male | 5,874 | 99.1 | (0.20) | 1,312 | 98.5 | (0.80) | 1,364 | 98.9 | (0.53) | 2,809 | 99.3 | (0.18) |
| Female | 5,741 | 96.6 | (0.41) | 1,273 | 94.6 | (1.37) | 1,321 | 95.8 | (1.21) | 2,790 | 96.9 | (0.49) |
| Adults (age 19-59) | 8,438 | 97.4 | (0.36) | 999 | 93.7 | (1.66) | 1,592 | 94.8 | (1.25) | 5,249 | ** 98.2 | (0.30) |
| Male | 4,357 | 99.0 | (0.19) | 432 | 97.6 | (1.24) | 832 | 98.3 | (0.54) | 2,805 | 99.3 | (0.20) |
| Female | 4,081 | 95.8 | (0.71) | 567 | 91.2 | (2.63) | 760 | 91.5 | (2.40) | 2,444 | 97.0 | (0.59) |
| Older adults (age 60+) | 4,491 | 93.4 | (0.75) | 327 | 87.8 | (3.68) | 935 | 88.4 | (2.01) | 2,778 | 94.5 | (0.84) |
| Male | 2,212 | 95.6 | (0.61) | 144 | 85.9 | (7.90) | 425 | 93.3 | (2.04) | 1,436 | 96.0 | (0.87) |
| Female | 2,279 | 91.7 | (1.25) | 183 | 89.0 | (3.44) | 510 | 85.9 | (2.85) | 1,342 | 93.2 | (1.38) |

Notes: Significant differences in means and proportions are noted by * (.05 level), ** (.01 level), or *** (.001 level). Differences are tested in comparison to FSP participants, identified as persons in households receiving food stamps in the past 12 months.

[1] The Dietary Reference Intakes (DRI) Estimated Average Requirement (EAR) is used to assess the adequacy of intakes for population groups. The EAR refers to protein per kg of body weight falling in the healthy range. Individuals with body weight outside the healthy range were assigned a reference weight corresponding to the weight closest to actual that yields a BMI in the healthy range. The reference weight was then used to measure protein per kg body weight. See Appendix A for details.

Source: NHANES 1999–2004 dietary recalls. Excludes pregnant and breastfeeding women and infants. 'Total Persons' includes persons with missing food stamp participation or income. Data reflect nutrient intake from foods and do not include the contribution of vitamin and mineral supplements. Usual intake was estimated using C-SIDE: Software for Intake Distribution Estimation. Estimates are age adjusted.

# Table B-30. Protein (% of energy intake)

| | Total Persons | | | Food Stamp Program Participants | | | Income-eligible Nonparticipants | | | Higher-income Nonparticipants | | |
|---|---|---|---|---|---|---|---|---|---|---|---|---|
| | Sample size | Mean | Standard error | Sample size | Mean | Standard error | Sample size | Mean | Standard error | Sample size | Mean | Standard error |
| **Mean Usual Intake** | | | | | | | | | | | | |
| All persons ......... | 25,165 | 14.8 | (0.07) | 4,017 | 14.6 | (0.25) | 5,368 | 14.6 | (0.16) | 13,934 | 14.9 | (0.08) |
| Male ......... | 12,743 | 15.0 | (0.09) | 1,934 | 14.9 | (0.28) | 2,700 | 14.9 | (0.22) | 7,201 | 15.0 | (0.11) |
| Female ......... | 12,422 | 14.7 | (0.10) | 2,083 | 14.4 | (0.37) | 2,668 | 14.3 | (0.22) | 6,733 | 14.8 | (0.11) |
| Children (age 1-18) ......... | 11,875 | 13.8 | (0.08) | 2,643 | 13.8 | (0.23) | 2,736 | 13.8 | (0.20) | 5,727 | 13.7 | (0.10) |
| Male ......... | 5,997 | 13.9 | (0.12) | 1,342 | 14.0 | (0.32) | 1,387 | 13.8 | (0.29) | 2,867 | 13.9 | (0.15) |
| Female ......... | 5,878 | 13.6 | (0.12) | 1,301 | 13.6 | (0.33) | 1,349 | 13.8 | (0.25) | 2,860 | 13.5 | (0.14) |
| Adults (age 19-59) ......... | 8,569 | 15.1 | (0.10) | 1,021 | 14.4 | (0.34) | 1,629 | 14.3 | (0.23) | 5,313 | 15.2 | (0.11) |
| Male ......... | 4,423 | 15.2 | (0.13) | 440 | 14.9 | (0.40) | 854 | 14.8 | (0.36) | 2,837 | 15.3 | (0.16) |
| Female ......... | 4,146 | 14.9 | (0.16) | 581 | 14.1 | (0.49) | 775 | 13.9 | (0.30) | 2,476 | 15.1 | (0.16) |
| Older adults (age 60+) .. | 4,721 | 15.9 | (0.15) | 353 | 15.8 | (0.55) | 1,003 | 16.1 | (0.30) | 2,894 | 15.8 | (0.16) |
| Male ......... | 2,323 | 16.0 | (0.19) | 152 | 15.5 | (0.74) | 459 | 16.6 | (0.48) | 1,497 | 15.9 | (0.22) |
| Female ......... | 2,398 | 15.8 | (0.22) | 201 | 16.0 | (0.76) | 544 | 15.9 | (0.38) | 1,397 | 15.7 | (0.23) |
| **Percent of Persons with Usual Intake Below the AMDR[1]** | | | | | | | | | | | | |
| All persons ......... | 25,165 | 1.6 | (0.16) | 4,017 | 3.9 | (0.80) | 5,368 | 2.6 | (0.53) | 13,934 | ** 1.2 | (0.16) |
| Male ......... | 12,743 | 0.8 | (0.16) | 1,934 | 1.8 u | (0.71) | 2,700 | 1.1 u | (0.34) | 7,201 | 0.8 u | (0.18) |
| Female ......... | 12,422 | 2.5 | (0.29) | 2,083 | 5.4 | (1.29) | 2,668 | 3.9 | (0.97) | 6,733 | ** 1.7 | (0.26) |
| Children (age 1-18) ......... | 11,875 | 1.3 | (0.21) | 2,643 | 1.9 u | (0.80) | 2,736 | 1.5 u | (0.57) | 5,727 | 1.3 | (0.23) |
| Male ......... | 5,997 | 0.6 u | (0.20) | 1,342 | 1.2 u | (0.96) | 1,387 | 0.8 u | (0.65) | 2,867 | 0.6 u | (0.22) |
| Female ......... | 5,878 | 2.1 | (0.37) | 1,301 | 2.6 u | (1.23) | 1,349 | 2.2 u | (0.92) | 2,860 | 2.0 | (0.42) |
| Adults (age 19-59) ......... | 8,569 | 2.2 | (0.28) | 1,021 | 6.6 | (1.61) | 1,629 | 4.4 | (1.02) | 5,313 | ** 1.4 | (0.24) |
| Male ......... | 4,423 | 1.2 | (0.26) | 440 | 2.7 u | (1.16) | 854 | 1.9 u | (0.68) | 2,837 | 1.0 u | (0.30) |
| Female ......... | 4,146 | 3.3 | (0.51) | 581 | 9.1 | (2.56) | 775 | 6.8 | (1.91) | 2,476 | ** 1.9 | (0.39) |
| Older adults (age 60+) .. | 4,721 | 0.2 u | (0.09) | 353 | 0.4 u | (0.39) | 1,003 | 0.2 u | (0.10) | 2,894 | 0.2 u | (0.09) |
| Male ......... | 2,323 | 0.0 u | (0.06) | 152 | 0.4 u | (0.62) | 459 | 0.0 u | (0.14) | 1,497 | 0.0 u | (0.01) |
| Female ......... | 2,398 | 0.3 u | (0.15) | 201 | 0.4 u | (0.50) | 544 | 0.3 u | (0.14) | 1,397 | 0.3 u | (0.17) |

See footnotes at end of table.

**Table B-30. (Continued)**

### Percent of Persons with Usual Intake Within the AMDR[1]

| | Total Persons | | | Food Stamp Program Participants | | | Income-eligible Nonparticipants | | | Higher-income Nonparticipants | | |
|---|---|---|---|---|---|---|---|---|---|---|---|---|
| | Sample size | Mean | Standard error | Sample size | Mean | Standard error | Sample size | Mean | Standard error | Sample size | Mean | Standard error |
| All persons | 25,165 | 98.3 | (0.16) | 4,017 | 96.1 | (0.80) | 5,368 | 97.4 | (0.53) | 13,934 | ** 98.8 | (0.16) |
| Male | 12,743 | 99.1 | (0.16) | 1,934 | 98.2 | (0.71) | 2,700 | 98.8 | (0.34) | 7,201 | 99.2 | (0.19) |
| Female | 12,422 | 97.5 | (0.29) | 2,083 | 94.6 | (1.29) | 2,668 | 96.1 | (0.97) | 6,733 | ** 98.3 | (0.26) |
| Children (age 1-18) | 11,875 | 98.5 | (0.21) | 2,643 | 98.0 | (0.80) | 2,736 | 98.4 | (0.58) | 5,727 | 98.6 | (0.24) |
| Male | 5,997 | 99.2 | (0.21) | 1,342 | 98.7 | (0.97) | 1,387 | 99.0 | (0.68) | 2,867 | 99.2 | (0.25) |
| Female | 5,878 | 97.8 | (0.37) | 1,301 | 97.3 | (1.24) | 1,349 | 97.7 | (0.92) | 2,860 | 97.9 | (0.43) |
| Adults (age 19-59) | 8,569 | 97.8 | (0.28) | 1,021 | 93.4 | (1.61) | 1,629 | 95.6 | (1.02) | 5,313 | ** 98.6 | (0.24) |
| Male | 4,423 | 98.8 | (0.26) | 440 | 97.3 | (1.16) | 854 | 98.1 | (0.68) | 2,837 | 99.0 | (0.30) |
| Female | 4,146 | 96.7 | (0.51) | 581 | 90.9 | (2.56) | 775 | 93.2 | (1.91) | 2,476 | ** 98.1 | (0.39) |
| Older adults (age 60+) | 4,721 | 99.8 | (0.09) | 353 | 99.6 | (0.39) | 1,003 | 99.8 | (0.10) | 2,894 | 99.8 | (0.09) |
| Male | 2,323 | 100.0 | (0.06) | 152 | 99.6 | (0.62) | 459 | 100.0 | (0.14) | 1,497 | 100.0 | (0.01) |
| Female | 2,398 | 99.7 | (0.15) | 201 | 99.6 | (0.50) | 544 | 99.7 | (0.14) | 1,397 | 99.7 | (0.17) |

### Percent of Persons with Usual Intake Above the AMDR[1]

| | Total Persons | | | Food Stamp Program Participants | | | Income-eligible Nonparticipants | | | Higher-income Nonparticipants | | |
|---|---|---|---|---|---|---|---|---|---|---|---|---|
| | Sample size | Mean | Standard error | Sample size | Mean | Standard error | Sample size | Mean | Standard error | Sample size | Mean | Standard error |
| All persons | 25,165 | 0.0 u | (0.01) | 4,017 | 0.0 u | (0.02) | 5,368 | 0.0 u | (0.03) | 13,934 | 0.0 u | (0.02) |
| Male | 12,743 | 0.0 u | (0.02) | 1,934 | 0.0 u | (0.02) | 2,700 | 0.0 u | (0.05) | 7,201 | 0.0 u | (0.03) |
| Female | 12,422 | 0.0 u | (0.01) | 2,083 | 0.0 u | (0.03) | 2,668 | 0.0 u | (0.03) | 6,733 | 0.0 u | (0.02) |
| Children (age 1-18) | 11,875 | 0.1 u | (0.04) | 2,643 | 0.1 u | (0.05) | 2,736 | 0.1 u | (0.11) | 5,727 | 0.1 u | (0.07) |
| Male | 5,997 | 0.2 u | (0.06) | 1,342 | 0.1 u | (0.07) | 1,387 | 0.1 u | (0.19) | 2,867 | 0.2 u | (0.12) |
| Female | 5,878 | 0.1 u | (0.05) | 1,301 | 0.1 u | (0.07) | 1,349 | 0.1 u | (0.10) | 2,860 | 0.1 u | (0.08) |
| Adults (age 19-59) | 8,569 | 0.0 | (0.00) | 1,021 | 0.0 | (0.00) | 1,629 | 0.0 | (0.00) | 5,313 | 0.0 | (0.00) |
| Male | 4,423 | 0.0 | (0.00) | 440 | 0.0 | (0.00) | 854 | 0.0 | (0.00) | 2,837 | 0.0 | (0.00) |
| Female | 4,146 | 0.0 | (0.00) | 581 | 0.0 | (0.00) | 775 | 0.0 | (0.00) | 2,476 | 0.0 | (0.00) |
| Older adults (age 60+) | 4,721 | 0.0 | (0.00) | 353 | 0.0 | (0.00) | 1,003 | 0.0 | (0.00) | 2,894 | 0.0 | (0.00) |
| Male | 2,323 | 0.0 | (0.00) | 152 | 0.0 | (0.00) | 459 | 0.0 | (0.00) | 1,497 | 0.0 | (0.00) |
| Female | 2,398 | 0.0 | (0.00) | 201 | 0.0 | (0.00) | 544 | 0.0 | (0.00) | 1,397 | 0.0 | (0.00) |

Notes: Significant differences in means and proportions are noted by * (.05 level), ** (.01 level), or *** (.001 level). Differences are tested in comparison to FSP participants, identified as persons in households receiving food stamps in the past 12 months.

u Denotes individual estimates not meeting the standards of reliability or precision due to inadequate cell size or large coefficient of variation.

[1] Acceptable Macronutrient Distribution Ranges (AMDR) are the ranges of intake for macronutrients, as a percent of total food energy, associated with reduced risk of chronic disease while providing intakes of essential nutrients.

Source: NHANES 1999–2004 dietary recalls. Excludes pregnant and breastfeeding women and infants. 'Total Persons' includes persons with missing food stamp participation or income. Data reflect nutrient intake from foods and do not include the contribution of vitamin and mineral supplements. Usual intake was estimated using C-SIDE: Software for Intake Distribution Estimation. Estimates are age adjusted.

# Table B-31. Carbohydrates (g)

| | Total Persons | | | Food Stamp Program Participants | | | Income-eligible Nonparticipants | | | Higher-income Nonparticipants | | |
|---|---|---|---|---|---|---|---|---|---|---|---|---|
| | Sample size | Mean | Standard error | Sample size | Mean | Standard error | Sample size | Mean | Standard error | Sample size | Mean | Standard error |
| **Mean Usual Intake** | | | | | | | | | | | | |
| All persons | 25,170 | 274 | (1.7) | 4,020 | 268 | (5.8) | 5,370 | 272 | (4.6) | 13,934 | 276 | (1.9) |
| Male | 12,747 | 310 | (2.8) | 1,936 | 302 | (10.4) | 2,702 | 313 | (7.9) | 7,201 | 311 | (2.9) |
| Female | 12,423 | 238 | (2.0) | 2,084 | 243 | (6.7) | 2,668 | 234 | (4.7) | 6,733 | 237 | (2.4) |
| Children (age 1-18) | 11,878 | 276 | (2.6) | 2,644 | 270 | (5.9) | 2,738 | 277 | (7.5) | 5,727 | 277 | (3.0) |
| Male | 6,000 | 301 | (4.2) | 1,343 | 293 | (9.0) | 1,389 | 303 | (12.4) | 2,867 | 303 | (4.6) |
| Female | 5,878 | 250 | (3.1) | 1,301 | 249 | (7.7) | 1,349 | 247 | (6.5) | 2,860 | 250 | (3.7) |
| Adults (age 19-59) | 8,570 | 288 | (2.6) | 1,022 | 290 | (9.9) | 1,629 | 298 | (7.5) | 5,313 | 286 | (2.9) |
| Male | 4,424 | 332 | (4.2) | 441 | 341 | (17.9) | 854 | 348 | (12.8) | 2,837 | 330 | (4.7) |
| Female | 4,146 | 242 | (3.1) | 581 | 257 | (11.3) | 775 | 249 | (7.9) | 2,476 | 237 | (3.3) |
| Older adults (age 60+) | 4,722 | 220 | (2.8) | 354 | 205 | (9.9) | 1,003 | 199 | (6.4) | 2,894 | 225 | (3.2) |
| Male | 2,323 | 247 | (4.9) | 152 | 220 | (16.1) | 459 | 234 | (16.1) | 1,497 | 249 | (4.6) |
| Female | 2,399 | 198 | (3.3) | 202 | 196 | (12.5) | 544 | 181 | (5.3) | 1,397 | 204 | (4.4) |
| **Percent of Persons with Usual Intake Greater than Estimated Average Requirement (EAR)[1]** | | | | | | | | | | | | |
| All persons | 25,170 | 99.4 | (0.06) | 4,020 | 98.7 | (0.39) | 5,370 | 98.9 | (0.23) | 13,934 | 99.6 | (0.06) |
| Male | 12,747 | 99.8 | (0.03) | 1,936 | 99.4 | (0.23) | 2,702 | 99.6 | (0.17) | 7,201 | 99.8 | (0.04) |
| Female | 12,423 | 99.1 | (0.12) | 2,084 | 98.2 | (0.62) | 2,668 | 98.4 | (0.38) | 6,733 | 99.4 | (0.11) |
| Children (age 1-18) | 11,878 | 99.8 | (0.04) | 2,644 | 99.7 | (0.14) | 2,738 | 99.8 | (0.09) | 5,727 | 99.8 | (0.06) |
| Male | 6,000 | 99.8 | (0.05) | 1,343 | 99.7 | (0.13) | 1,389 | 99.8 | (0.14) | 2,867 | 99.9 | (0.08) |
| Female | 5,878 | 99.8 | (0.06) | 1,301 | 99.7 | (0.23) | 1,349 | 99.8 | (0.08) | 2,860 | 99.8 | (0.09) |
| Adults (age 19-59) | 8,570 | 99.4 | (0.11) | 1,022 | 98.8 | (0.48) | 1,629 | 99.4 | (0.20) | 5,313 | 99.6 | (0.09) |
| Male | 4,424 | 99.9 | (0.05) | 441 | 99.7 | (0.27) | 854 | 99.8 | (0.13) | 2,837 | 100.0 | (0.06) |
| Female | 4,146 | 98.9 | (0.21) | 581 | 98.2 | (0.78) | 775 | 98.9 | (0.37) | 2,476 | 99.1 | (0.18) |
| Older adults (age 60+) | 4,722 | 98.9 | (0.16) | 354 | 97.1 | (1.61) | 1,003 | 97.1 | (0.88) | 2,894 | 99.3 | (0.12) |
| Male | 2,323 | 99.4 | (0.13) | 152 | 98.0 | (1.17) | 459 | 98.6 | (0.62) | 1,497 | 99.5 | (0.16) |
| Female | 2,399 | 98.6 | (0.27) | 202 | 96.6 | (2.49) | 544 | 96.4 | (1.29) | 1,397 | 99.2 | (0.18) |

Notes: Significant differences in means and proportions are noted by * (.05 level), ** (.01 level), or *** (.001 level). Differences are tested in comparison to FSP participants, identified as persons in households receiving food stamps in the past 12 months.

[1] The Dietary Reference Intakes (DRI) Estimated Average Requirement (EAR) is used to assess the adequacy of intakes for population groups.

Source: NHANES 1999-2004 dietary recalls. Excludes pregnant and breastfeeding women and infants. 'Total Persons' includes persons with missing food stamp participation or income. Data reflect nutrient intake from foods and do not include the contribution of vitamin and mineral supplements. Usual intake was estimated using C-SIDE: Software for Intake Distribution Estimation. Estimates are age adjusted.

# Table B-32. Carbohydrate (% of energy intake)

| | Total Persons | | | Food Stamp Program Participants | | | Income-eligible Nonparticipants | | | Higher-income Nonparticipants | | |
|---|---|---|---|---|---|---|---|---|---|---|---|---|
| | Sample size | Mean | Standard error | Sample size | Mean | Standard error | Sample size | Mean | Standard error | Sample size | Mean | Standard error |
| **Mean Usual Intake** | | | | | | | | | | | | |
| All persons ........... | 25,165 | 51.4 | (0.16) | 4,017 | 52.4 | (0.47) | 5,368 | 52.7 | (0.39) | 13,934 | ** 51.1 | (0.19) |
| Male ........... | 12,743 | 50.5 | (0.21) | 1,934 | 51.5 | (0.76) | 2,700 | 51.6 | (0.61) | 7,201 | 50.4 | (0.26) |
| Female ........... | 12,422 | 52.3 | (0.24) | 2,083 | 53.1 | (0.60) | 2,668 | 53.6 | (0.50) | 6,733 | 51.9 | (0.28) |
| Children (age 1-18) ....... | 11,875 | 54.9 | (0.19) | 2,643 | 54.2 | (0.50) | 2,736 | 54.5 | (0.41) | 5,727 | 55.2 | (0.26) |
| Male ........... | 5,997 | 54.8 | (0.24) | 1,342 | 54.2 | (0.72) | 1,387 | 54.4 | (0.56) | 2,867 | 55.2 | (0.36) |
| Female ........... | 5,878 | 55.0 | (0.29) | 1,301 | 54.2 | (0.68) | 1,349 | 54.6 | (0.62) | 2,860 | 55.3 | (0.37) |
| Adults (age 19-59) ......... | 8,569 | 50.0 | (0.26) | 1,021 | 52.0 | (0.62) | 1,629 | 52.5 | (0.63) | 5,313 | *** 49.3 | (0.30) |
| Male ........... | 4,423 | 48.9 | (0.33) | 440 | 50.1 | (0.98) | 854 | 51.1 | (0.87) | 2,837 | 48.4 | (0.40) |
| Female ........... | 4,146 | 51.2 | (0.40) | 581 | 53.2 | (0.80) | 775 | 53.8 | (0.91) | 2,476 | ** 50.2 | (0.46) |
| Older adults (age 60+) .. | 4,721 | 50.6 | (0.34) | 353 | 52.0 | (1.41) | 1,003 | 51.5 | (0.67) | 2,894 | 50.3 | (0.39) |
| Male ........... | 2,323 | 49.2 | (0.44) | 152 | 52.3 | (2.27) | 459 | 50.1 | (1.36) | 1,497 | 48.9 | (0.49) |
| Female ........... | 2,398 | 51.8 | (0.50) | 201 | 51.9 | (1.79) | 544 | 52.3 | (0.73) | 1,397 | 51.6 | (0.60) |
| **Percent of Persons with Usual Intake Below the AMDR[1]** | | | | | | | | | | | | |
| All persons ........... | 25,165 | 16.4 | (0.73) | 4,017 | 13.0 | (1.81) | 5,368 | 11.6 | (1.45) | 13,934 | * 17.6 | (0.91) |
| Male ........... | 12,743 | 19.9 | (1.15) | 1,934 | 16.3 | (3.14) | 2,700 | 15.6 | (2.68) | 7,201 | 20.8 | (1.35) |
| Female ........... | 12,422 | 13.1 | (0.89) | 2,083 | 10.7 | (2.15) | 2,668 | 8.4 | (1.37) | 6,733 | 14.4 | (1.18) |
| Children (age 1-18) ....... | 11,875 | 1.8 | (0.24) | 2,643 | 2.7 | (0.70) | 2,736 | 2.5 | (0.62) | 5,727 | 1.5 | (0.35) |
| Male ........... | 5,997 | 1.5 | (0.28) | 1,342 | 2.6 u | (0.93) | 1,387 | 2.6 u | (0.96) | 2,867 | 1.2 u | (0.40) |
| Female ........... | 5,878 | 2.0 | (0.39) | 1,301 | 2.9 u | (1.09) | 1,349 | 2.4 u | (0.78) | 2,860 | 1.8 u | (0.55) |
| Adults (age 19-59) ......... | 8,569 | 24.9 | (1.18) | 1,021 | 19.0 | (2.34) | 1,629 | 16.1 | (2.46) | 5,313 | ** 27.6 | (1.50) |
| Male ........... | 4,423 | 29.8 | (1.73) | 440 | 25.7 | (4.19) | 854 | 21.3 | (4.35) | 2,837 | * 31.9 | (2.19) |
| Female ........... | 4,146 | 19.9 | (1.60) | 581 | 14.6 | (2.74) | 775 | 11.0 | (2.38) | 2,476 | * 22.7 | (2.02) |
| Older adults (age 60+) .. | 4,721 | 20.7 | (1.39) | 353 | 17.1 | (4.99) | 1,003 | 16.7 | (2.72) | 2,894 | 21.6 | (1.59) |
| Male ........... | 2,323 | 28.7 | (2.21) | 152 | 21.5 u | (7.50) | 459 | 27.5 | (6.16) | 1,497 | 28.9 | (2.28) |
| Female ........... | 2,398 | 14.4 | (1.77) | 201 | 14.5 u | (6.60) | 544 | 11.2 | (2.66) | 1,397 | 15.2 | (2.21) |

See footnotes at end of table.

## Table B-32. (Continued)

| | Total Persons | | | Food Stamp Program Participants | | | Income-eligible Nonparticipants | | | Higher-income Nonparticipants | | |
|---|---|---|---|---|---|---|---|---|---|---|---|---|
| | Sample size | Mean | Standard error | Sample size | Mean | Standard error | Sample size | Mean | Standard error | Sample size | Mean | Standard error |
| **Percent of Persons with Usual Intake Within the AMDR[1]** | | | | | | | | | | | | |
| All persons | 25,165 | 82.1 | (0.74) | 4,017 | 83.9 | (1.94) | 5,368 | 86.0 | (1.55) | 13,934 | 81.2 | (0.93) |
| Male | 12,743 | 79.3 | (1.16) | 1,934 | 81.6 | (3.23) | 2,700 | 83.0 | (2.72) | 7,201 | 78.4 | (1.36) |
| Female | 12,422 | 84.8 | (0.93) | 2,083 | 85.2 | (2.41) | 2,668 | 88.2 | (1.69) | 6,733 | 84.0 | (1.21) |
| Children (age 1-18) | 11,875 | 96.6 | (0.33) | 2,643 | 95.7 | (0.89) | 2,736 | 96.1 | (0.81) | 5,727 | 96.8 | (0.46) |
| Male | 5,997 | 97.2 | (0.38) | 1,342 | 96.2 | (1.17) | 1,387 | 96.3 | (1.12) | 2,867 | 97.4 | (0.57) |
| Female | 5,878 | 96.0 | (0.55) | 1,301 | 94.9 | (1.42) | 1,349 | 95.8 | (1.24) | 2,860 | 96.2 | (0.72) |
| Adults (age 19-59) | 8,569 | 72.6 | (1.22) | 1,021 | 75.6 | (2.70) | 1,629 | 79.2 | (2.73) | 5,313 | 70.8 | (1.52) |
| Male | 4,423 | 68.6 | (1.75) | 440 | 71.4 | (4.37) | 854 | 75.7 | (4.44) | 2,837 | 66.7 | (2.22) |
| Female | 4,146 | 76.8 | (1.70) | 581 | 78.3 | (3.42) | 775 | 82.6 | (3.21) | 2,476 | 75.4 | (2.06) |
| Older adults (age 60+) | 4,721 | 77.5 | (1.43) | 353 | 77.8 | (5.53) | 1,003 | 81.0 | (2.87) | 2,894 | 76.8 | (1.64) |
| Male | 2,323 | 69.6 | (2.24) | 152 | 70.1 | (8.96) | 459 | 69.2 | (6.39) | 1,497 | 70.0 | (2.30) |
| Female | 2,398 | 83.6 | (1.86) | 201 | 82.5 | (7.04) | 544 | 87.0 | (2.86) | 1,397 | 82.9 | (2.33) |
| **Percent of Persons with Usual Intake Above the AMDR[1]** | | | | | | | | | | | | |
| All persons | 25,165 | 1.5 | (0.15) | 4,017 | 3.1 u | (0.71) | 5,368 | 2.3 | (0.56) | 13,934 | ** 1.2 | (0.15) |
| Male | 12,743 | 0.8 | (0.11) | 1,934 | 2.0 u | (0.78) | 2,700 | 1.4 u | (0.42) | 7,201 | 0.8 u | (0.15) |
| Female | 12,422 | 2.2 | (0.27) | 2,083 | 4.0 | (1.10) | 2,668 | 3.3 u | (1.00) | 6,733 | * 1.6 | (0.27) |
| Children (age 1-18) | 11,875 | 1.6 | (0.23) | 2,643 | 1.6 u | (0.56) | 2,736 | 1.4 u | (0.53) | 5,727 | 1.7 | (0.31) |
| Male | 5,997 | 1.2 | (0.26) | 1,342 | 1.2 u | (0.70) | 1,387 | 1.2 u | (0.57) | 2,867 | 1.4 | (0.41) |
| Female | 5,878 | 2.0 | (0.39) | 1,301 | 2.2 u | (0.91) | 1,349 | 1.8 u | (0.97) | 2,860 | 1.9 | (0.47) |
| Adults (age 19-59) | 8,569 | 2.4 | (0.31) | 1,021 | 5.4 | (1.33) | 1,629 | 4.7 | (1.18) | 5,313 | ** 1.6 | (0.27) |
| Male | 4,423 | 1.7 | (0.26) | 440 | 2.8 u | (1.25) | 854 | 3.0 | (0.89) | 2,837 | 1.4 | (0.34) |
| Female | 4,146 | 3.2 | (0.56) | 581 | 7.1 | (2.05) | 775 | 6.4 u | (2.16) | 2,476 | * 1.9 | (0.42) |
| Older adults (age 60+) | 4,721 | 1.9 | (0.36) | 353 | 5.1 u | (2.40) | 1,003 | 2.3 u | (0.90) | 2,894 | 1.5 | (0.42) |
| Male | 2,323 | 1.7 | (0.37) | 152 | 8.4 u | (4.90) | 459 | 3.3 u | (1.71) | 1,497 | 1.1 | (0.30) |
| Female | 2,398 | 2.0 | (0.57) | 201 | 3.1 u | (2.44) | 544 | 1.8 u | (1.04) | 1,397 | 1.9 u | (0.74) |

Notes: Significant differences in means and proportions are noted by * (.05 level), ** (.01 level), or *** (.001 level). Differences are tested in comparison to FSP participants, identified as persons in households receiving food stamps in the past 12 months.

u Denotes individual estimates not meeting the standards of reliability or precision due to inadequate cell size or large coefficient of variation.

[1] Acceptable Macronutrient Distribution Ranges (AMDR) are the ranges of intake for macronutrients, as a percent of total food energy, associated with reduced risk of chronic disease while providing intakes of essential nutrients.

Source: NHANES 1999-2004 dietary recalls. Excludes pregnant and breastfeeding women and infants. 'Total Persons' includes persons with missing food stamp participation or income. Data reflect nutrient intake from foods and do not include the contribution of vitamin and mineral supplements. Usual intake was estimated using C-SIDE: Software for Intake Distribution Estimation. Estimates are age adjusted.

# Table B-33. Cholesterol (mg)

| | Total Persons | | | Food Stamp Program Participants | | | Income-eligible Nonparticipants | | | Higher-income Nonparticipants | | |
|---|---|---|---|---|---|---|---|---|---|---|---|---|
| | Sample size | Mean | Standard error | Sample size | Mean | Standard error | Sample size | Mean | Standard error | Sample size | Mean | Standard error |
| **Mean Usual Intake** | | | | | | | | | | | | |
| All persons | 25,170 | 267 | (3.2) | 4,020 | 270 | (9.8) | 5,370 | 265 | (7.3) | 13,934 | 266 | (3.3) |
| Male | 12,747 | 312 | (4.8) | 1,936 | 326 | (16.1) | 2,702 | 317 | (12.3) | 7,201 | 309 | (5.4) |
| Female | 12,423 | 222 | (4.0) | 2,084 | 231 | (12.0) | 2,668 | 220 | (8.6) | 6,733 | 218 | (3.5) |
| Children (age 1-18) | 11,878 | 222 | (3.4) | 2,644 | 231 | (7.4) | 2,738 | 231 | (7.3) | 5,727 | 214 | (4.2) |
| Male | 6,000 | 246 | (5.6) | 1,343 | 255 | (11.7) | 1,389 | 250 | (10.9) | 2,867 | 241 | (7.2) |
| Female | 5,878 | 197 | (3.8) | 1,301 | 210 | (9.5) | 1,349 | 209 | (9.6) | 2,860 | 185 | (4.3) |
| Adults (age 19-59) | 8,570 | 295 | (4.8) | 1,022 | 290 | (14.3) | 1,629 | 289 | (11.6) | 5,313 | 297 | (6.8) |
| Male | 4,424 | 352 | (8.6) | 441 | 369 | (24.7) | 854 | 350 | (17.8) | 2,837 | 352 | (12.2) |
| Female | 4,146 | 235 | (3.9) | 581 | 239 | (17.2) | 775 | 231 | (15.1) | 2,476 | 235 | (4.9) |
| Older adults (age 60+) | 4,722 | 244 | (9.9) | 354 | 258 | (33.3) | 1,003 | 228 | (10.9) | 2,894 | 246 | (7.1) |
| Male | 2,323 | 281 | (10.3) | 152 | 285 | (49.3) | 459 | 295 | (23.0) | 1,497 | 280 | (10.8) |
| Female | 2,399 | 215 | (15.7) | 202 | 242 | (44.4) | 544 | 194 | (11.5) | 1,397 | 217 | (9.3) |
| **Percent of Persons Meeting Dietary Guidelines Recommendation[1]** | | | | | | | | | | | | |
| All persons | 25,170 | 68.2 | (1.18) | 4,020 | 67.2 | (3.00) | 5,370 | 69.3 | (2.18) | 13,934 | 68.3 | (1.20) |
| Male | 12,747 | 52.8 | (1.69) | 1,936 | 48.9 | (4.65) | 2,702 | 52.4 | (3.50) | 7,201 | 53.4 | (2.02) |
| Female | 12,423 | 83.8 | (1.63) | 2,084 | 80.0 | (3.82) | 2,668 | 84.1 | (2.72) | 6,733 | 84.7 | (1.13) |
| Children (age 1-18) | 11,878 | 85.1 | (1.26) | 2,644 | 83.4 | (2.50) | 2,738 | 83.4 | (2.66) | 5,727 | 86.7 | (1.62) |
| Male | 6,000 | 77.7 | (2.25) | 1,343 | 76.1 | (4.35) | 1,389 | 77.3 | (4.34) | 2,867 | 79.0 | (3.11) |
| Female | 5,878 | 93.0 | (1.03) | 1,301 | 89.7 | (2.75) | 1,349 | 89.9 | (2.82) | 2,860 | 95.1 | (0.92) |
| Adults (age 19-59) | 8,570 | 58.1 | (1.52) | 1,022 | 59.2 | (4.76) | 1,629 | 60.2 | (3.57) | 5,313 | 57.4 | (2.43) |
| Male | 4,424 | 38.0 | (2.55) | 441 | 33.0 | (7.33) | 854 | 40.4 | (5.07) | 2,837 | 37.7 | (4.21) |
| Female | 4,146 | 79.1 | (1.60) | 581 | 76.5 | (6.24) | 775 | 79.3 | (5.03) | 2,476 | 79.5 | (2.04) |
| Older adults (age 60+) | 4,722 | 75.0 | (3.20) | 354 | 70.3 | (9.88) | 1,003 | 79.7 | (3.05) | 2,894 | 74.4 | (2.48) |
| Male | 2,323 | 63.8 | (3.21) | 152 | 62.7 | (14.30) | 459 | 59.9 | (6.45) | 1,497 | 64.0 | (3.43) |
| Female | 2,399 | 83.8 | (5.11) | 202 | 74.9 | (13.30) | 544 | 89.7 | (3.24) | 1,397 | 83.6 | (3.56) |

Notes: Significant differences in means and proportions are noted by * (.05 level), ** (.01 level), or *** (.001 level). Differences are tested in comparison to FSP participants, identified as persons in households receiving food stamps in the past 12 months.

[1] Recommended intake of cholesterol is less than or equal to 300 mg per day.

Source: NHANES 1999–2004 dietary recalls. Excludes pregnant and breastfeeding women and infants. 'Total Persons' includes persons with missing food stamp participation or income. Data reflect nutrient intake from foods and do not include the contribution of vitamin and mineral supplements. Usual intake was estimated using C-SIDE: Software for Intake Distribution Estimation. Estimates are age adjusted.

# APPENDIX C: OTHER DETAILED TABLES

## LIST OF TABLES

# Table C-1. Mean Percent of Energy From Solid Fats, Alcoholic Beverages, and Added Sugars (SoFAAS) - All Persons[1]

| | Total Persons | | | Food Stamp Program Participants | | | Income-eligible Nonparticipants | | | Higher-income Nonparticipants | | |
|---|---|---|---|---|---|---|---|---|---|---|---|---|
| | Sample size | Mean percent of calories | Standard Error | Sample size | Mean percent of calories | Standard Error | Sample size | Mean percent of calories | Standard Error | Sample size | Mean percent of calories | Standard Error |
| **Both sexes** | | | | | | | | | | | | |
| Daily intake ............ | 16,415 | 38.3 | (0.36) | 2,301 | 40.6 | (0.74) | 3,575 | ***38.6 | (0.59) | 9,094 | ***38.0 | (0.32) |
| Breakfast ............. | 13,087 | 34.3 | (0.44) | 1,712 | 37.7 | (1.08) | 2,782 | 35.8 | (0.64) | 7,424 | ***33.7 | (0.49) |
| Lunch ............... | 12,892 | 32.6 | (0.33) | 1,747 | 34.8 | (0.87) | 2,736 | *32.8 | (0.78) | 7,320 | **32.2 | (0.30) |
| Dinner ............... | 14,240 | 31.7 | (0.36) | 1,944 | 31.6 | (0.88) | 2,922 | 31.7 | (0.51) | 8,149 | 31.8 | (0.37) |
| Snacks .............. | 14,391 | 50.8 | (0.54) | 2,011 | 54.5 | (1.14) | 3,067 | *51.6 | (0.89) | 8,065 | ***50.2 | (0.62) |
| **Male** | | | | | | | | | | | | |
| Daily intake ............ | 8,298 | 39.3 | (0.38) | 1,098 | 40.6 | (0.92) | 1,810 | *38.9 | (0.78) | 4,681 | 39.2 | (0.32) |
| Breakfast ............. | 6,571 | 35.2 | (0.51) | 827 | 37.8 | (1.49) | 1,409 | 36.2 | (0.80) | 3,764 | 34.8 | (0.59) |
| Lunch ............... | 6,397 | 33.0 | (0.37) | 858 | 34.1 | (1.55) | 1,343 | 32.4 | (0.84) | 3,663 | 32.8 | (0.38) |
| Dinner ............... | 7,160 | 32.6 | (0.36) | 935 | 31.1 | (1.05) | 1,472 | 32.9 | (0.66) | 4,158 | *32.7 | (0.33) |
| Snacks .............. | 7,246 | 52.8 | (0.55) | 959 | 56.0 | (1.47) | 1,539 | **51.9 | (1.24) | 4,132 | 52.8 | (0.56) |
| **Female** | | | | | | | | | | | | |
| Daily intake ............ | 8,117 | 37.4 | (0.42) | 1,203 | 40.7 | (0.78) | 1,765 | **38.3 | (0.59) | 4,413 | ***36.7 | (0.45) |
| Breakfast ............. | 6,516 | 33.4 | (0.50) | 885 | 37.9 | (1.18) | 1,373 | 35.7 | (1.02) | 3,660 | ***32.6 | (0.64) |
| Lunch ............... | 6,495 | 32.2 | (0.45) | 889 | 35.4 | (1.28) | 1,393 | *33.0 | (1.03) | 3,657 | **31.6 | (0.41) |
| Dinner ............... | 7,080 | 30.7 | (0.49) | 1,009 | 32.1 | (1.01) | 1,450 | 30.5 | (0.82) | 3,991 | 30.8 | (0.56) |
| Snacks .............. | 7,145 | 48.9 | (0.62) | 1,052 | 53.7 | (1.39) | 1,528 | 51.5 | (1.27) | 3,933 | ***47.3 | (0.81) |

Notes: Significant differences in means and proportions are noted by * (.05 level), ** (.01 level), or *** (.001 level). Differences are tested in comparison to FSP participants, identified as persons in households receiving food stamps in the past 12 months.

[1] Calories from solid fats and added sugars were identified from the Pyramid Servings Database compiled by USDA, CNPP. Calories from alcoholic beverages include calories from carbohydrate in beer and wine, and calories from alcohol in all alcoholic beverages except cooking wine.

Sources: NHANES 1999–2002 dietary recalls and MyPyramid Equivalents Database for USDA Survey Food Codes, 1994-2002, Version 1.0, October 2006. Excludes pregnant and breastfeeding women and infants. 'Total Persons' includes persons with missing food stamp participation or income. Percents are age adjusted to account for different age distributions of Food Stamp participants and nonparticipants.

# Table C-1. Mean Percent of Energy From Solid Fats, Alcoholic Beverages, and Added Sugars (SoFAAS) - Children (age 2–18)[1]

| | Total Persons | | | Food Stamp Program Participants | | | Income-eligible Nonparticipants | | | Higher-income Nonparticipants | | |
|---|---|---|---|---|---|---|---|---|---|---|---|---|
| | Sample size | Mean percent of calories | Standard Error | Sample size | Mean percent of calories | Standard Error | Sample size | Mean percent of calories | Standard Error | Sample size | Mean percent of calories | Standard Error |
| **Both sexes** | | | | | | | | | | | | |
| Daily intake | 7,581 | 39.1 | (0.35) | 1,495 | 39.0 | (0.77) | 1,799 | 39.5 | (0.54) | 3,682 | 39.1 | (0.37) |
| Breakfast | 5,958 | 36.2 | (0.53) | 1,154 | 36.1 | (1.12) | 1,380 | 38.0 | (0.88) | 2,933 | 35.8 | (0.57) |
| Lunch | 6,316 | 34.9 | (0.46) | 1,216 | 35.2 | (0.81) | 1,487 | 35.3 | (0.84) | 3,132 | 34.6 | (0.51) |
| Dinner | 6,518 | 33.4 | (0.39) | 1,282 | 32.9 | (0.86) | 1,476 | 33.0 | (0.50) | 3,258 | 33.9 | (0.47) |
| Snacks | 6,792 | 48.0 | (0.64) | 1,337 | 47.1 | (1.39) | 1,591 | 49.0 | (1.22) | 3,322 | 48.1 | (0.73) |
| **Male** | | | | | | | | | | | | |
| Daily intake | 3,822 | 39.3 | (0.51) | 758 | 38.5 | (1.14) | 918 | 40.0 | (0.77) | 1,828 | 39.5 | (0.45) |
| Breakfast | 3,034 | 36.6 | (0.66) | 601 | 33.8 | (1.43) | 717 | 38.1 ** | (0.73) | 1,455 | 36.8 | (0.88) |
| Lunch | 3,182 | 35.1 | (0.49) | 629 | 34.6 | (1.08) | 759 | 36.0 | (1.11) | 1,540 | 34.8 | (0.63) |
| Dinner | 3,255 | 33.6 | (0.56) | 654 | 32.4 | (1.02) | 753 | 33.6 | (0.68) | 1,586 | 34.3 | (0.68) |
| Snacks | 3,389 | 48.1 | (0.83) | 670 | 46.4 | (2.15) | 800 | 48.3 | (1.41) | 1,639 | 48.6 | (0.93) |
| **Female** | | | | | | | | | | | | |
| Daily intake | 3,759 | 38.8 | (0.34) | 737 | 39.6 | (0.85) | 881 | 39.0 | (0.68) | 1,854 | 38.6 | (0.40) |
| Breakfast | 2,924 | 35.8 | (0.60) | 553 | 38.5 | (1.44) | 663 | 37.7 | (1.45) | 1,478 | 34.8 | (0.65) |
| Lunch | 3,134 | 34.6 | (0.56) | 587 | 35.8 | (1.02) | 728 | 34.4 | (0.96) | 1,592 | 34.2 | (0.58) |
| Dinner | 3,263 | 33.1 | (0.39) | 628 | 33.6 | (1.19) | 723 | 32.1 | (0.72) | 1,672 | 33.5 | (0.48) |
| Snacks | 3,403 | 48.0 | (0.75) | 667 | 48.0 | (1.34) | 791 | 49.8 | (1.61) | 1,683 | 47.6 | (0.92) |

Notes: Significant differences in means and proportions are noted by * (.05 level), ** (.01 level), or *** (.001 level). Differences are tested in comparison to FSP participants, identified as persons in households receiving food stamps in the past 12 months.

[1] Calories from solid fats and added sugars were identified from the Pyramid Servings Database compiled by USDA, CNPP. Calories from alcoholic beverages include calories from carbohydrate in beer and wine, and calories from alcohol in all alcoholic beverages except cooking wine.

Sources: NHANES 1999–2002 dietary recalls and MyPyramid Equivalents Database for USDA Survey Food Codes, 1994-2002, Version 1.0, October 2006. Excludes pregnant and breastfeeding women and infants. 'Total Persons' includes persons with missing food stamp participation or income. Percents are age adjusted to account for different age distributions of Food Stamp participants and nonparticipants.

# Table C-1. Mean Percent of Energy From Solid Fats, Alcoholic Beverages, and Added Sugars (SoFAAS) - Adults (age 19–59)[1]

| | Total Persons | | | Food Stamp Program Participants | | | Income-eligible Nonparticipants | | | Higher-income Nonparticipants | | |
|---|---|---|---|---|---|---|---|---|---|---|---|---|
| | Sample size | Mean percent of calories | Standard Error | Sample size | Mean percent of calories | Standard Error | Sample size | Mean percent of calories | Standard Error | Sample size | Mean percent of calories | Standard Error |
| **Both sexes** | | | | | | | | | | | | |
| Daily intake | 5,774 | 39.6 | (0.46) | 592 | 43.3 | (0.93) | 1,124 | ***40.3 | (0.82) | 3,587 | ***39.1 | (0.41) |
| Breakfast | 4,365 | 35.4 | (0.59) | 382 | 40.3 | (1.60) | 835 | 37.3 | (1.03) | 2,800 | ***34.8 | (0.66) |
| Lunch | 4,296 | 32.7 | (0.46) | 399 | 36.7 | (1.16) | 806 | **33.2 | (1.03) | 2,756 | ***32.3 | (0.43) |
| Dinner | 5,017 | 31.9 | (0.47) | 496 | 32.4 | (0.99) | 913 | 32.4 | (0.67) | 3,220 | 31.8 | (0.51) |
| Snacks | 5,079 | 53.9 | (0.72) | 504 | 59.7 | (1.58) | 960 | *55.2 | (1.12) | 3,210 | ***52.9 | (0.83) |
| **Male** | | | | | | | | | | | | |
| Daily intake | 2,964 | 40.7 | (0.51) | 244 | 43.1 | (1.23) | 594 | ***40.0 | (1.00) | 1,903 | *40.6 | (0.49) |
| Breakfast | 2,179 | 36.4 | (0.73) | 149 | 41.2 | (2.17) | 435 | *36.7 | (1.37) | 1,433 | *35.8 | (0.81) |
| Lunch | 2,158 | 33.1 | (0.60) | 173 | 35.1 | (2.09) | 406 | 32.3 | (1.22) | 1,420 | 32.9 | (0.65) |
| Dinner | 2,569 | 33.2 | (0.51) | 207 | 31.2 | (1.52) | 474 | 33.9 | (0.87) | 1,705 | 33.0 | (0.51) |
| Snacks | 2,613 | 56.3 | (0.75) | 213 | 62.1 | (1.99) | 504 | ***55.4 | (1.78) | 1,698 | **56.1 | (0.74) |
| **Female** | | | | | | | | | | | | |
| Daily intake | 2,810 | 38.4 | (0.58) | 348 | 43.4 | (1.10) | 530 | **40.5 | (0.93) | 1,684 | ***37.4 | (0.60) |
| Breakfast | 2,186 | 34.5 | (0.69) | 233 | 40.1 | (1.75) | 400 | 37.8 | (1.51) | 1,367 | ***33.6 | (0.92) |
| Lunch | 2,138 | 32.3 | (0.63) | 226 | 37.6 | (1.87) | 400 | *33.8 | (1.50) | 1,336 | **31.6 | (0.57) |
| Dinner | 2,448 | 30.6 | (0.69) | 289 | 33.1 | (1.15) | 439 | 30.8 | (1.10) | 1,515 | 30.6 | (0.78) |
| Snacks | 2,466 | 51.3 | (0.91) | 291 | 58.0 | (1.90) | 456 | 55.1 | (1.62) | 1,512 | ***49.1 | (1.23) |

Notes: Significant differences in means and proportions are noted by * (.05 level), ** (.01 level), or *** (.001 level). Differences are tested in comparison to FSP participants, identified as persons in households receiving food stamps in the past 12 months.

[1] Calories from solid fats and added sugars were identified from the Pyramid Servings Database compiled by USDA, CNPP. Calories from alcoholic beverages include calories from carbohydrate in beer and wine, and calories from alcohol in all alcoholic beverages except cooking wine.

Sources: NHANES 1999–2002 dietary recalls and MyPyramid Equivalents Database for USDA Survey Food Codes, 1994–2002, Version 1.0, October 2006. Excludes pregnant and breastfeeding women and infants. 'Total Persons' includes persons with missing food stamp participation or income. Percents are age adjusted to account for different age distributions of Food Stamp participants and nonparticipants.

# Table C-1. Mean Percent of Energy From Solid Fats, Alcoholic Beverages, and Added Sugars (SoFAAS) - Older Adults (age 60+)[1]

| | Total Persons | | | Food Stamp Program Participants | | | Income-eligible Nonparticipants | | | Higher-income Nonparticipants | | |
|---|---|---|---|---|---|---|---|---|---|---|---|---|
| | Sample size | Mean percent of calories | Standard Error | Sample size | Mean percent of calories | Standard Error | Sample size | Mean percent of calories | Standard Error | Sample size | Mean percent of calories | Standard Error |
| **Both sexes** | | | | | | | | | | | | |
| Daily intake ............ | 3,060 | 32.7 | (0.33) | 214 | 33.8 | (1.53) | 652 | 32.0 | (0.72) | 1,825 | 32.7 | (0.39) |
| Breakfast ............ | 2,764 | 27.4 | (0.56) | 176 | 31.0 | (2.06) | 567 | 28.1 | (1.22) | 1,691 | 27.0 | (0.67) |
| Lunch ............ | 2,280 | 28.6 | (0.46) | 132 | 27.6 | (2.15) | 443 | 28.5 | (1.25) | 1,432 | 28.3 | (0.45) |
| Dinner ............ | 2,705 | 28.3 | (0.42) | 166 | 27.0 | (1.88) | 533 | 28.1 | (0.93) | 1,671 | 28.4 | (0.50) |
| Snacks ............ | 2,520 | 44.5 | (0.64) | 170 | 48.0 | (2.88) | 516 | 43.5 | (1.44) | 1,533 | 44.0 | (0.53) |
| **Male** | | | | | | | | | | | | |
| Daily intake ............ | 1,512 | 34.1 | (0.37) | 96 | 35.1 | (1.99) | 298 | 33.8 | (0.94) | 950 | 34.0 | (0.49) |
| Breakfast ............ | 1,358 | 29.0 | (0.66) | 77 | 33.4 | (3.73) | 257 | 31.9 | (1.31) | 876 | 28.3 | (0.87) |
| Lunch ............ | 1,057 | 29.4 | (0.58) | 56 | 29.3 | (3.32) | 178 | 27.8 | (1.32) | 703 | 29.3 | (0.58) |
| Dinner ............ | 1,336 | 29.4 | (0.48) | 74 | 28.7 | (1.55) | 245 | 28.6 | (1.62) | 867 | 29.4 | (0.59) |
| Snacks ............ | 1,244 | 47.7 | (0.87) | 76 | 49.6 | (3.96) | 235 | 44.9 | (1.98) | 795 | 47.6 | (1.11) |
| **Female** | | | | | | | | | | | | |
| Daily intake ............ | 1,548 | 31.6 | (0.52) | 118 | 33.0 | (1.88) | 354 | 30.6 | (0.75) | 875 | 31.6 | (0.59) |
| Breakfast ............ | 1,406 | 26.2 | (0.75) | 99 | 29.7 | (1.98) | 310 | 25.9 | (1.76) | 815 | 25.9 | (0.87) |
| Lunch ............ | 1,223 | 28.0 | (0.65) | 76 | 26.8 | (2.45) | 265 | 28.6 | (1.55) | 729 | 27.6 | (0.62) |
| Dinner ............ | 1,369 | 27.4 | (0.55) | 92 | 26.0 | (2.96) | 288 | 27.5 | (1.23) | 804 | * 27.5 | (0.65) |
| Snacks ............ | 1,276 | 41.9 | (0.84) | 94 | 47.0 | (3.07) | 281 | 42.5 | (2.19) | 738 | 40.9 | (0.90) |

Notes: Significant differences in means and proportions are noted by * (.05 level), ** (.01 level), or *** (.001 level). Differences are tested in comparison to FSP participants, identified as persons in households receiving food stamps in the past 12 months.

[1] Calories from solid fats and added sugars were identified from the Pyramid Servings Database compiled by USDA, CNPP. Calories from alcoholic beverages include calories from carbohydrate in beer and wine, and calories from alcohol in all alcoholic beverages except cooking wine.

Sources: NHANES 1999–2002 dietary recalls and MyPyramid Equivalents Database for USDA Survey Food Codes, 1994-2002, Version 1.0, October 2006. Excludes pregnant and breastfeeding women and infants. 'Total Persons' includes persons with missing food stamp participation or income. Percents are age adjusted to account for different age distributions of Food Stamp participants and nonparticipants.

# Table C-2. Mean Energy Density of Foods: Daily Intake and By Meal - All Persons[1]

| | Total Persons | | | Food Stamp Program Participants | | | Income-eligible Nonparticipants | | | Higher-income Nonparticipants | | |
|---|---|---|---|---|---|---|---|---|---|---|---|---|
| | Sample size | Mean energy density | Standard Error | Sample size | Mean energy density | Standard Error | Sample size | Mean energy density | Standard Error | Sample size | Mean energy density | Standard Error |
| **Both sexes** | | | | | | | | | | | | |
| Daily intake ............ | 25,138 | 1.69 | (0.01) | 4,010 | 1.73 | (0.03) | 5,361 | 1.69 | (0.02) | 13,924 | 1.68 | (0.01) |
| Breakfast ............ | 19,480 | 1.69 | (0.02) | 2,960 | 1.68 | (0.04) | 4,082 | 1.73 | (0.04) | 10,994 | 1.68 | (0.02) |
| Lunch ............ | 19,440 | 2.05 | (0.02) | 3,021 | 2.10 | (0.04) | 4,033 | 2.05 | (0.04) | 11,015 | 2.05 | (0.01) |
| Dinner ............ | 21,958 | 1.82 | (0.01) | 3,430 | 1.83 | (0.03) | 4,458 | 1.84 | (0.02) | 12,505 | 1.81 | (0.01) |
| Snacks ............ | 20,391 | 2.59 | (0.03) | 3,311 | 2.61 | (0.07) | 4,266 | 2.54 | (0.05) | 11,339 | 2.59 | (0.03) |
| **Male** | | | | | | | | | | | | |
| Daily intake ............ | 12,729 | 1.74 | (0.01) | 1,931 | 1.73 | (0.03) | 2,695 | 1.75 | (0.02) | 7,195 | 1.74 | (0.01) |
| Breakfast ............ | 9,817 | 1.70 | (0.03) | 1,433 | 1.69 | (0.06) | 2,068 | 1.74 | (0.05) | 5,614 | 1.70 | (0.03) |
| Lunch ............ | 9,666 | 2.10 | (0.02) | 1,475 | 2.14 | (0.06) | 1,967 | 2.02 | (0.04) | 5,552 | 2.11 | (0.02) |
| Dinner ............ | 11,059 | 1.85 | (0.02) | 1,645 | 1.78 | (0.04) | 2,230 | ** 1.91 | (0.03) | 6,423 | 1.85 | (0.02) |
| Snacks ............ | 10,133 | 2.62 | (0.03) | 1,589 | 2.50 | (0.09) | 2,105 | 2.57 | (0.07) | 5,722 | 2.62 | (0.04) |
| **Female** | | | | | | | | | | | | |
| Daily intake ............ | 12,409 | 1.64 | (0.01) | 2,079 | 1.73 | (0.03) | 2,666 | * 1.64 | (0.03) | 6,729 | ***1.63 | (0.02) |
| Breakfast ............ | 9,663 | 1.67 | (0.02) | 1,527 | 1.67 | (0.04) | 2,014 | 1.72 | (0.05) | 5,380 | 1.66 | (0.03) |
| Lunch ............ | 9,774 | 2.00 | (0.02) | 1,546 | 2.07 | (0.04) | 2,066 | 2.06 | (0.06) | 5,463 | 1.99 | (0.02) |
| Dinner ............ | 10,899 | 1.78 | (0.02) | 1,785 | 1.86 | (0.03) | 2,228 | 1.79 | (0.04) | 6,082 | * 1.77 | (0.02) |
| Snacks ............ | 10,258 | 2.55 | (0.04) | 1,722 | 2.66 | (0.08) | 2,161 | 2.52 | (0.06) | 5,617 | 2.55 | (0.04) |

Notes: Significant differences in means and proportions are noted by * (.05 level), ** (.01 level), or *** (.001 level). Differences are tested in comparison to FSP participants, identified as persons in households receiving food stamps in the past 12 months.

[1] Energy density is measured as calories per 100 grams of solid food. Beverages (fluid milk, juice drinks, soft drinks, coffee, tea, and alcoholic beverages) are not included in the analyses.

Source: NHANES 1999–2004 sample of persons with complete dietary recalls, excluding pregnant and breastfeeding women. 'Total Persons' includes persons with missing food stamp participation or income are age adjusted to account for different age distributions of food stamp participants and nonparticipants.

# Table C-2. Mean Energy Density of Foods: Daily Intake and By Meal - Children (age 1–18)[1]

| | Total Persons | | | Food Stamp Program Participants | | | Income-eligible Nonparticipants | | | Higher-income Nonparticipants | | |
|---|---|---|---|---|---|---|---|---|---|---|---|---|
| | Sample size | Mean energy density | Standard Error | Sample size | Mean energy density | Standard Error | Sample size | Mean energy density | Standard Error | Sample size | Mean energy density | Standard Error |
| **Both sexes** | | | | | | | | | | | | |
| Daily intake | 11,862 | 1.98 | (0.02) | 2,637 | 1.96 | (0.03) | 2,732 | 1.95 | (0.03) | 5,726 | 2.00 | (0.02) |
| Breakfast | 9,162 | 1.98 | (0.02) | 2,026 | 1.90 | (0.05) | 2,072 | 1.93 | (0.04) | 4,457 | *2.02 | (0.03) |
| Lunch | 9,744 | 2.28 | (0.03) | 2,140 | 2.24 | (0.05) | 2,210 | 2.23 | (0.04) | 4,790 | 2.31 | (0.03) |
| Dinner | 10,284 | 1.98 | (0.02) | 2,298 | 1.90 | (0.04) | 2,277 | 1.99 | (0.03) | 5,077 | *2.00 | (0.02) |
| Snacks | 10,139 | 2.88 | (0.03) | 2,282 | 2.97 | (0.08) | 2,305 | 2.88 | (0.07) | 4,902 | 2.86 | (0.04) |
| **Male** | | | | | | | | | | | | |
| Daily intake | 5,990 | 2.00 | (0.02) | 1,339 | 2.00 | (0.05) | 1,383 | 2.00 | (0.04) | 2,867 | 2.01 | (0.02) |
| Breakfast | 4,659 | 1.97 | (0.03) | 1,041 | 1.91 | (0.06) | 1,067 | 1.95 | (0.05) | 2,237 | 1.98 | (0.04) |
| Lunch | 4,910 | 2.30 | (0.03) | 1,100 | 2.27 | (0.07) | 1,114 | 2.29 | (0.05) | 2,380 | 2.32 | (0.02) |
| Dinner | 5,170 | 2.00 | (0.03) | 1,168 | 1.93 | (0.05) | 1,161 | 2.01 | (0.04) | 2,519 | *2.02 | (0.03) |
| Snacks | 5,035 | 2.89 | (0.04) | 1,150 | 2.99 | (0.10) | 1,139 | 2.94 | (0.08) | 2,412 | 2.85 | (0.06) |
| **Female** | | | | | | | | | | | | |
| Daily intake | 5,872 | 1.96 | (0.02) | 1,298 | 1.93 | (0.04) | 1,349 | 1.90 | (0.04) | 2,859 | 1.97 | (0.02) |
| Breakfast | 4,503 | 2.00 | (0.03) | 985 | 1.90 | (0.07) | 1,005 | 1.91 | (0.05) | 2,220 | *2.05 | (0.03) |
| Lunch | 4,834 | 2.26 | (0.03) | 1,040 | 2.21 | (0.07) | 1,096 | 2.16 | (0.06) | 2,410 | 2.30 | (0.04) |
| Dinner | 5,114 | 1.96 | (0.02) | 1,130 | 1.88 | (0.04) | 1,116 | 1.96 | (0.05) | 2,558 | 1.98 | (0.03) |
| Snacks | 5,104 | 2.86 | (0.04) | 1,132 | 2.94 | (0.10) | 1,166 | 2.80 | (0.08) | 2,490 | 2.86 | (0.05) |

Notes: Significant differences in means and proportions are noted by * (.05 level), ** (.01 level), or *** (.001 level). Differences are tested in comparison to FSP participants, identified as persons in households receiving food stamps in the past 12 months.

[1] Energy density is measured as calories per 100 grams of solid food. Beverages (fluid milk, juice drinks, soft drinks, coffee, tea, and alcoholic beverages) are not included in the analyses.

Source: NHANES 1999–2004 sample of persons with complete dietary recalls, excluding pregnant and breastfeeding women. 'Total Persons' includes persons with missing food stamp participation or income are age adjusted to account for different age distributions of food stamp participants and nonparticipants.

# Table C-2. Mean Energy Density of Foods: Daily Intake and By Meal - Adults (age 19–59)[1]

| | Total Persons | | | Food Stamp Program Participants | | | Income-eligible Nonparticipants | | | Higher-income Nonparticipants | | |
|---|---|---|---|---|---|---|---|---|---|---|---|---|
| | Sample size | Mean energy density | Standard Error | Sample size | Mean energy density | Standard Error | Sample size | Mean energy density | Standard Error | Sample size | Mean energy density | Standard Error |
| **Both sexes** | | | | | | | | | | | | |
| Daily intake | 8,559 | 1.66 | (0.02) | 1,020 | 1.74 | (0.04) | 1,627 | 1.69 | (0.03) | 5,307 | ** 1.64 | (0.02) |
| Breakfast | 6,141 | 1.65 | (0.03) | 648 | 1.70 | (0.06) | 1,145 | 1.75 | (0.06) | 3,927 | 1.62 | (0.04) |
| Lunch | 6,261 | 2.03 | (0.02) | 653 | 2.11 | (0.05) | 1,157 | 2.07 | (0.05) | 4,028 | 2.02 | (0.02) |
| Dinner | 7,473 | 1.84 | (0.02) | 849 | 1.90 | (0.04) | 1,340 | 1.86 | (0.03) | 4,781 | * 1.82 | (0.02) |
| Snacks | 6,647 | 2.54 | (0.04) | 775 | 2.55 | (0.08) | 1,225 | 2.51 | (0.07) | 4,175 | 2.54 | (0.05) |
| **Male** | | | | | | | | | | | | |
| Daily intake | 4,419 | 1.72 | (0.02) | 440 | 1.74 | (0.04) | 854 | 1.75 | (0.03) | 2,833 | 1.71 | (0.02) |
| Breakfast | 3,111 | 1.67 | (0.04) | 271 | 1.73 | (0.09) | 605 | 1.74 | (0.08) | 2,037 | 1.66 | (0.04) |
| Lunch | 3,155 | 2.09 | (0.02) | 280 | 2.19 | (0.09) | 585 | 2.00 | (0.05) | 2,085 | 2.10 | (0.03) |
| Dinner | 3,836 | 1.87 | (0.02) | 358 | 1.83 | (0.05) | 690 | 1.94 | (0.04) | 2,542 | 1.86 | (0.02) |
| Snacks | 3,353 | 2.60 | (0.05) | 338 | 2.50 | (0.11) | 630 | 2.54 | (0.09) | 2,160 | 2.60 | (0.06) |
| **Female** | | | | | | | | | | | | |
| Daily intake | 4,140 | 1.59 | (0.02) | 580 | 1.75 | (0.04) | 773 | * 1.63 | (0.04) | 2,474 | *** 1.56 | (0.02) |
| Breakfast | 3,030 | 1.63 | (0.04) | 377 | 1.69 | (0.07) | 540 | 1.76 | (0.09) | 1,890 | 1.58 | (0.05) |
| Lunch | 3,106 | 1.98 | (0.03) | 373 | 2.06 | (0.06) | 572 | 2.13 | (0.08) | 1,943 | 1.94 | (0.02) |
| Dinner | 3,637 | 1.80 | (0.02) | 491 | 1.95 | (0.04) | 650 | 1.79 | (0.07) | 2,239 | *** 1.77 | (0.03) |
| Snacks | 3,294 | 2.49 | (0.05) | 437 | 2.58 | (0.11) | 595 | 2.50 | (0.09) | 2,015 | 2.49 | (0.06) |

Notes: Significant differences in means and proportions are noted by * (.05 level), ** (.01 level), or *** (.001 level). Differences are tested in comparison to FSP participants, identified as persons in households receiving food stamps in the past 12 months.

[1] Energy density is measured as calories per 100 grams of solid food. Beverages (fluid milk, juice drinks, soft drinks, coffee, tea, and alcoholic beverages) are not included in the analyses.

Source: NHANES 1999–2004 sample of persons with complete dietary recalls, excluding pregnant and breastfeeding women. 'Total Persons' includes persons with missing food stamp participation or income are age adjusted to account for different age distributions of food stamp participants and nonparticipants.

# Table C-2. Mean Energy Density of Foods: Daily Intake and By Meal - Older Adults (age 60+)[1]

| | Total Persons | | | Food Stamp Program Participants | | | Income-eligible Nonparticipants | | | Higher-income Nonparticipants | | |
|---|---|---|---|---|---|---|---|---|---|---|---|---|
| | Sample size | Mean energy density | Standard Error | Sample size | Mean energy density | Standard Error | Sample size | Mean energy density | Standard Error | Sample size | Mean energy density | Standard Error |
| **Both sexes** | | | | | | | | | | | | |
| Daily intake | 4,717 | 1.34 | (0.01) | 353 | 1.34 | (0.05) | 1,002 | 1.31 | (0.02) | 2,891 | 1.35 | (0.01) |
| Breakfast | 4,177 | 1.35 | (0.03) | 286 | 1.26 | (0.10) | 865 | 1.35 | (0.04) | 2,610 | 1.36 | (0.03) |
| Lunch | 3,435 | 1.76 | (0.03) | 228 | 1.84 | (0.08) | 666 | 1.69 | (0.05) | 2,197 | 1.76 | (0.03) |
| Dinner | 4,201 | 1.50 | (0.02) | 283 | 1.41 | (0.05) | 841 | * 1.55 | (0.03) | 2,647 | 1.49 | (0.02) |
| Snacks | 3,605 | 2.28 | (0.04) | 254 | 2.26 | (0.16) | 736 | 2.15 | (0.09) | 2,262 | 2.32 | (0.05) |
| **Male** | | | | | | | | | | | | |
| Daily intake | 2,320 | 1.40 | (0.01) | 152 | 1.29 | (0.07) | 458 | 1.36 | (0.03) | 1,495 | 1.42 | (0.02) |
| Breakfast | 2,047 | 1.38 | (0.03) | 121 | 1.23 | (0.09) | 396 | 1.41 | (0.07) | 1,340 | 1.39 | (0.04) |
| Lunch | 1,601 | 1.84 | (0.03) | 95 | 1.78 | (0.13) | 268 | 1.69 | (0.08) | 1,087 | 1.85 | (0.03) |
| Dinner | 2,053 | 1.54 | (0.02) | 119 | 1.33 | (0.07) | 379 | *** 1.63 | (0.05) | 1,362 | ** 1.53 | (0.02) |
| Snacks | 1,745 | 2.26 | (0.05) | 101 | 1.75 | (0.19) | 336 | 2.09 | (0.10) | 1,150 | ** 2.33 | (0.06) |
| **Female** | | | | | | | | | | | | |
| Daily intake | 2,397 | 1.30 | (0.02) | 201 | 1.38 | (0.05) | 544 | 1.28 | (0.02) | 1,396 | 1.30 | (0.02) * |
| Breakfast | 2,130 | 1.33 | (0.03) | 165 | 1.27 | (0.14) | 469 | 1.31 | (0.05) | 1,270 | 1.32 | (0.04) |
| Lunch | 1,834 | 1.70 | (0.03) | 133 | 1.88 | (0.11) | 398 | 1.69 | (0.07) | 1,110 | 1.69 | (0.04) |
| Dinner | 2,148 | 1.47 | (0.02) | 164 | 1.46 | (0.06) | 462 | 1.52 | (0.04) | 1,285 | 1.46 | (0.03) |
| Snacks | 1,860 | 2.29 | (0.06) | 153 | 2.52 | (0.21) | 400 | 2.16 | (0.11) | 1,112 | 2.31 | (0.06) |

Notes: Significant differences in means and proportions are noted by * (.05 level), ** (.01 level), or *** (.001 level). Differences are tested in comparison to FSP participants, identified as persons in households receiving food stamps in the past 12 months.

[1] Energy density is measured as calories per 100 grams of solid food. Beverages (fluid milk, juice drinks, soft drinks, coffee, tea, and alcoholic beverages) are not included in the analyses.

Source: NHANES 1999–2004 sample of persons with complete dietary recalls, excluding pregnant and breastfeeding women. 'Total Persons' includes persons with missing food stamp participation or income are age adjusted to account for different age distributions of food stamp participants and nonparticipants.

## Table C-3. Distribution of Body Weight for Food Stamp Participants and Nonparticipants

| | Total Persons | | Food Stamp Program Participants | | Income-eligible Nonparticipants | | Higher-income Nonparticipants | |
|---|---|---|---|---|---|---|---|---|
| | Percent | Standard Error | Percent | Standard Error | Percent | Standard Error | Percent | Standard Error |
| **Both sexes** | | | | | | | | |
| **All persons** | | | | | | | | |
| Low BMI | 2.3 | (0.13) | 2.7 | (0.33) | † 2.7 | (0.40) | † 2.1 | (0.16) |
| Healthy weight | 41.8 | (0.57) | 39.1 | (1.83) | 41.7 | (1.00) | 42.2 | (0.62) |
| At risk of overweight / overweight[1] | 29.3 | (0.53) | 25.2 | (1.49) | 27.6 | (1.14) | 30.3 | (0.61) |
| Overweight / obese[2] | 26.6 | (0.63) | 33.0 | (1.88) | 28.0 | (1.03) | 25.4 | (0.71) |
| *Sample size* | 23,759 | | 3,674 | | 5,016 | | 13,311 | |
| **Children (age 2–18)** | | | | | | | | |
| Low BMI | 3.3 | (0.25) | 4.0 | (0.68) | 3.6 | (0.52) | † 3.1 | (0.33) |
| Healthy weight | 65.9 | (0.96) | 62.8 | (1.94) | 63.0 | (1.76) | 67.8 | (1.20) |
| At risk of overweight | 15.2 | (0.56) | 14.9 | (1.23) | 16.7 | (1.19) | 14.8 | (0.74) |
| Overweight | 15.6 | (0.72) | 18.4 | (1.68) | 16.7 | (1.29) | 14.3 | (0.86) |
| *Sample size* | 10,830 | | 2,348 | | 2,489 | | 5,284 | |
| **Adults (age 19–59)** | | | | | | | | |
| Low BMI | 2.2 | (0.17) | 2.5 | (0.56) | † 2.6 | (0.62) | † 1.9 | (0.21) |
| Healthy weight | 35.2 | (0.73) | 32.8 | (2.65) | 36.1 | (1.33) | 35.0 | (0.83) |
| Overweight | 32.5 | (0.79) | 26.5 | (1.93) | 29.3 | (1.72) | 34.2 | (0.89) |
| Obese | 30.2 | (0.88) | 38.1 | (2.37) | 32.0 | (1.36) | 28.8 | (1.03) |
| *Sample size* | 8,438 | | 999 | | 1,592 | | 5,249 | |
| **Older adults (age 60+)** | | | | | | | | |
| Low BMI | 1.5 | (0.26) | 1.4 u | (0.85) | † 1.8 u | (0.65) | 1.2 | (0.27) |
| Healthy weight | 28.7 | (0.89) | 25.4 | (3.77) | 29.4 | (1.94) | 28.8 | (0.97) |
| Overweight | 39.0 | (1.04) | 36.2 | (5.20) | 37.8 | (2.18) | 39.7 | (1.14) |
| Obese | 30.8 | (0.86) | 37.0 | (5.70) | 30.9 | (2.13) | 30.2 | (1.02) |
| *Sample size* | 4,491 | | 327 | | 935 | | 2,778 | |
| **Males** | | | | | | | | |
| **All persons** | | | | | | | | |
| Low BMI | 2.0 | (0.17) | 2.6 | (0.44) | † 3.1 | (0.62) | † 1.5 | (0.15) |
| Healthy weight | 39.1 | (0.70) | 45.6 | (2.75) | 40.3 | (1.19) | 38.4 | (0.83) |
| At risk of overweight / overweight[1] | 33.8 | (0.64) | 27.8 | (2.17) | 31.2 | (1.40) | 35.0 | (0.72) |
| Overweight / obese[2] | 25.2 | (0.66) | 24.0 | (1.78) | 25.3 | (1.12) | 25.2 | (0.78) |
| *Sample size* | 12,034 | | 1,765 | | 2,520 | | 6,877 | |
| **Children (age 2–18)** | | | | | | | | |
| Low BMI | 3.7 | (0.34) | 4.3 | (0.68) | 4.4 | (0.80) | † 3.4 | (0.46) |
| Healthy weight | 64.4 | (1.29) | 62.5 | (2.15) | 60.0 | (2.97) | 66.5 | (1.64) |
| At risk of overweight | 15.3 | (0.86) | 14.8 | (1.88) | 17.4 | (2.31) | 14.7 | (0.94) |
| Overweight | 16.5 | (0.89) | 18.3 | (2.15) | 18.2 | (1.44) | 15.4 | (1.27) |
| *Sample size* | 5,465 | | 1,189 | | 1,263 | | 2,636 | |
| **Adults (age 19–59)** | | | | | | | | |
| Low BMI | 1.5 | (0.26) | 2.1 u | (0.80) | 3.0 u | (1.02) | † 0.9 | (0.15) |
| Healthy weight | 31.7 | (1.05) | 41.8 | (4.04) | 34.6 | (1.66) | 29.9 | (1.20) |
| Overweight | 39.0 | (0.96) | 30.9 | (3.23) | 34.1 | (2.11) | 41.2 | (1.17) |
| Obese | 27.7 | (1.04) | 25.3 | (2.93) | 28.3 | (1.74) | 28.0 | (1.20) |
| *Sample size* | 4,357 | | 432 | | 832 | | 2,805 | |
| **Older adults (age 60+)** | | | | | | | | |
| Low BMI | 0.8 | (0.18) | 1.8 u | (1.29) | 1.8 u | (0.85) | † 0.6 u | (0.18) |
| Healthy weight | 26.6 | (1.14) | 33.6 | (5.00) | 30.7 | (2.95) | 25.5 | (1.34) |
| Overweight | 43.3 | (1.39) | 36.7 | (5.05) | 41.7 | (3.19) | 43.7 | (1.69) |
| Obese | 29.2 | (1.22) | 28.0 | (5.26) | 25.8 | (3.22) | 30.2 | (1.51) |
| *Sample size* | 2,212 | | 144 | | 425 | | 1,436 | |

See footnotes at end of table.

## Table C-3. (Continued)

| | Total Persons | | Food Stamp Program Participants | | Income-eligible Nonparticipants | | Higher-income Nonparticipants | |
|---|---|---|---|---|---|---|---|---|
| | Percent | Standard Error | Percent | Standard Error | Percent | Standard Error | Percent | Standard Error |
| **Females** | | | | | | | | |
| **All persons** | | | | | | | | |
| Low BMI | 2.7 | (0.21) | 2.7 | (0.52) | † 2.2 | (0.51) | † 2.9 | (0.29) |
| Healthy weight | 44.5 | (0.92) | 34.9 | (2.01) | 43.3 | (1.54) | 46.4 | (1.04) |
| At risk of overweight / overweight[1] | 24.7 | (0.81) | 23.5 | (1.85) | 24.3 | (1.54) | 25.2 | (0.90) |
| Overweight / obese[2] | 28.1 | (0.82) | 38.9 | (2.42) | 30.2 | (1.55) | 25.6 | (0.99) |
| *Sample size* | 11,725 | | 1,909 | | 2,496 | | 6,434 | |
| **Children (age 2–18)** | | | | | | | | |
| Low BMI | 2.9 | (0.35) | 3.6 u | (1.09) | † 2.6 | (0.74) | † 2.8 | (0.48) |
| Healthy weight | 67.4 | (1.20) | 63.0 | (2.70) | 66.6 | (2.04) | 69.1 | (1.35) |
| At risk of overweight | 15.2 | (0.64) | 14.9 | (1.69) | 15.8 | (1.37) | 14.9 | (0.87) |
| Overweight | 14.6 | (0.85) | 18.5 | (2.25) | 15.0 | (1.82) | 13.1 | (0.93) |
| *Sample size* | 5,365 | | 1,159 | | 1,226 | | 2,648 | |
| **Adults (age 19–59)** | | | | | | | | |
| Low BMI | 2.8 | (0.32) | 2.8 | (0.83) | † 2.2 u | (0.84) | † 3.2 | (0.43) |
| Healthy weight | 38.7 | (1.14) | 26.9 | (2.60) | 37.4 | (1.97) | 40.9 | (1.44) |
| Overweight | 25.7 | (1.12) | 23.7 | (2.28) | 24.8 | (2.26) | 26.4 | (1.20) |
| Obese | 32.7 | (1.09) | 46.6 | (2.87) | 35.6 | (1.90) | 29.6 | (1.41) |
| *Sample size* | 4,081 | | 567 | | 760 | | 2,444 | |
| **Older adults (age 60+)** | | | | | | | | |
| Low BMI | 1.9 | (0.43) | 1.2 u | (1.17) | † 1.6 u | (0.77) | † 1.8 | (0.46) |
| Healthy weight | 30.4 | (1.31) | 20.4 | (4.67) | 29.2 | (2.69) | 31.7 | (1.34) |
| Overweight | 35.7 | (1.34) | 35.6 | (6.26) | 35.3 | (3.26) | 36.3 | (1.53) |
| Obese | 32.0 | (1.10) | 42.9 | (6.99) | 33.9 | (2.99) | 30.2 | (1.31) |
| *Sample size* | 2,279 | | 183 | | 510 | | 1,342 | |

Notes: Significant differences in distributions are noted by †. Differences are tested in comparison to FSP participants using chi-square tests.

[U] Denotes individual estimates not meeting the standards of reliability or precision due to inadequate cell size or large coefficient of variation.

[1] Category includes children at risk of overweight and overweight adults.

[2] Category includes overweight children and obese adults.

For children, low BMI is defined by BMI-for-age less than the 5th percentile of the CDC BMI-for-age growth chart; healthy weight is defined by BMI-for-age between the 5th and 85th percentiles; overweight is defined by BMI-for-age between the 85th and 95th percentiles; and obese is defined by BMI-for-age above the 95th percentile of the BMI-for-age growth chart.

For adults, low BMI is defined as BMI < 18.5; healthy weight is defined by $18.5 \leq BMI < 25$; overweight is defined by $25 \leq BMI < 30$; and obese is defined by BMI $\leq 30$.

Source: NHANES 1999–2004 persons with complete dietary recalls. Excludes pregnant and breastfeeding women and infants. 'Total Persons' includes persons with missing food stamp participation or income. Percents are age adjusted to account for different age distributions of Food Stamp participants and nonparticipants

# Table C-4. Percent of Persons Reporting All Three Main Meals (Breakfast, Lunch, and Dinner)

| | Total Persons | | | Food Stamp Program Participants | | | Income-eligible Nonparticipants | | | Higher-income Nonparticipants | | |
|---|---|---|---|---|---|---|---|---|---|---|---|---|
| | Sample size | Percent | Standard Error | Sample size | Percent | Standard Error | Sample size | Percent | Standard Error | Sample size | Percent | Standard Error |
| All persons ............ | 25,170 | 58.8 | (0.86) | 4,020 | 44.2 | (1.41) | 5,370 | * 48.5 | (1.53) | 13,934 | *** 63.2 | (0.87) |
| Males ................. | 12,747 | 56.8 | (0.99) | 1,936 | 43.7 | (2.01) | 2,702 | 44.7 | (1.63) | 7,201 | *** 60.5 | (1.04) |
| Females ............... | 12,423 | 60.7 | (0.93) | 2,084 | 44.4 | (1.91) | 2,668 | * 51.1 | (1.95) | 6,733 | *** 66.1 | (0.95) |
| Children (age 1–18) ...... | 11,878 | 64.9 | (0.95) | 2,644 | 59.7 | (2.00) | 2,738 | 56.9 | (1.65) | 5,727 | *** 68.6 | (1.14) |
| Males ................. | 6,000 | 64.9 | (1.14) | 1,343 | 60.9 | (2.61) | 1,389 | 56.9 | (2.73) | 2,867 | ** 68.5 | (1.30) |
| Females ............... | 5,878 | 64.8 | (1.08) | 1,301 | 58.6 | (2.44) | 1,349 | 56.7 | (1.96) | 2,860 | *** 68.8 | (1.38) |
| Adults (age 19–59) ...... | 8,570 | 54.3 | (1.01) | 1,022 | 38.8 | (2.28) | 1,629 | 43.7 | (2.39) | 5,313 | *** 58.8 | (1.00) |
| Males ................. | 4,424 | 52.2 | (1.19) | 441 | 38.2 | (3.08) | 854 | 40.1 | (2.84) | 2,837 | *** 55.8 | (1.22) |
| Females ............... | 4,146 | 56.6 | (1.17) | 581 | 39.1 | (2.78) | 775 | 47.2 | (3.08) | 2,476 | *** 62.7 | (1.14) |
| Older adults (age 60+) .. | 4,722 | 64.6 | (1.27) | 354 | 38.2 | (3.82) | 1,003 | ** 51.4 | (2.98) | 2,894 | *** 69.6 | (1.38) |
| Males ................. | 2,323 | 60.0 | (1.54) | 152 | 35.8 | (4.20) | 459 | 41.1 | (2.91) | 1,497 | *** 64.5 | (1.53) |
| Females ............... | 2,399 | 68.1 | (1.53) | 202 | 40.1 | (5.51) | 544 | 55.6 | (3.62) | 1,397 | *** 73.9 | (1.71) |

Notes: Significant differences in means and proportions are noted by * (.05 level), ** (.01 level), or *** (.001 level). Differences are tested in comparison to FSP participants, identified as persons in households receiving food stamps in the past 12 months.

Source: NHANES 1999–2004 sample of persons with complete dietary recalls, excluding pregnant and breastfeeding women. 'Total Persons' includes persons with missing food stamp participation or income are age adjusted to account for different age distributions of food stamp participants and nonparticipants.

# Table C-5. Percent of Persons Reporting Each Meal: Breakfast, Lunch, and Dinner

## Percent of Persons Eating Breakfast

| | Total Persons | | | Food Stamp Program Participants | | | Income-eligible Nonparticipants | | | Higher-income Nonparticipants | | |
|---|---|---|---|---|---|---|---|---|---|---|---|---|
| | Sample size | Percent | Std Error | Sample size | Percent | Std Error | Sample size | Percent | Std Error | Sample size | Percent | Std Error |
| All persons | 25,170 | 80.1 | (0.59) | 4,020 | 73.6 | (0.93) | 5,370 | 76.2 | (1.37) | 13,934 | ***81.8 | (0.64) |
| Males | 12,747 | 79.4 | (0.64) | 1,936 | 73.6 | (1.60) | 2,702 | 76.8 | (1.60) | 7,201 | 80.6 | (0.73) |
| Females | 12,423 | 80.8 | (0.71) | 2,084 | 73.5 | (1.21) | 2,668 | 75.7 | (1.66) | 6,733 | 83.4 | (0.81) |
| Children (age 1–18) | 11,878 | 81.6 | (0.77) | 2,644 | 78.0 | (1.26) | 2,738 | 78.8 | (1.32) | 5,727 | 83.0 | (0.98) |
| Males | 6,000 | 82.2 | (0.77) | 1,343 | 77.9 | (1.91) | 1,389 | 79.4 | (1.51) | 2,867 | 83.8 | (0.94) |
| Females | 5,878 | 80.9 | (1.00) | 1,301 | 78.2 | (1.50) | 1,349 | 78.0 | (2.06) | 2,860 | ˙82.0 | (1.26) |
| Adults (age 19–59) | 8,570 | 76.0 | (0.76) | 1,022 | 68.4 | (1.59) | 1,629 | 71.4 | (2.16) | 5,313 | ***78.0 | (0.77) |
| Males | 4,424 | 74.9 | (0.85) | 441 | 69.5 | (2.39) | 854 | 72.2 | (2.66) | 2,837 | 75.9 | (0.92) |
| Females | 4,146 | 77.4 | (0.95) | 581 | 67.8 | (2.23) | 775 | 70.9 | (2.51) | 2,476 | ***80.7 | (1.06) |
| Older adults (age 60+) | 4,722 | 91.9 | (0.53) | 354 | 84.4 | (2.19) | 1,003 | 88.1 | (1.42) | 2,894 | ***93.3 | (0.60) |
| Males | 2,323 | 91.0 | (0.69) | 152 | 81.2 | (4.36) | 459 | 88.7 | (1.97) | 1,497 | 91.8 | (0.78) |
| Females | 2,399 | 92.6 | (0.71) | 202 | 86.2 | (2.55) | 544 | 87.6 | (1.96) | 1,397 | 94.6 | (0.84) |

## Percent of Persons Eating Lunch

| | Total Persons | | | Food Stamp Program Participants | | | Income-eligible Nonparticipants | | | Higher-income Nonparticipants | | |
|---|---|---|---|---|---|---|---|---|---|---|---|---|
| | Sample size | Percent | Std Error | Sample size | Percent | Std Error | Sample size | Percent | Std Error | Sample size | Percent | Std Error |
| All persons | 25,170 | 79.5 | (0.58) | 4,020 | 69.1 | (1.60) | 5,370 | **74.8 | (1.20) | 13,934 | **82.0 | (0.59) |
| Males | 12,747 | 77.7 | (0.66) | 1,936 | 69.0 | (2.28) | 2,702 | 70.1 | (1.72) | 7,201 | *79.9 | (0.76) |
| Females | 12,423 | 81.1 | (0.75) | 2,084 | 69.0 | (1.90) | 2,668 | ***78.1 | (1.33) | 6,733 | 84.4 | (0.70) |
| Children (age 1–18) | 11,878 | 85.4 | (0.63) | 2,644 | 82.8 | (1.24) | 2,738 | 82.0 | (1.04) | 5,727 | ***87.3 | (0.76) |
| Males | 6,000 | 85.6 | (0.76) | 1,343 | 84.5 | (1.61) | 1,389 | 82.1 | (1.51) | 2,867 | 86.8 | (0.96) |
| Females | 5,878 | 85.3 | (0.70) | 1,301 | 81.1 | (1.69) | 1,349 | 82.0 | (1.69) | 2,860 | ***87.7 | (0.88) |
| Adults (age 19–59) | 8,570 | 77.5 | (0.72) | 1,022 | 66.0 | (2.43) | 1,629 | *73.2 | (1.81) | 5,313 | **80.2 | (0.75) |
| Males | 4,424 | 75.6 | (0.83) | 441 | 65.0 | (3.88) | 854 | 68.4 | (2.53) | 2,837 | *77.9 | (0.94) |
| Females | 4,146 | 79.5 | (1.01) | 581 | 66.4 | (2.62) | 775 | ***77.5 | (2.34) | 2,476 | 83.0 | (0.93) |
| Older adults (age 60+) | 4,722 | 76.9 | (1.00) | 354 | 58.4 | (3.88) | 1,003 | *68.6 | (2.18) | 2,894 | ***80.1 | (1.16) |
| Males | 2,323 | 72.5 | (1.34) | 152 | 58.3 | (4.81) | 459 | 56.8 | (2.34) | 1,497 | ***75.8 | (1.43) |
| Females | 2,399 | 80.1 | (1.12) | 202 | 58.8 | (5.18) | 544 | *73.9 | (2.64) | 1,397 | ***83.8 | (1.38) |

See footnotes at end of table.

## Table C-5. (Continued)

| | Total Persons | | | Food Stamp Program Participants | | | Income-eligible Nonparticipants | | | Higher-income Nonparticipants | | |
|---|---|---|---|---|---|---|---|---|---|---|---|---|
| | Sample size | Percent | Std Error | Sample size | Percent | Std Error | Sample size | Percent | Std Error | Sample size | Percent | Std Error |
| **Percent of Persons Eating Dinner** | | | | | | | | | | | | |
| All persons .......... | 25,170 | 90.8 | (0.33) | 4,020 | 85.3 | (1.10) | 5,370 | 86.5 | (0.81) | 13,934 | ***92.6 | (0.37) |
| Males .......... | 12,747 | 90.3 | (0.42) | 1,936 | 83.6 | (1.67) | 2,702 | 85.7 | (1.12) | 7,201 | ***92.0 | (0.51) |
| Females .......... | 12,423 | 91.4 | (0.39) | 2,084 | 86.6 | (1.52) | 2,668 | 87.4 | (1.07) | 6,733 | ***93.3 | (0.40) |
| Children (age 1–18) ...... | 11,878 | 91.0 | (0.45) | 2,644 | 88.6 | (1.25) | 2,738 | 87.6 | (1.65) | 5,727 | **92.9 | (0.47) |
| Males .......... | 6,000 | 90.2 | (0.77) | 1,343 | 87.4 | (1.68) | 1,389 | 86.9 | (2.55) | 2,867 | **92.4 | (0.71) |
| Females .......... | 5,878 | 91.9 | (0.46) | 1,301 | 89.8 | (1.34) | 1,349 | 88.4 | (1.57) | 2,860 | *93.4 | (0.49) |
| Adults (age 19–59) ...... | 8,570 | 90.6 | (0.40) | 1,022 | 85.0 | (1.58) | 1,629 | 86.0 | (1.04) | 5,313 | ***92.3 | (0.51) |
| Males .......... | 4,424 | 90.3 | (0.59) | 441 | 83.7 | (2.55) | 854 | 85.4 | (1.50) | 2,837 | **91.8 | (0.73) |
| Females .......... | 4,146 | 90.9 | (0.47) | 581 | 85.9 | (2.16) | 775 | 86.8 | (1.51) | 2,476 | 92.9 | (0.52) |
| Older adults (age 60+) .. | 4,722 | 91.6 | (0.68) | 354 | 81.0 | (2.91) | 1,003 | 86.5 | (1.94) | 2,894 | ***93.3 | (0.69) |
| Males .......... | 2,323 | 90.6 | (1.09) | 152 | 77.3 | (5.52) | 459 | 84.9 | (2.16) | 1,497 | *92.0 | (1.26) |
| Females .......... | 2,399 | 92.3 | (0.78) | 202 | 83.3 | (3.79) | 544 | 87.4 | (2.36) | 1,397 | **94.3 | (0.65) |

Notes: Significant differences in means and proportions are noted by * (.05 level), ** (.01 level), or *** (.001 level). Differences are tested in comparison to FSP participants, identified as persons in households receiving food stamps in the past 12 months.

Source: NHANES 1999–2004 sample of persons with complete dietary recalls, excluding pregnant and breastfeeding women. 'Total Persons' includes persons with missing food stamp participation or income are age adjusted to account for different age distributions of food stamp participants and nonparticipants.

## Table C-6. Average Number of Snacks Consumed

| | Total Persons | | | Food Stamp Program Participants | | | Income-eligible Nonparticipants | | | Higher-income Nonparticipants | | |
|---|---|---|---|---|---|---|---|---|---|---|---|---|
| | Sample size | Mean | Std Error | Sample size | Mean | Std Error | Sample size | Mean | Std Error | Sample size | Mean | Std Error |
| All persons ............. | 25,170 | 2.3 | (0.02) | 4,020 | 2.2 | (0.06) | 5,370 | 2.2 | (0.04) | 13,934 | ** 2.4 | (0.02) |
| Males ................... | 12,747 | 2.3 | (0.03) | 1,936 | 2.2 | (0.07) | 2,702 | 2.2 | (0.05) | 7,201 | 2.4 | (0.03) |
| Females ............... | 12,423 | 2.3 | (0.02) | 2,084 | 2.2 | (0.07) | 2,668 | 2.2 | (0.06) | 6,733 | ** 2.4 | (0.03) |
| Children (age 1–18) ...... | 11,878 | 2.5 | (0.03) | 2,644 | 2.4 | (0.07) | 2,738 | 2.5 | (0.03) | 5,727 | 2.5 | (0.03) |
| Males ................... | 6,000 | 2.5 | (0.03) | 1,343 | 2.4 | (0.10) | 1,389 | 2.5 | (0.07) | 2,867 | 2.5 | (0.04) |
| Females ............... | 5,878 | 2.5 | (0.03) | 1,301 | 2.4 | (0.07) | 1,349 | 2.4 | (0.06) | 2,860 | 2.5 | (0.04) |
| Adults (age 19–59) ...... | 8,570 | 2.3 | (0.03) | 1,022 | 2.2 | (0.08) | 1,629 | 2.2 | (0.07) | 5,313 | 2.4 | (0.04) |
| Males ................... | 4,424 | 2.3 | (0.04) | 441 | 2.3 u | (0.10) | 854 | 2.2 | (0.08) | 2,837 | 2.4 | (0.04) |
| Females ............... | 4,146 | 2.3 | (0.04) | 581 | 2.1 u | (0.10) | 775 | 2.2 | (0.08) | 2,476 | * 2.4 | (0.05) |
| Older adults (age 60+) .. | 4,722 | 2.0 | (0.03) | 354 | 1.8 u | (0.09) | 1,003 | 1.8 | (0.06) | 2,894 | ** 2.1 | (0.04) |
| Males ................... | 2,323 | 2.0 | (0.04) | 152 | 1.6 u | (0.11) | 459 | 1.7 u | (0.09) | 1,497 | *** 2.1 | (0.04) |
| Females ............... | 2,399 | 2.0 | (0.04) | 202 | 1.9 u | (0.13) | 544 | 1.8 u | (0.06) | 1,397 | 2.1 | (0.05) |

Notes: Significant differences in means are noted by * (.05 level), ** (.01 level), or *** (.001 level). Differences are tested in comparison to FSP participants.
u Denotes individual estimates not meeting the standards of reliability or precision due to inadequate cell size or large coefficient of variation.

Source: NHANES 1999–2004 sample of persons with complete dietary recalls, excluding pregnant and breastfeeding women. 'Total Persons' includes persons with missing food stamp participation or income are age adjusted to account for different age distributions of food stamp participants and nonparticipants.

## Table C-7. Mean Nutrient Rich (NR) Score: Daily Intake and By Meal - All Persons[1]

| | Total Persons | | | Food Stamp Program Participants | | | Income-eligible Nonparticipants | | | Higher-income Nonparticipants | | |
|---|---|---|---|---|---|---|---|---|---|---|---|---|
| | Sample size | Mean score | Standard Error | Sample size | Mean score | Standard Error | Sample size | Mean score | Standard Error | Sample size | Mean score | Standard Error |
| **Both sexes** | | | | | | | | | | | | |
| Daily intake | 25,161 | 94.4 | (0.56) | 4,016 | 90.1 | (1.09) | 5,366 | 90.9 | (0.67) | 13,933 | ***95.6 | (0.58) |
| Breakfast | 20,179 | 140.9 | (1.81) | 3,073 | 131.1 | (3.32) | 4,218 | 125.6 | (2.03) | 11,405 | ***145.5 | (2.11) |
| Lunch | 19,694 | 93.8 | (0.55) | 3,063 | 89.3 | (1.20) | 4,090 | 93.6* | (1.36) | 11,152 | ***94.1 | (0.66) |
| Dinner | 22,067 | 98.4 | (0.48) | 3,445 | 95.6 | (1.22) | 4,486 | 95.9 | (1.02) | 12,561 | **99.3 | (0.61) |
| Snacks | 22,252 | 74.0 | (0.80) | 3,567 | 69.2 | (1.73) | 4,679 | 72.6 | (1.90) | 12,403 | **74.6 | (0.92) |
| **Male** | | | | | | | | | | | | |
| Daily intake | 12,741 | 93.2 | (0.56) | 1,934 | 90.7 | (1.44) | 2,698 | 91.0 | (1.07) | 7,201 | *93.8 | (0.56) |
| Breakfast | 10,138 | 141.7 | (2.15) | 1,485 | 134.1 | (4.76) | 2,123 | 126.0 | (2.72) | 5,809 | '146.2 | (2.46) |
| Lunch | 9,795 | 92.4 | (0.63) | 1,493 | 91.8 | (2.40) | 1,997 | 94.2 | (1.96) | 5,625 | 91.9 | (0.79) |
| Dinner | 11,113 | 97.2 | (0.60) | 1,650 | 97.5 | (2.10) | 2,242 | 95.7 | (1.57) | 6,455 | 97.7 | (0.69) |
| Snacks | 11,220 | 71.7 | (1.05) | 1,712 | 69.4 | (3.05) | 2,331 | 73.5 | (3.74) | 6,385 | 71.2 | (1.12) |
| **Female** | | | | | | | | | | | | |
| Daily intake | 12,420 | 95.5 | (0.65) | 2,082 | 89.6 | (1.30) | 2,668 | 90.6 | (0.81) | 6,732 | ***97.4 | (0.73) |
| Breakfast | 10,041 | 140.2 | (2.01) | 1,588 | 128.6 | (3.61) | 2,095 | 124.6 | (2.60) | 5,596 | ***144.8 | (2.45) |
| Lunch | 9,899 | 95.1 | (0.71) | 1,570 | 87.9 | (1.56) | 2,093 | 93.1** | (1.83) | 5,527 | **96.3 | (0.84) |
| Dinner | 10,954 | 99.5 | (0.68) | 1,795 | 94.4 | (1.55) | 2,244 | 96.0 | (1.32) | 6,106 | ***101.0 | (0.88) |
| Snacks | 11,032 | 76.3 | (0.85) | 1,855 | 69.2 | (2.23) | 2,348 | 71.5 | (1.82) | 6,018 | ***78.5 | (1.19) |

Notes: Significant differences in means and proportions are noted by * (.05 level), ** (.01 level), or *** (.001 level). Differences are tested in comparison to FSP participants, identified as persons in households receiving food stamps in the past 12 months.

[1] The nutrient rich score is based on the Naturally Nutrient Rich (NNR) score proposed by Drenowski (2005), but does not exclude fortified foods.

Source: NHANES 1999-2004 sample of persons with complete dietary recalls, excluding pregnant and breastfeeding women. 'Total Persons' includes persons with missing food stamp participation or income are age adjusted to account for different age distributions of food stamp participants and nonparticipants.

# Table C-7. Mean Nutrient Rich (NR) Score: Daily Intake and By Meal - Children (age 1-18)[1]

| | Total Persons | | | Food Stamp Program Participants | | | Income-eligible Nonparticipants | | | Higher-income Nonparticipants | | |
|---|---|---|---|---|---|---|---|---|---|---|---|---|
| | Sample size | Mean score | Standard Error | Sample size | Mean score | Standard Error | Sample size | Mean score | Standard Error | Sample size | Mean score | Standard Error |
| **Both sexes** | | | | | | | | | | | | |
| Daily intake | 11,871 | 93.5 | (0.60) | 2,642 | 93.0 | (0.95) | 2,734 | 92.0 | (1.05) | 5,726 | 94.1 | (0.69) |
| Breakfast | 9,427 | 150.6 | (1.80) | 2,092 | 146.5 | (2.90) | 2,141 | 142.8 | (3.30) | 4,576 | 154.4 | (2.43) |
| Lunch | 9,855 | 87.0 | (0.59) | 2,162 | 88.2 | (1.19) | 2,241 | 88.2 | (1.03) | 4,841 | 86.4 | (0.90) |
| Dinner | 10,345 | 93.2 | (0.80) | 2,306 | 92.4 | (1.81) | 2,291 | 90.8 | (1.17) | 5,109 | 94.1 | (1.03) |
| Snacks | 10,760 | 72.5 | (0.95) | 2,400 | 71.3 | (1.57) | 2,455 | 73.1 | (2.06) | 5,211 | 72.5 | (1.27) |
| **Male** | | | | | | | | | | | | |
| Daily intake | 5,995 | 94.2 | (0.79) | 1,342 | 94.0 | (1.30) | 1,385 | 92.2 | (1.43) | 2,867 | 94.9 | (0.87) |
| Breakfast | 4,777 | 151.6 | (2.03) | 1,074 | 149.9 | (3.29) | 1,093 | 142.1 | (4.05) | 2,289 | 155.1 | (2.53) |
| Lunch | 4,970 | 87.1 | (0.75) | 1,108 | 88.6 | (1.99) | 1,131 | 87.8 | (1.34) | 2,412 | 86.6 | (1.13) |
| Dinner | 5,196 | 93.4 | (1.04) | 1,171 | 92.4 | (3.12) | 1,166 | 91.9 | (1.90) | 2,534 | 94.0 | (1.33) |
| Snacks | 5,373 | 73.0 | (1.25) | 1,204 | 71.3 | (1.95) | 1,223 | 72.8 | (2.73) | 2,587 | 73.1 | (1.47) |
| **Female** | | | | | | | | | | | | |
| Daily intake | 5,876 | 92.8 | (0.64) | 1,300 | 92.1 | (1.39) | 1,349 | 91.9 | (1.09) | 2,859 | 93.3 | (0.72) |
| Breakfast | 4,650 | 149.5 | (2.30) | 1,018 | 143.1 | (4.55) | 1,048 | 143.6 | (4.39) | 2,287 | 153.8 | (3.14) |
| Lunch | 4,885 | 86.9 | (0.93) | 1,054 | 87.8 | (1.25) | 1,110 | 89.0 | (1.99) | 2,429 | 86.2 | (1.26) |
| Dinner | 5,149 | 93.1 | (0.78) | 1,135 | 92.4 | (1.87) | 1,125 | 89.7 | (1.10) | 2,575 | 94.2 | (1.00) |
| Snacks | 5,387 | 71.9 | (1.14) | 1,196 | 71.2 | (2.10) | 1,232 | 73.8 | (2.02) | 2,624 | 72.0 | (1.80) |

Notes: Significant differences in means and proportions are noted by * (.05 level), ** (.01 level), or *** (.001 level). Differences are tested in comparison to FSP participants, identified as persons in households receiving food stamps in the past 12 months.

[1] The nutrient rich score is based on the Naturally Nutrient Rich (NNR) score proposed by Drenowski (2005), but does not exclude fortified foods. Total sample of persons with complete dietary recalls, excluding pregnant and breastfeeding women.

Source: NHANES 1999-2004

# Table C-7. Mean Nutrient Rich (NR) Score: Daily Intake and By Meal - Adults (age 19-59)[1]

| | Total Persons | | | Food Stamp Program Participants | | | Income-eligible Nonparticipants | | | Higher-income Nonparticipants | | |
|---|---|---|---|---|---|---|---|---|---|---|---|---|
| | Sample size | Mean score | Standard Error | Sample size | Mean score | Standard Error | Sample size | Mean score | Standard Error | Sample size | Mean score | Standard Error |
| **Both sexes** | | | | | | | | | | | | |
| Daily intake | 8,569 | 91.0 | (0.67) | 1,021 | 85.9 | (1.83) | 1,629 | 86.2 | (0.97) | 5,313 | ***92.4 | (0.70) |
| Breakfast | 6,473 | 134.0 | (2.40) | 686 | 126.0 | (5.11) | 1,192 | *113.9 | (2.48) | 4,153 | *138.9 | (3.01) |
| Lunch | 6,363 | 93.5 | (0.76) | 672 | 86.6 | (1.95) | 1,174 | 93.1 | (2.24) | 4,088 | ***93.9 | (0.80) |
| Dinner | 7,514 | 97.6 | (0.68) | 855 | 94.4 | (1.91) | 1,352 | 94.5 | (1.50) | 4,801 | *98.9 | (0.87) |
| Snacks | 7,538 | 71.8 | (1.10) | 885 | 64.7 | (2.24) | 1,403 | 68.6 | (3.35) | 4,726 | **72.7 | (1.21) |
| **Male** | | | | | | | | | | | | |
| Daily intake | 4,423 | 89.1 | (0.66) | 440 | 86.9 | (2.49) | 854 | 87.1 | (1.64) | 2,837 | 89.7 | (0.62) |
| Breakfast | 3,271 | 134.2 | (3.10) | 287 | 130.3 | (7.42) | 626 | *114.5 | (3.26) | 2,149 | 139.1 | (3.61) |
| Lunch | 3,206 | 91.6 | (0.94) | 290 | 90.1 | (3.95) | 593 | 95.9 | (3.40) | 2,116 | 90.7 | (1.02) |
| Dinner | 3,861 | 96.2 | (0.76) | 360 | 98.4 | (3.44) | 696 | 95.1 | (2.42) | 2,557 | 96.5 | (0.81) |
| Snacks | 3,902 | 68.6 | (1.50) | 391 | 63.7 | (3.48) | 732 | 72.4 | (6.27) | 2,521 | 67.3 | (1.54) |
| **Female** | | | | | | | | | | | | |
| Daily intake | 4,146 | 92.8 | (0.86) | 581 | 85.3 | (2.11) | 775 | 85.3 | (1.26) | 2,476 | **95.6 | (1.04) |
| Breakfast | 3,202 | 133.8 | (2.61) | 399 | 122.8 | (5.61) | 566 | 113.1 | (3.60) | 2,004 | *138.7 | (3.58) |
| Lunch | 3,157 | 95.3 | (0.98) | 382 | 84.9 | (2.33) | 581 | *90.9 | (2.62) | 1,972 | ***97.2 | (1.09) |
| Dinner | 3,653 | 99.0 | (1.10) | 495 | 91.8 | (1.98) | 656 | 94.2 | (1.97) | 2,244 | ***101.5 | (1.45) |
| Snacks | 3,636 | 75.2 | (1.28) | 494 | 65.4 | (3.07) | 671 | 65.0 | (2.72) | 2,205 | ***79.0 | (1.76) |

Notes: Significant differences in means and proportions are noted by * (.05 level), ** (.01 level), or *** (.001 level). Differences are tested in comparison to FSP participants, identified as persons in households receiving food stamps in the past 12 months.

[1] The nutrient rich score is based on the Naturally Nutrient Rich (NNR) score proposed by Drenowski (2005), but does not exclude fortified foods.

Source: NHANES 1999-2004 sample of persons with complete dietary recalls, excluding pregnant and breastfeeding women. 'Total Persons' includes persons with missing food stamp participation or income are age adjusted to account for different age distributions of food stamp participants and nonparticipants.

# Table C-7. Mean Nutrient Rich (NR) Score: Daily Intake and By Meal - Older Adults (age 60+)[1]

| | Total Persons | | | Food Stamp Program Participants | | | Income-eligible Nonparticipants | | | Higher-income Nonparticipants | | |
|---|---|---|---|---|---|---|---|---|---|---|---|---|
| | Sample size | Mean score | Standard Error | Sample size | Mean score | Standard Error | Sample size | Mean score | Standard Error | Sample size | Mean score | Standard Error |
| **Both sexes** | | | | | | | | | | | | |
| Daily intake ............ | 4,721 | 107.5 | (0.61) | 353 | 99.8 | (2.65) | 1,003 | 104.8 | (1.17) | 2,894 | ** 108.7 | (0.79) |
| Breakfast ............ | 4,279 | 149.6 | (2.05) | 295 | 124.1 | (5.60) | 885 | * 137.2 | (4.14) | 2,676 | *** 154.1 | (2.54) |
| Lunch ............ | 3,476 | 105.8 | (1.21) | 229 | 99.8 | (3.29) | 675 | 102.7 | (2.99) | 2,223 | * 106.9 | (1.51) |
| Dinner ............ | 4,208 | 109.1 | (0.70) | 284 | 105.4 | (2.69) | 843 | 108.3 | (2.45) | 2,651 | 108.9 | (0.86) |
| Snacks ............ | 3,954 | 84.2 | (1.23) | 282 | 81.5 | (6.08) | 821 | 84.9 | (2.84) | 2,466 | 84.7 | (1.31) |
| **Male** | | | | | | | | | | | | |
| Daily intake ............ | 2,323 | 105.7 | (0.82) | 152 | 98.7 | (3.07) | 459 | 102.3 | (1.77) | 1,497 | * 106.9 | (0.95) |
| Breakfast ............ | 2,090 | 151.8 | (2.98) | 124 | 122.1 | (6.66) | 404 | 138.6 | (7.52) | 1,371 | *** 156.8 | (3.67) |
| Lunch ............ | 1,619 | 103.6 | (1.68) | 95 | 103.8 | (6.96) | 273 | 98.1 | (2.34) | 1,097 | 104.4 | (1.99) |
| Dinner ............ | 2,056 | 106.7 | (0.82) | 119 | 102.4 | (2.93) | 380 | 103.5 | (3.27) | 1,364 | 107.6 | (0.99) |
| Snacks ............ | 1,945 | 80.7 | (1.45) | 117 | 86.7 | (11.27) | 376 | 78.4 | (3.66) | 1,277 | 81.6 | (1.89) |
| **Female** | | | | | | | | | | | | |
| Daily intake ............ | 2,398 | 109.0 | (0.95) | 201 | 100.5 | (3.30) | 544 | 106.0 | (1.74) | 1,397 | *¹ 110.3 | (1.24) |
| Breakfast ............ | 2,189 | 147.6 | (2.95) | 171 | 125.4 | (7.25) | 481 | 133.7 | (4.46) | 1,305 | * 151.7 | (3.98) |
| Lunch ............ | 1,857 | 107.4 | (1.49) | 134 | 97.4 | (3.94) | 402 | 105.8 | (4.27) | 1,126 | ** 109.0 | (1.82) |
| Dinner ............ | 2,152 | 111.0 | (1.07) | 165 | 107.1 | (3.93) | 463 | 111.2 | (2.72) | 1,287 | 110.1 | (1.44) |
| Snacks ............ | 2,009 | 86.9 | (1.85) | 165 | 79.3 | (6.23) | 445 | 88.4 | (3.91) | 1,189 | 87.4 | (2.04) |

Notes: Significant differences in means and proportions are noted by * (.05 level), ** (.01 level), or *** (.001 level). Differences are tested in comparison to FSP participants, identified as persons in households receiving food stamps in the past 12 months.

[1] The nutrient rich score is based on the Naturally Nutrient Rich (NNR) score proposed by Drenowski (2005), but does not exclude fortified foods.

Source: NHANES 1999-2004 sample of persons with complete dietary recalls, excluding pregnant and breastfeeding women. 'Total Persons' includes persons with missing food stamp participation or income age adjusted to account for different age distributions of food stamp participants and nonparticipants.

## Table C-8. Food Choices within Food Groups

| | All Persons | | | | Children (age 1–18) | | | |
|---|---|---|---|---|---|---|---|---|
| | Percent of persons consuming on the intake day | | | | | | | |
| | Total Persons | Food Stamp Program Partic. | Income-eligible Nonpartic. | Higher-income Nonpartic. | Total Persons | Food Stamp Program Partic. | Income-eligible Nonpartic. | Higher-income Nonpartic. |
| Sample size | 25,170 | 4,020 | 5,370 | 13,934 | 11,878 | 2,644 | 2,738 | 5,727 |
| **Grains** | 76.7 | 71.7 | 74.9 | ***77.8 | 80.9 | 77.0 | 77.6 | ***82.8 |
| *Types of grains, among those eating any* | | | | | | | | |
| Whole grains | 27.8 | 19.0 | 20.0 | ***30.9 | 28.5 | 22.3 | 24.0 | ***32.1 |
| Not whole grain | 94.8 | 94.7 | *96.6 | 94.4 | 94.8 | 96.1 | 95.3 | *94.1 |
| Bread | 33.6 | 33.7 | 33.5 | 33.7 | 26.8 | 25.8 | 29.2 | 26.4 |
| Rolls | 8.1 | 6.5 | 7.0 | *8.5 | 6.8 | 7.3 | 7.8 | 6.4 |
| English muffin | 1.5 | 0.4 u | 0.3 | ***1.9 | 0.5 | 0.0 u | 0.0 u | ***0.8 |
| Bagels | 5.5 | 3.1 | 2.9 | ***6.2 | 5.2 | 3.4 | 3.3 | 5.7 |
| Biscuits, scones, croissants | 5.7 | 8.7 | **5.1 | **5.5 | 4.0 | 3.4 | 4.0 | 4.2 |
| Muffins | 3.2 | 1.3 | 2.2 | ***3.6 | 2.3 | 1.9 | 2.6 | 2.4 |
| Cornbread | 3.6 | 4.9 | 4.5 | *3.2 | 2.2 | 3.2 | 2.2 | *1.9 |
| Corn tortillas | 4.1 | 5.1 | **8.5 | *2.9 | 3.6 | 3.9 | **7.5 | *2.2 |
| Flour tortillas | 5.8 | 6.6 | 8.8 | 5.1 | 4.7 | 5.4 | 7.0 | 3.8 |
| Taco shells | 2.0 | 1.9 | 2.6 | 1.7 | 1.6 | 2.3 | 3.0 | *1.0 |
| Crackers | 17.8 | 15.2 | 17.6 | *18.7 | 19.3 | 16.0 | 13.1 | ***22.2 |
| Breakfast/granola bar | 3.7 | 1.4 | 1.9 | ***4.5 | 4.9 | 1.6 u | 3.3 | ***6.2 |
| Pancakes, waffles, French toast | 7.9 | 5.6 | 6.8 | ***8.8 | 12.0 | 7.8 | 8.9 | ***14.5 |
| Cold cereal | 33.7 | 29.6 | 28.8 | ***35.1 | 51.0 | 52.3 | 49.4 | 51.4 |
| Hot cereal | 7.8 | 8.2 | 7.8 | 7.7 | 5.1 | 6.1 | *4.0 | 5.2 |
| Rice | 13.4 | 16.5 | 17.0 | **11.9 | 10.8 | 13.3 | 13.3 | 9.6 |
| Pasta | 6.2 | 5.3 | 5.7 | 6.4 | 6.4 | 5.0 | 5.9 | 6.6 |
| **Vegetables** | 67.2 | 58.7 | **63.4 | ***68.7 | 59.2 | 60.6 | 58.8 | 58.6 |
| *Types of vegetables, among those eating any* | | | | | | | | |
| Raw vegetables | 39.5 | 27.9 | **33.7 | ***42.1 | 28.1 | 21.9 | 26.4 | **30.7 |
| Raw lettuce/greens | 4.4 | 2.8 | 4.3 | **4.3 | 3.2 | 3.1 | 4.1 | 2.9 |
| Raw carrots | 4.6 | 2.2 | 3.4 | *5.4 | 6.9 | 3.4 | 5.6 | ***9.0 |
| Raw tomatoes | 7.2 | 5.6 | 7.6 | 7.2 | 4.1 | 2.9 | 4.6 | 3.8 |
| Raw cabbage/coleslaw | 3.0 | 2.6 | 3.2 | 2.9 | 0.8 | 0.6 | 1.3 u | 0.8 |
| Other raw (high nutrients) [1] | 3.2 | 2.7 | 2.9 | 3.2 | 2.1 | 2.4 | 1.6 | 2.1 |
| Other raw (low nutrients) [1] | 6.8 | 6.8 | 6.5 | 6.8 | 5.3 | 4.9 | 5.6 | 5.0 |
| Salads (w/greens) | 21.4 | 11.4 | *14.9 | ***23.7 | 12.2 | 9.3 | 10.4 | *13.5 |
| Cooked vegetables, excluding potatoes | 51.7 | 51.6 | 55.3 | 51.2 | 45.3 | 47.7 | 47.0 | 43.7 |
| Cooked green beans | 9.0 | 11.0 | 9.1 | *8.6 | 8.7 | 11.1 | 6.4 | 8.7 |
| Cooked corn | 9.8 | 11.6 | 10.1 | 9.4 | 11.3 | 15.3 | *11.2 | **10.0 |
| Cooked peas | 2.6 | 2.6 | 3.0 | 2.5 | 2.6 | 3.2 | 2.1 | 2.6 |
| Cooked carrots | 4.1 | 3.6 | 4.2 | 4.1 | 3.6 | 4.4 | 2.9 | 3.7 |
| Cooked broccoli | 5.3 | 4.1 | 5.1 | 5.5 | 4.4 | 5.2 | 3.5 | 4.6 |
| Cooked tomatoes | 14.2 | 12.3 | *15.5 | 14.5 | 11.8 | 8.0 | ***14.6 | **11.6 |
| Cooked mixed | 4.3 | 3.1 | *5.5 | 4.1 | 3.3 | 3.5 | 4.6 | 2.7 |
| Cooked starchy | 0.5 | 1.3 | 0.9 | 0.4 | 0.2 | 0.2 u | 0.6 u | 0.1 u |
| Other cooked deep yellow | 1.9 | 1.7 | 2.6 | 1.8 | 1.1 | 1.0 u | 1.7 | 1.0 |
| Other cooked dark green | 2.8 | 4.2 | *2.8 | *2.7 | 1.5 | 1.7 | 1.8 | 1.2 |
| Other cooked (high nutrients) [1] | 5.0 | 3.0 | 5.0 | ***5.1 | 2.9 | 3.2 | 3.5 | 2.6 |
| Other cooked (low nutrients) [1] | 9.3 | 8.7 | 9.1 | 9.8 | 4.2 | 3.2 | 5.6 | 4.3 |
| Other fried | 2.4 | 2.4 | 2.6 | 2.3 | 1.1 | 1.0 u | 1.0 | 1.2 |
| Cooked potatoes | 50.3 | 55.0 | 52.3 | **49.4 | 58.2 | 60.6 | 59.6 | 57.3 |

See footnotes at end of table.

## Table C-8. (Continued)

| | Adults (age 19–59) | | | | Older Adults (age 60+) | | | |
|---|---|---|---|---|---|---|---|---|
| | Percent of persons consuming on the intake day | | | | | | | |
| | Total Persons | Food Stamp Program Partic. | Income-eligible Nonpartic. | Higher-income Nonpartic. | Total Persons | Food Stamp Program Partic. | Income-eligible Nonpartic. | Higher-income Nonpartic. |
| Sample size | 8,570 | 1,022 | 1,629 | 5,313 | 4,722 | 354 | 1,003 | 2,894 |
| **Grains** | 71.3 | 66.1 | 69.5 | **72.2 | 88.5 | 83.1 | 88.5 | *89.1 |
| ***Types of grains, among those eating any*** | | | | | | | | |
| Whole grains | 24.8 | 15.4 | 15.9 | ***27.5 | 37.2 | 26.3 | 27.2 | ***40.9 |
| Not whole grain | 94.6 | 93.7 | *97.3 | 94.2 | 95.6 | 96.3 u | 96.4 | 95.5 |
| Bread | 32.3 | 33.4 | 31.3 | 32.5 | 48.8 | 47.1 | 48.3 | 49.1 |
| Rolls | 8.4 | 6.4 | 6.4 | 8.9 | 9.3 | 5.4 | 7.7 | *10.6 |
| English muffin | 1.6 | 0.5 u | 0.2 u | **1.9 | 2.7 | 1.0 u | 0.8 u | *3.3 |
| Bagels | 6.2 | 2.9 | 3.4 | ***7.0 | 3.5 | 3.8 u | 0.3 u | 4.3 |
| Biscuits, scones, croissants | 6.1 | 10.4 | **4.7 | *5.9 | 7.1 | 11.6 | 8.0 | 6.5 |
| Muffins | 3.3 | 1.1 u | *2.0 | ***3.8 | 4.0 | 1.3 u | 1.8 | ***4.5 |
| Cornbread | 3.6 | 6.2 | *3.2 | 3.4 | 5.7 | 3.1 | ***11.9 | 4.7 |
| Corn tortillas | 5.1 | 6.0 | **10.4 | 3.9 | 1.3 | 3.6 u | 3.5 | *0.5 |
| Flour tortillas | 7.3 | 7.9 | 11.2 | 6.5 | 2.3 | 4.0 u | 3.6 | 2.1 |
| Taco shells | 2.5 | 2.0 u | *3.1 | 2.3 | 0.7 | 1.0 u | 0.6 u | 0.7 |
| Crackers | 15.9 | 12.3 | **19.2 | 16.0 | 22.2 | 24.5 | 19.5 | 22.8 |
| Breakfast/granola bar | 3.7 | 1.4 u | 1.7 | ***4.4 | 1.8 | 0.9 u | 0.5 u | 2.0 |
| Pancakes, waffles, French toast | 6.7 | 5.4 | 6.6 | 6.9 | 5.5 | 3.0 u | 4.4 | *6.3 |
| Cold cereal | 25.9 | 21.6 | 18.7 | **27.6 | 33.5 | 21.1 | *30.2 | ***35.2 |
| Hot cereal | 6.6 | 5.9 | 6.3 | 6.7 | 15.9 | 19.8 | 17.9 | 14.9 |
| Rice | 15.4 | 18.4 | 19.6 | *13.7 | 10.9 | 15.2 | 14.0 | 9.4 |
| Pasta | 6.6 | 5.6 | 6.6 | 6.8 | 4.5 | 4.9 | 2.9 | 4.8 |
| **Vegetables** | 69.1 | 58.3 | *64.1 | ***71.6 | 73.1 | 56.9 | **67.6 | ***74.6 |
| ***Types of vegetables, among those eating any*** | | | | | | | | |
| Raw vegetables | 41.8 | 28.9 | 34.2 | ***44.8 | 49.4 | 33.8 | 42.8 | ***50.7 |
| Raw lettuce/greens | 5.4 | 3.0 | 4.7 | **5.5 | 2.8 | 1.6 u | 3.4 | 2.4 |
| Raw carrots | 4.2 | 2.1 | 3.0 | *4.6 | 2.6 | 0.8 u | 1.3 u | 2.8 |
| Raw tomatoes | 8.0 | 6.7 | 8.6 | 7.9 | 9.6 | 6.4 u | 8.8 | 10.2 |
| Raw cabbage/coleslaw | 3.1 | 3.9 | 2.4 | 3.1 | 5.8 | 0.9 u | ***8.2 | ***5.4 |
| Other raw (high nutrients) [1] | 3.9 | 3.5 | 3.8 | 3.9 | 2.4 | 0.3 u | 2.1 | 2.4 |
| Other raw (low nutrients) [1] | 7.2 | 6.9 | 7.0 | 7.4 | 7.5 | 9.7 | 6.2 | 7.4 |
| Salads (w/greens) | 23.4 | 11.2 | 15.1 | ***26.5 | 28.9 | 16.0 | 20.9 | ***30.2 |
| Cooked vegetables, excluding potatoes | 52.4 | 50.5 | 57.7 | 52.1 | 59.3 | 61.8 | 59.7 | 59.8 |
| Cooked green beans | 7.7 | 10.4 | 8.7 | 7.2 | 13.8 | 13.1 | 14.6 | 12.9 |
| Cooked corn | 9.2 | 11.1 | 9.8 | 9.0 | 9.3 | 7.4 | 9.4 | 9.6 |
| Cooked peas | 2.3 | 1.8 | 2.8 | 2.1 | 4.0 | 4.6 u | 4.9 | 3.9 |
| Cooked carrots | 4.0 | 2.6 u | 4.2 | 4.2 | 5.1 | 6.0 u | 6.1 | 4.5 |
| Cooked broccoli | 5.4 | 3.5 | 5.5 | 5.7 | 6.2 | 4.6 u | 6.1 | 6.2 |
| Cooked tomatoes | 17.4 | 14.6 | *19.2 | 17.8 | 7.2 | 11.2 | 5.1 | 7.4 |
| Cooked mixed | 4.2 | 2.4 | **6.0 | 4.1 | 6.1 | 5.1 u | 5.1 | 6.5 |
| Cooked starchy | 0.7 | 1.7 u | 1.2 u | 0.5 u | 0.5 | 1.5 u | 0.6 u | 0.4 u |
| Other cooked deep yellow | 1.8 | 1.7 | 2.5 | 1.7 | 3.6 | 3.0 u | 4.2 | 3.6 |
| Other cooked dark green | 2.8 | 4.0 | 2.5 | 2.8 | 4.8 | 9.0 | 5.4 | 4.5 |
| Other cooked (high nutrients) [1] | 5.3 | 3.1 | 4.7 | **5.7 | 7.4 | 2.3 u | *7.9 | ***7.3 |
| Other cooked (low nutrients) [1] | 10.6 | 8.2 | 9.2 | 11.4 | 13.2 | 19.4 | 14.0 | 12.9 |
| Other fried | 3.0 | 2.8 u | 3.3 | 2.9 | 2.2 | 3.0 u | 2.8 u | 2.0 |
| Cooked potatoes | 48.8 | 55.8 | *50.1 | **47.8 | 43.3 | 43.5 | 48.7 | 42.3 |

See footnotes at end of table.

## Table C-8. (Continued)

| | All Persons | | | | Children (age 1–18) | | | |
|---|---|---|---|---|---|---|---|---|
| | Percent of persons consuming on the intake day | | | | | | | |
| | Total Persons | Food Stamp Program Partic. | Income-eligible Nonpartic. | Higher-income Nonpartic. | Total Persons | Food Stamp Program Partic. | Income-eligible Nonpartic. | Higher-income Nonpartic. |
| Cooked potatoes-not fried ........ | 23.0 | 27.3 | 24.2 | ** 22.3 | 19.2 | 20.8 | 21.6 | 17.7 |
| Cooked potatoes-fried .............. | 30.0 | 31.7 | 30.8 | 29.4 | 42.1 | 43.0 | 42.1 | 42.2 |
| Vegetable juice ......................... | 1.4 | 1.4 | 1.1 | 1.4 | 0.2 | 0.2 u | 0.4 u | 0.2 |
| **Fruit and 100% fruit juice** ........ | 53.8 | 45.4 | * 49.9 | *** 55.5 | 57.8 | 55.7 | 55.0 | 59.1 |
| *Types of fruit, among those eating any* | | | | | | | | |
| Any whole fruit ................................ | 70.5 | 66.1 | 70.5 | * 71.5 | 66.0 | 62.0 | 63.8 | * 68.5 |
| Fresh fruit ...................................... | 62.8 | 55.0 | * 62.5 | ** 64.1 | 56.5 | 53.3 | 53.2 | 59.5 |
| Fresh orange ............................... | 7.0 | 6.6 | * 9.0 | 6.4 | 7.5 | 8.9 | 12.6 | ** 5.5 |
| Fresh other citrus ...................... | 2.3 | 1.4 | 2.2 | * 2.4 | 0.8 | 0.6 | 0.9 u | 0.8 |
| Fresh apple .................................. | 17.0 | 12.1 | ** 16.8 | *** 17.9 | 19.9 | 18.4 | 16.5 | 22.0 |
| Fresh banana ............................... | 23.3 | 21.1 | 22.5 | 23.4 | 14.8 | 14.7 | 16.2 | 14.6 |
| Fresh melon ................................. | 6.3 | 4.0 | 5.6 | 6.6 | 4.6 | 5.8 | 1.9 | 5.0 |
| Fresh watermelon ....................... | 4.2 | 4.3 | 4.4 | 4.1 | 3.8 | 3.8 | 3.0 | 4.0 |
| Fresh grapes ............................... | 8.9 | 7.2 | 8.1 | 9.4 | 8.4 | 5.9 | 5.8 | ** 10.0 |
| Fresh peach/nectarine .............. | 4.8 | 4.4 | 4.5 | 5.2 | 3.3 | 3.2 | 2.4 | 3.8 |
| Fresh pear .................................... | 2.6 | 1.9 | 3.8 | 2.6 | 1.7 | 1.3 | 2.6 | 1.6 |
| Fresh berries ............................... | 7.2 | 2.2 | * 3.8 | *** 8.8 | 6.4 | 2.1 | 1.8 | *** 8.8 |
| Other fresh fruit ......................... | 6.8 | 5.5 | 5.5 | 7.2 | 5.7 | 4.8 | 4.3 | 6.5 |
| Avocado/guacamole ................. | 2.9 | 2.2 | 3.4 | 2.9 | 1.4 | 0.7 | * 2.1 | 1.3 |
| Lemon/lime - any form .............. | 2.3 | 1.6 | 2.6 | 2.3 | 1.0 | 0.6 | 1.8 | 0.8 |
| Canned or frozen fruit, total .......... | 10.9 | 11.9 | 9.3 | 11.3 | 14.4 | 14.6 | 14.0 | 14.3 |
| Canned or frozen in syrup .......... | 7.5 | 9.0 | 6.6 | 7.6 | 9.0 | 9.5 | 9.2 | 8.4 |
| Canned or frozen, no syrup ........ | 3.8 | 3.2 | 3.2 | 4.1 | 5.5 | 5.2 | 4.8 | 6.0 |
| Applesauce,canned/frozen apples ................................ | 3.1 | 2.6 | 2.9 | 3.4 | 5.0 | 2.9 | * 6.0 | ** 5.2 |
| Canned/frozen peaches ........... | 2.2 | 3.0 | * 1.4 | 2.3 | 2.8 | 3.1 | 2.1 | 2.8 |
| Canned/frozen pineapple ........ | 1.7 | 2.0 | 1.4 | 1.7 | 2.3 | 4.0 u | 2.0 | 2.1 |
| Other canned/frozen ................. | 4.6 | 4.7 | 4.1 | 4.9 | 5.3 | 5.2 | 4.2 | 5.4 |
| 100% Fruit juice ......................... | 52.3 | 56.0 | * 48.7 | 52.0 | 62.6 | 67.4 | 63.9 | ** 60.0 |
| Non-citrus juice ......................... | 19.1 | 25.3 | * 18.6 | ** 18.2 | 33.9 | 36.0 | 34.9 | 32.5 |
| Citrus juice ................................. | 36.8 | 35.3 | 33.3 | 37.2 | 34.2 | 38.2 | 34.4 | 32.5 |
| Dried fruit ...................................... | 4.1 | 3.0 | 3.7 | 4.2 | 1.6 | 0.4 u | * 1.4 | ** 1.8 |
| **Milk & milk products** .............. | 64.5 | 59.3 | 59.4 | *** 66.4 | 79.0 | 78.7 | 74.4 | 80.7 |
| *Types of milk, among those eating any* | | | | | | | | |
| Cow's milk, total ........................... | 53.4 | 50.8 | 49.7 | * 54.8 | 72.5 | 73.4 | 69.1 | 73.4 |
| Unflavored white milk, total .......... | 49.8 | 47.2 | 45.5 | ** 51.3 | 65.2 | 65.3 | 60.8 | 66.5 |
| Unflavored whole milk, .............. | 24.5 | 45.5 | *** 33.2 | *** 19.5 | 34.1 | 54.0 | *** 40.4 | *** 26.3 |
| Unflavored non-whole, total ........ | 33.6 | 19.3 | ** 24.8 | *** 38.3 | 37.3 | 20.9 | ** 28.8 | *** 45.0 |
| 2% milk, unflavored .............. | 28.7 | 22.9 | 27.7 | ** 30.3 | 32.0 | 21.6 | ** 31.2 | * 35.5 |
| 1% milk, unflavored .............. | 9.4 | 3.8 | 6.2 | *** 10.9 | 8.8 | 2.6 | * 5.7 | *** 11.3 |
| Skim milk, unflavored ............ | 15.0 | 6.1 | 8.5 | *** 17.6 | 8.6 | 3.8 | 2.7 | ** 11.6 |
| Unflavored, fat not specified ....... | 1.9 | 3.2 | 2.7 | 1.4 | 3.5 | 5.6 | 4.5 | * 2.6 |
| Flavored milk, total ..................... | 7.3 | 7.0 | 8.1 | 7.2 | 17.5 | 18.1 | 19.4 | 16.9 |

See footnotes at end of table.

## Table C-8. (Continued)

| | Adults (age 19–59) | | | | Older Adults (age 60+) | | | |
|---|---|---|---|---|---|---|---|---|
| | Percent of persons consuming on the intake day | | | | | | | |
| | Total Persons | Food Stamp Program Partic. | Income-eligible Nonpartic. | Higher-income Nonpartic. | Total Persons | Food Stamp Program Partic. | Income-eligible Nonpartic. | Higher-income Nonpartic. |
| Cooked potatoes-not fried | 22.1 | 29.1 | *22.0 | **21.9 | 31.8 | 30.8 | 35.5 | 31.2 |
| Cooked potatoes-fried | 29.4 | 31.6 | 30.4 | 28.4 | 13.0 | 14.4 | 15.2 | 12.6 |
| Vegetable juice | 1.3 | 2.0 | 1.2 u | 1.2 | 3.5 | 1.2 u | 2.3 u | **3.9 |
| **Fruit and 100% fruit juice** | 47.2 | 38.2 | **44.6 | ***48.8 | 70.3 | 54.2 | 59.9 | ***73.3 |
| *Types of fruit, among those eating any* | | | | | | | | |
| Any whole fruit | 69.5 | 64.8 | 70.9 | 70.1 | 80.9 | 76.8 | 80.0 | 81.2 |
| Fresh fruit | 63.4 | 51.5 | ***65.1 | **64.2 | 70.9 | 68.9 | 68.7 | 71.3 |
| Fresh orange | 6.5 | 5.8 | 7.8 | 6.3 | 7.7 | 5.4 u | 7.6 | 7.9 |
| Fresh other citrus | 2.5 | 1.6 u | 3.0 | 2.5 | 4.0 | 2.0 u | 2.1 | 4.3 |
| Fresh apple | 16.3 | 9.3 | ***17.6 | ***16.4 | 15.4 | 11.7 | 14.5 | 16.4 |
| Fresh banana | 24.0 | 19.3 | 23.6 | 24.5 | 33.9 | 36.9 | 28.2 | **33.9 |
| Fresh melon | 5.9 | 3.3 u | 6.1 | 6.0 | 10.4 | 4.0 u | 9.7 | **11.1 |
| Fresh watermelon | 4.4 | 3.6 | 5.1 | 4.2 | 4.2 | 7.4 u | 5.0 u | 3.8 |
| Fresh grapes | 8.8 | 7.3 | 10.0 | 8.8 | 9.8 | 9.4 | 5.6 | 10.9 |
| Fresh peach/nectarine | 5.2 | 4.9 | 4.2 | 5.6 | 6.1 | 4.9 u | 8.6 | 5.9 |
| Fresh pear | 2.9 | 2.5 u | 4.0 | 2.7 | 3.4 | 1.2 u | 4.7 | *3.6 |
| Fresh berries | 7.7 | 2.0 u | **5.1 | *9.0 | 7.0 | 2.9 u | 3.2 | *8.2 |
| Other fresh fruit | 7.0 | 5.3 | 6.3 | 7.4 | 7.8 | 6.7 u | 4.8 | 8.0 |
| Avocado/guacamole | 4.1 | 3.1 | 4.6 | 4.2 | 1.3 | 1.3 u | 1.5 u | 1.2 |
| Lemon/lime - any form | 3.1 | 1.3 u | 3.3 | ^3.2 | 1.9 | 4.0 u | 1.6 u | 1.6 |
| Canned or frozen fruit, total | 7.3 | 9.9 | 5.5 | 7.7 | 17.4 | 14.4 | 15.0 | 18.6 |
| Canned or frozen in syrup | 5.3 | 8.4 | 4.5 | 5.5 | 12.2 | 10.4 | 10.2 | 13.2 |
| Canned or frozen, no syrup | 2.3 | 1.7 u | 1.6 | 2.5 | 6.1 | 5.4 | 5.9 | 6.3 |
| Applesauce,canned/frozen apples | 1.8 | 2.1 u | 0.5 u | 2.1 | 4.9 | 4.1 u | 6.2 | 4.8 |
| Canned/frozen peaches | 1.2 | 3.5 | 0.7 u | 1.0 | 5.0 | 1.4 u | 2.4 | ***5.8 |
| Canned/frozen pineapple | 1.2 | 1.4 u | 0.8 u | 1.3 | 2.3 | 0.6 u | 2.3 u | **2.4 |
| Other canned/frozen | 3.7 | 2.9 u | 3.8 | 4.0 | 6.7 | 9.6 | 5.3 | 7.1 |
| 100% Fruit juice | 48.4 | 53.1 | **44.1 | 48.4 | 49.3 | 48.0 | 41.0 | 51.4 |
| Non-citrus juice | 14.8 | 24.8 | **13.4 | **14.0 | 10.5 | 10.4 | 10.6 | 10.4 |
| Citrus juice | 36.4 | 33.0 | 32.8 | 37.2 | 42.2 | 38.9 | 33.6 | 44.3 |
| Dried fruit | 4.5 | 4.3 u | 4.6 u | 4.5 | 6.6 | 2.2 u | 4.3 | **7.3 |
| **Milk & milk products** | 56.6 | 49.3 | 51.2 | ***58.9 | 68.8 | 63.1 | 63.9 | *70.2 |
| *Types of milk, among those eating any* | | | | | | | | |
| Cow's milk, total | 43.3 | 40.0 | 39.7 | *45.0 | 58.0 | 52.6 | 53.8 | 59.2 |
| Unflavored white milk, total | 40.8 | 37.4 | 36.5 | *42.4 | 56.9 | 52.0 | 52.4 | 58.2 |
| Unflavored whole milk, | 22.2 | 44.4 | **31.2 | ***18.1 | 17.2 | 36.3 | 28.6 | ***13.6 |
| Unflavored non-whole, total | 28.5 | 15.7 | 20.1 | ***32.2 | 45.4 | 28.8 | 34.7 | ***49.2 |
| 2% milk, unflavored | 26.5 | 21.8 | 25.2 | 27.4 | 31.3 | 28.6 | 31.3 | 31.7 |
| 1% milk, unflavored | 8.6 | 4.1 | 6.0 | **9.5 | 13.5 | 4.7 | 8.1 | ***15.1 |
| Skim milk, unflavored | 15.9 | 5.2 | 9.1 | ***18.3 | 22.4 | 12.4 | 15.2 | ***24.8 |
| Unflavored, fat not specified | 1.3 | 1.7 u | 1.9 | 1.0 | 1.4 | 4.6 | 2.4 | 0.9 |
| Flavored milk, total | 4.1 | 3.8 | 4.6 | 4.2 | 2.0 | 0.5 u | *2.3 | **2.0 |

See footnotes at end of table.

## Table C-8. (Continued)

| | All Persons | | | | Children (age 1–18) | | | |
|---|---|---|---|---|---|---|---|---|
| | Total Persons | Food Stamp Program Partic. | Income-eligible Nonpartic. | Higher-income Nonpartic. | Total Persons | Food Stamp Program Partic. | Income-eligible Nonpartic. | Higher-income Nonpartic. |
| | Percent of persons consuming on the intake day | | | | | | | |
| Flavored, whole milk | 3.7 | 3.7 | 5.6 | 3.3 | 7.1 | 6.8 | 8.5 | 6.9 |
| Flavored non-whole, total | 4.0 | 3.4 | 4.1 | 4.2 | 7.3 | 6.6 | 8.0 | 7.3 |
| 2% milk, flavored | 2.0 | 1.3 | 2.0 | 2.0 | 3.9 | 4.5 | 5.2 | 3.4 |
| 1% milk, flavored | 1.0 | 0.6 u | 1.4 | 1.1 | 2.0 | 1.1 | 2.0 | *2.2 |
| Skim milk, flavored | 1.0 | 1.4 | 0.7 u | 1.1 | 1.5 | 1.0 u | 0.7 u | 1.8 |
| Flavored, fat not specified | 3.0 | 3.8 | 3.5 | 2.8 | 8.2 | 9.8 | 10.3 | 7.2 |
| Soymilk | 1.6 | 0.8 | 0.8 | *1.9 | 0.4 | 0.5 u | 0.4 u | 0.5 |
| Dry or evaporated milk | 3.7 | 2.9 | *4.3 | 3.7 | 3.1 | 2.0 | **4.3 | 3.1 |
| Yogurt | 7.0 | 3.6 | 4.1 | ***7.9 | 6.8 | 3.1 | 4.5 | ***8.4 |
| Cheese | 32.3 | 27.4 | 27.9 | **33.6 | 26.0 | 22.9 | 24.1 | *27.3 |
| **Meat and meat alternates** | 68.0 | 67.1 | 69.4 | 67.6 | 61.3 | 60.4 | 64.4 | 59.8 |
| *Types of meat, among those eating any* | | | | | | | | |
| Beef | 14.7 | 13.8 | 15.4 | 14.4 | 14.2 | 14.4 | 15.8 | 12.8 |
| Ground beef | 5.8 | 6.1 | 6.1 | 5.5 | 6.0 | 6.6 | 6.8 | 5.6 |
| Pork | 10.5 | 12.7 | 11.8 | **9.7 | 8.3 | 10.1 | 8.4 | 7.8 |
| Ham | 2.6 | 2.6 | 2.1 | 2.6 | 2.2 | 3.5 | 2.7 | 1.7 |
| Lamb and misc. meats | 1.3 | 1.7 | 1.9 | 1.1 | 1.0 | 1.0 u | 2.0 u | 0.8 |
| Chicken | 34.8 | 39.6 | *32.4 | *34.5 | 41.6 | 46.0 | *39.0 | 41.8 |
| Turkey | 2.3 | 2.5 | 1.8 | 2.4 | 1.9 | 1.8 | 1.3 | 1.7 |
| Organ meats | 0.6 | 0.7 | *0.7 | 0.5 | 0.3 | 0.3 u | 0.2 u | 0.2 u |
| Hot dogs | 2.9 | 2.0 | *3.8 | 2.9 | 6.1 | 5.7 | 7.0 | 5.9 |
| Cold cuts | 4.4 | 3.8 | 5.1 | 4.5 | 4.9 | 3.4 | 5.0 | **5.4 |
| Fish | 9.0 | 7.3 | 8.9 | 9.1 | 7.0 | 7.0 | 6.8 | 7.2 |
| Shellfish | 4.8 | 4.3 | 3.8 | 4.9 | 2.8 | 3.2 | 2.8 | 3.0 |
| Bacon/sausage | 14.0 | 14.3 | 12.4 | 14.3 | 12.4 | 14.6 | *9.8 | 12.9 |
| Eggs | 21.9 | 25.8 | 25.1 | **20.6 | 19.1 | 21.7 | 22.3 | *16.9 |
| Beans | 8.4 | 10.8 | 12.3 | **7.1 | 6.5 | 8.1 | 11.0 | **4.2 |
| Baked/refried beans | 7.0 | 5.9 | 6.5 | 7.3 | 5.6 | 5.2 | 5.1 | 5.9 |
| Soy products | 1.2 | 0.4 u | 1.3 | *1.3 | 0.6 | 0.0 u | 1.3 u | **0.6 |
| Protein/meal enhancement | 3.8 | 2.6 | 2.5 | *4.3 | 1.0 | 0.4 u | 0.8 u | *1.1 |
| Nuts | 9.8 | 4.1 | **7.2 | ***11.0 | 4.4 | 2.0 | 5.4 | ***5.0 |
| Peanut/almond butter | 4.7 | 3.0 | 4.1 | *5.1 | 3.7 | 2.5 | 2.9 | 4.3 |
| Seeds | 1.4 | 1.2 | 1.0 | 1.6 | 1.3 | 1.0 | 1.1 | 1.5 |
| **Mixed dishes** | 81.6 | 78.2 | 78.9 | ***82.7 | 86.2 | 86.2 | 84.4 | 86.8 |
| *Types of mixed dishes, among those eating any* | | | | | | | | |
| Tomato sauce & meat (no pasta) | 1.7 | 2.1 | 1.6 | 1.7 | 2.1 | 2.4 | 2.5 | 1.9 |
| Chili con carne | 1.8 | 2.8 | 1.6 | 1.8 | 1.2 | 1.7 u | 1.0 | 1.2 |
| Meat mixtures w/ red meat | 7.6 | 9.4 | 8.2 | *7.1 | 5.0 | 6.0 | 6.1 | *4.3 |
| Meat mixtures w/ chicken/turkey | 5.8 | 5.1 | 6.3 | 5.7 | 4.2 | 4.8 | 4.1 | 3.6 |
| Meat mixtures w/ fish | 1.4 | 0.9 | 1.7 | 1.4 | 0.9 | 0.6 | 1.7 | 0.8 |
| Hamburgers/cheeseburgers | 15.7 | 15.4 | 15.7 | 15.5 | 17.3 | 17.9 | 16.8 | 17.2 |
| Other sandwiches | 50.6 | 48.7 | 47.5 | 51.8 | 48.2 | 47.8 | 44.5 | 49.6 |
| Hot dogs | 5.1 | 5.4 | 4.7 | 5.2 | 7.7 | 8.4 | 7.6 | 7.2 |
| Luncheon meat | 15.9 | 15.7 | 13.9 | 16.3 | 14.8 | 16.3 | 13.3 | 14.6 |
| Beef,pork,ham | 4.2 | 2.6 | 3.9 | ***4.5 | 2.3 | 2.3 | 2.0 | 2.5 |
| Chicken,turkey | 5.4 | 3.0 | **5.2 | ***5.9 | 4.7 | 4.5 | 5.0 | 4.9 |
| Cheese (no meat) | 2.8 | 2.1 | 2.9 | 2.9 | 3.8 | 3.0 | 4.4 | 3.9 |
| Fish | 2.8 | 2.4 | 2.7 | 2.8 | 1.7 | 1.0 | 2.4 | 1.6 |
| Peanut butter | 4.6 | 4.7 | 4.2 | 5.0 | 8.1 | 6.7 | 6.9 | *9.2 |
| Breakfast sandwiches | 5.1 | 6.0 | 4.7 | 5.0 | 3.4 | 5.7 | 2.6 | 3.1 |

See footnotes at end of table.

## Table C-8. (Continued)

| | Adults (age 19–59) | | | | Older Adults (age 60+) | | | |
|---|---|---|---|---|---|---|---|---|
| | Percent of persons consuming on the intake day | | | | | | | |
| | Total Persons | Food Stamp Program Partic. | Income-eligible Nonpartic. | Higher-income Nonpartic. | Total Persons | Food Stamp Program Partic. | Income-eligible Nonpartic. | Higher-income Nonpartic. |
| Flavored, whole milk | 2.9 | 3.3 | 5.5 | 2.3 | 1.0 | 0.2 u | ***1.5 u | **0.9 |
| Flavored non-whole, total | 3.3 | 2.8 u | 3.1 | 3.6 | 1.4 | 0.1 u | 1.4 u | 1.7 |
| 2% milk, flavored | 1.5 | 0.2 u | *1.0 | ***1.8 | 0.6 | 0.1 u | 0.7 u | *0.6 u |
| 1% milk, flavored | 0.7 | 0.6 u | 1.4 u | 0.8 | 0.4 | 0.0 | 0.2 u | 0.5 u |
| Skim milk, flavored | 1.0 | 2.0 u | 0.7 u | 0.9 | 0.5 | 0.0 | 0.5 u | **0.6 |
| Flavored, fat not specified | 1.3 | 1.9 | 1.2 | 1.5 | 0.5 | 0.6 u | 0.8 u | 0.4 u |
| Soymilk | 1.8 | 0.7 u | 0.5 u | *2.2 | 2.5 | 1.5 u | 2.2 | 2.7 |
| Dry or evaporated milk | 3.6 | 1.8 | *3.8 | **3.7 | 4.8 | 8.0 | 6.1 | 4.4 |
| Yogurt | 7.3 | 4.1 | 4.1 | ***8.0 | 6.1 | 2.6 u | 3.5 | **6.7 |
| Cheese | 36.3 | 31.9 | 31.0 | 37.4 | 28.5 | 18.2 | 23.2 | **30.2 |
| **Meat and meat alternates** | 69.1 | 68.3 | 69.8 | 69.0 | 75.3 | 73.6 | 75.8 | 74.7 |
| ***Types of meat, among those eating any*** | | | | | | | | |
| Beef | 15.2 | 15.3 | 15.4 | 15.3 | 13.9 | 7.7 | *14.6 | **13.6 |
| Ground beef | 6.1 | 6.9 | 6.0 | 5.8 | 4.8 | 2.7 u | 5.5 | 4.6 |
| Pork | 11.8 | 13.3 | 14.1 | 10.8 | 9.2 | 14.6 | 9.2 | 9.0 |
| Ham | 2.3 | 2.4 | 1.4 | 2.4 | 4.4 | 1.8 u | 3.2 | **4.9 |
| Lamb and misc. meats | 1.4 | 1.7 | *1.9 | 1.3 | 1.6 | 2.6 u | 1.8 | 1.1 |
| Chicken | 34.4 | 40.7 | **31.6 | 33.8 | 25.4 | 25.3 | 24.9 | 25.0 |
| Turkey | 2.3 | 2.4 | 1.4 | 2.5 | 3.0 | 3.9 | 3.6 | 3.0 |
| Organ meats | 0.6 | 0.9 u | 0.8 u | 0.5 | 0.9 | 0.8 u | 1.0 u | 1.0 |
| Hot dogs | 1.8 | 0.5 u | *2.8 | *2.0 | 1.5 | 1.2 u | 2.3 | 1.4 |
| Cold cuts | 4.2 | 3.5 | 4.9 | 4.2 | 4.2 | 5.5 u | 5.6 | 3.9 |
| Fish | 9.4 | 7.5 | 9.0 | 9.4 | 11.2 | 7.0 | *11.6 | 11.5 |
| Shellfish | 5.8 | 5.3 | 4.4 | 5.8 | 4.5 | 2.6 u | 3.7 | 4.7 |
| Bacon/sausage | 13.5 | 13.0 | 11.9 | 13.8 | 18.1 | 18.5 | 18.2 | 18.2 |
| Eggs | 21.4 | 24.4 | 24.8 | 20.4 | 28.2 | 37.4 | 30.8 | *27.5 |
| Beans | 9.3 | 11.2 | 12.2 | 8.4 | 8.4 | 13.3 | 14.6 | ***7.0 |
| Baked/refried beans | 8.2 | 7.4 | 7.3 | 8.5 | 5.2 | 1.6 | **5.5 | ***5.4 |
| Soy products | 1.4 | 0.7 u | 1.1 | 1.7 | 1.1 | 0.0 | 1.7 u | ***1.1 |
| Protein/meal enhancement | 4.8 | 3.5 | 3.2 | 5.3 | 5.0 | 2.8 u | 2.9 | *5.5 |
| Nuts | 11.0 | 4.6 | *8.2 | ***12.3 | 14.2 | 5.3 | 7.1 | **16.1 |
| Peanut/almond butter | 4.1 | 2.2 u | 3.7 | **4.5 | 8.0 | 7.0 u | 7.0 | 8.4 |
| Seeds | 1.7 | 1.5 u | 1.2 | 1.9 | 0.8 | 0.7 u | 0.2 u | 1.0 |
| **Mixed dishes** | 81.1 | 75.8 | 78.3 | **82.3 | 75.9 | 73.9 | 71.9 | 77.3 |
| ***Types of mixed dishes, among those eating any*** | | | | | | | | |
| Tomato sauce & meat (no pasta) | 1.5 | 2.2 | 1.5 u | 1.4 | 2.0 | 1.7 u | 0.7 u | 2.2 |
| Chili con carne | 2.0 | 3.3 | 1.6 | 2.1 | 2.1 | 2.6 u | 2.6 | 1.9 |
| Meat mixtures w/ red meat | 7.6 | 8.8 | 8.2 | 7.1 | 11.4 | 16.5 | 10.8 | 11.6 |
| Meat mixtures W/ chicken/turkey | 6.2 | 4.5 | 7.1 | 6.3 | 6.7 | 7.7 | 7.2 | 6.9 |
| Meat mixtures W/ fish | 1.4 | 0.9 u | 1.7 | 1.5 | 1.8 | 1.4 u | 1.7 | 2.0 |
| Hamburgers/cheeseburgers | 16.8 | 16.2 | 17.2 | 16.4 | 9.5 | 8.7 | 10.3 | 9.4 |
| Other sandwiches | 50.7 | 49.4 | 47.7 | 51.7 | 54.3 | 47.9 | 51.1 | 55.4 |
| Hot dogs | 4.4 | 4.0 | 3.6 | 4.7 | 3.7 | 5.7 u | 4.0 | 3.7 |
| Luncheon meat | 16.1 | 15.0 | 14.2 | 16.7 | 16.9 | 17.2 | 13.4 | 17.7 |
| Beef,pork,ham | 5.0 | 3.3 | 4.4 | *5.5 | 4.6 | 0.9 u | *5.0 | **4.6 |
| Chicken,turkey | 6.3 | 2.8 | **6.0 | ***6.8 | 3.8 | 1.5 u | 2.8 | *4.1 |
| Cheese (no meat) | 2.2 | 1.8 | 1.9 | 2.3 | 3.5 | 1.6 u | 3.7 | *3.5 |
| Fish | 3.0 | 3.2 | 3.0 | 2.9 | 3.7 | 1.8 u | 2.4 | *4.4 |
| Peanut butter | 3.4 | 4.0 | 3.2 | 3.5 | 3.4 | 3.9 u | 3.4 | 3.6 |
| Breakfast sandwiches | 6.0 | 6.6 | 5.5 | 5.9 | 4.8 | 4.6 u | 5.0 | 4.9 |

See footnotes at end of table.

## Table C-8. (Continued)

| | All Persons | | | | Children (age 1–18) | | | |
|---|---|---|---|---|---|---|---|---|
| | Percent of persons consuming on the intake day | | | | | | | |
| | Total Persons | Food Stamp Program Partic. | Income-eligible Nonpartic. | Higher-income Nonpartic. | Total Persons | Food Stamp Program Partic. | Income-eligible Nonpartic. | Higher-income Nonpartic. |
| Pizza (no meat) | 4.8 | 3.8 | 3.8 | *5.2 | 8.2 | 5.3 | 6.6 | ***9.6 |
| Pizza w/ meat | 11.3 | 11.6 | 10.0 | 11.6 | 16.2 | 15.8 | 15.4 | 16.6 |
| Mexican entrees | 8.5 | 6.5 | *9.6 | *8.7 | 8.5 | 6.4 | ***11.0 | 8.2 |
| Macaroni & cheese | 6.5 | 8.4 | *5.7 | 6.4 | 10.0 | 11.3 | *7.4 | 10.8 |
| Pasta dishes, Italian style | 8.0 | 8.6 | 6.2 | 8.2 | 10.0 | 11.7 | 8.6 | 9.8 |
| Rice dishes | 7.8 | 6.5 | *9.1 | 7.6 | 6.5 | 5.4 | **8.8 | 6.1 |
| Other grain mixtures | 6.2 | 4.5 | 5.1 | *6.6 | 4.9 | 3.9 | 4.6 | 5.1 |
| Meat soup | 3.5 | 3.6 | 5.2 | 3.1 | 2.6 | 2.5 | 3.9 | 2.0 |
| Bean soup | 1.3 | 1.1 | 1.2 | 1.3 | 0.6 | 0.3 u | 1.0 u | 0.6 |
| Grain soups | 5.7 | 8.2 | 7.5 | **4.9 | 8.2 | 11.2 | 10.6 | **6.7 |
| Vegetables mixtures (inc soup) | 5.7 | 4.6 | 5.5 | 5.7 | 3.3 | 2.7 | 4.4 | 3.1 |
| **Beverages excluding milk and 100% fruit juice** | 90.4 | 90.5 | 89.9 | 90.5 | 80.1 | 82.0 | 81.6 | 79.1 |
| *Types of beverages, among those drinking any* | | | | | | | | |
| Coffee | 40.8 | 37.1 | 37.2 | **41.8 | 3.2 | 5.5 | 3.0 | 2.7 |
| Tea | 22.3 | 18.3 | 21.7 | **23.1 | 13.9 | 13.3 | 14.4 | 14.1 |
| Beer | 11.4 | 9.6 | 9.8 | *11.9 | 0.8 | 0.6 | 1.2 | 0.8 |
| Wine | 5.1 | 1.3 | 1.6 | ***6.3 | 0.4 | 0.4 u | 0.2 u | 0.4 |
| Liquor | 4.7 | 3.2 | 2.2 | **5.3 | 0.4 | 0.2 u | 0.3 | 0.4 |
| Noncarbonated, sweetened drinks | 25.1 | 26.4 | 24.5 | 25.0 | 46.3 | 43.8 | 43.6 | 47.9 |
| Noncarbonated, low-calorie/sugar free drinks | 1.6 | 1.2 | 1.1 | 1.8 | 1.6 | 1.3 | 1.4 | 1.8 |
| Any soda | 65.2 | 67.5 | 67.1 | 64.6 | 69.5 | 70.7 | 70.0 | 68.6 |
| Soda, regular | 51.3 | 59.0 | 58.4 | ***48.8 | 64.7 | 66.5 | 66.3 | 63.5 |
| Soda, sugar-free | 16.2 | 10.2 | 11.0 | ***18.1 | 6.8 | 6.4 | 5.2 | 7.1 |
| **Sweets and desserts** | 79.2 | 75.8 | 75.8 | **80.6 | 79.5 | 78.6 | 74.6 | 81.2 |
| *Types of sweets, among those eating any* | | | | | | | | |
| Sugar and sugar substitutes | 33.1 | 36.6 | 35.4 | 32.6 | 11.1 | 14.0 | 10.5 | 10.4 |
| Syrups/sweet toppings | 12.6 | 8.4 | 10.0 | ***14.0 | 16.5 | 10.5 | 13.3 | ***19.4 |
| Jelly | 6.9 | 5.8 | 4.6 | *7.4 | 4.0 | 4.2 | 3.0 | 4.3 |
| Jello | 1.7 | 1.3 | 1.6 | 1.8 | 2.2 | 2.4 | 2.1 | 2.2 |
| Candy | 35.7 | 32.2 | 33.6 | **36.2 | 43.8 | 43.0 | 44.3 | 43.5 |
| Ice cream | 22.2 | 18.6 | 19.1 | ***23.5 | 24.6 | 21.5 | 21.4 | *26.5 |
| Pudding | 3.2 | 3.8 | 2.9 | 3.2 | 2.8 | 3.6 | 2.2 | 2.9 |
| Ice/popsicles | 3.1 | 3.0 | 3.0 | 3.1 | 7.7 | 8.4 | *6.1 | 7.7 |
| Sweet rolls | 4.0 | 5.0 | 5.0 | 3.7 | 3.7 | 4.1 | 5.8 | 3.1 |
| Cake/cupcakes | 13.1 | 13.6 | 11.0 | 13.4 | 11.9 | 13.4 | 10.9 | 11.7 |
| Cookies | 32.8 | 27.3 | 29.5 | ***34.2 | 40.2 | 39.2 | 39.0 | 40.9 |
| Pies/cobblers | 5.1 | 4.9 | 4.5 | 5.3 | 2.3 | 2.6 | 2.2 | 2.4 |
| Pastries | 4.8 | 3.3 | 4.2 | **5.2 | 6.2 | 4.0 | 4.2 | *7.2 |
| Doughnuts | 5.8 | 5.0 | *8.0 | 5.5 | 5.1 | 4.6 | 6.5 | 4.9 |
| **Salty snacks** | 35.2 | 32.4 | 31.0 | **36.4 | 46.2 | 47.6 | 46.0 | 45.8 |
| *Types of salty snacks, among those eating any* | | | | | | | | |
| Corn-based salty snacks | 37.1 | 34.2 | 35.5 | 37.6 | 43.1 | 43.1 | 42.7 | 43.0 |
| Pretzels/party mix | 19.1 | 15.9 | 17.4 | 19.6 | 18.1 | 12.9 | 17.5 | **20.1 |
| Popcorn | 15.7 | 9.6 | 11.2 | ***17.9 | 15.4 | 10.8 | 7.0 | ***19.6 |
| Potato chips | 40.1 | 50.0 | 46.6 | **37.5 | 38.8 | 46.5 | 45.5 | ***34.4 |

See footnotes at end of table

## Table C-8. (Continued)

| | Adults (age 19–59) | | | | Older Adults (age 60+) | | | |
|---|---|---|---|---|---|---|---|---|
| | Percent of persons consuming on the intake day | | | | | | | |
| | Total Persons | Food Stamp Program Partic. | Income-eligible Nonpartic. | Higher-income Nonpartic. | Total Persons | Food Stamp Program Partic. | Income-eligible Nonpartic. | Higher-income Nonpartic. |
| Pizza (no meat) | 4.2 | 3.9 | 3.4 | 4.4 | 1.2 | 1.0 u | 1.0 u | 1.1 |
| Pizza w/ meat | 11.0 | 12.5 | 9.6 | 11.3 | 4.4 | 1.9 u | 3.5 | 4.7 |
| Mexican entrees | 10.0 | 8.1 | 10.5 | 10.5 | 3.3 | 1.4 u | 3.9 | 3.3 |
| Macaroni & cheese | 5.4 | 7.8 | 5.1 | 5.0 | 4.9 | 5.9 u | 5.5 | 4.6 |
| Pasta dishes, Italian style | 7.4 | 7.5 | 4.4 | 7.9 | 7.2 | 7.3 | 8.3 | 6.8 |
| Rice dishes | 9.2 | 7.6 | 9.9 | 9.2 | 4.8 | 4.4 | 6.2 | 4.6 |
| Other grain mixtures | 7.2 | 5.4 | 5.8 | 7.6 | 4.8 | 2.4 u | 3.5 | 5.3 |
| Meat soup | 3.6 | 3.6 | 5.7 | 3.3 | 4.5 | 5.0 u | 5.7 | 4.1 |
| Bean soup | 1.3 | 1.3 u | 1.3 u | 1.3 | 2.2 | 1.7 u | 1.2 u | 2.5 |
| Grain soups | 5.0 | 7.5 | 7.1 | 4.2 | 4.5 | 5.8 u | 4.2 | 4.3 |
| Vegetables mixtures (inc soup) | 5.2 | 3.7 | 4.9 | 5.2 | 11.0 | 10.8 | 9.1 | 11.5 |
| **Beverages excluding milk and 100% fruit juice** | 94.0 | 93.1 | 93.2 | 94.5 | 94.0 | 95.0 | 91.8 | 94.4 |
| *Types of beverages, among those drinking any* | | | | | | | | |
| Coffee | 47.7 | 42.2 | 40.6 | 49.6 | 76.1 | 69.1 | 78.0 | 76.6 |
| Tea | 23.6 | 19.2 | 22.0 | 24.7 | 30.7 | 23.2 | 31.8 | 31.6 |
| Beer | 17.6 | 14.7 | 15.2 | 18.4 | 6.6 | 6.1 | 4.8 | 7.2 |
| Wine | 6.6 | 1.8 | 2.2 | 8.2 | 7.3 | 0.7 u | 1.9 | 9.0 |
| Liquor | 6.1 | 4.8 | 3.2 | 6.6 | 6.9 | 2.2 u | 1.9 | 8.4 |
| Noncarbonated, sweetened drinks | 18.9 | 23.0 | 19.7 | 18.2 | 12.8 | 10.6 | 11.3 | 12.6 |
| Noncarbonated, low-calorie/sugar free drinks | 1.3 | 1.0 u | 1.0 | 1.4 | 2.4 | 1.9 u | 1.0 u | 2.9 |
| Any soda | 69.6 | 70.7 | 73.4 | 69.0 | 43.1 | 51.4 | 41.9 | 43.2 |
| Soda, regular | 52.9 | 62.9 | 64.3 | 49.6 | 24.6 | 33.5 | 27.5 | 22.7 |
| Soda, sugar-free | 19.6 | 9.5 | 12.4 | 22.2 | 19.3 | 18.2 | 15.3 | 21.2 |
| **Sweets and desserts** | 77.0 | 72.3 | 74.2 | 78.2 | 86.4 | 83.3 | 82.9 | 87.7 |
| *Types of sweets, among those eating any* | | | | | | | | |
| Sugar and sugar substitutes | 39.2 | 41.4 | 41.0 | 38.9 | 46.8 | 55.7 | 54.3 | 46.1 |
| Syrups/sweet toppings | 11.3 | 8.2 | 9.3 | 12.1 | 11.2 | 6.1 | 7.5 | 12.2 |
| Jelly | 5.9 | 5.2 | 4.0 | 6.1 | 14.9 | 10.5 | 9.0 | 16.7 |
| Jello | 1.0 | 0.6 u | 1.1 | 1.2 | 3.0 | 2.1 u | 2.4 | 3.2 |
| Candy | 34.5 | 32.1 | 32.0 | 35.4 | 27.1 | 15.8 | 23.3 | 27.9 |
| Ice cream | 20.2 | 16.9 | 16.8 | 21.3 | 25.3 | 19.5 | 23.2 | 26.6 |
| Pudding | 3.0 | 4.1 | 3.3 | 2.9 | 4.2 | 2.7 u | 2.8 | 4.4 |
| Ice/popsicles | 1.7 | 1.2 u | 2.1 | 1.6 | 0.8 | 0.8 u | 0.9 u | 0.9 |
| Sweet rolls | 4.1 | 5.4 | 4.4 | 4.0 | 4.0 | 4.8 | 5.6 | 3.7 |
| Cake/cupcakes | 13.2 | 14.0 | 10.9 | 13.5 | 15.0 | 12.4 | 11.6 | 16.0 |
| Cookies | 29.2 | 23.4 | 25.5 | 30.9 | 33.6 | 22.1 | 28.5 | 35.4 |
| Pies/cobblers | 5.1 | 5.6 | 4.2 | 5.4 | 9.4 | 6.3 | 8.9 | 9.7 |
| Pastries | 4.5 | 3.5 | 4.6 | 4.7 | 3.5 | 1.6 u | 2.6 | 3.6 |
| Doughnuts | 6.5 | 5.0 | 9.7 | 5.9 | 4.6 | 5.9 | 4.9 | 5.0 |
| **Salty snacks** | 34.4 | 29.7 | 29.3 | 36.0 | 20.8 | 17.8 | 14.5 | 23.1 |
| *Types of salty snacks, among those eating any* | | | | | | | | |
| Corn-based salty snacks | 38.0 | 31.7 | 36.6 | 38.8 | 24.6 | 27.9 | 19.9 | 24.7 |
| Pretzels/party mix | 19.1 | 17.7 | 16.0 | 18.8 | 20.8 | 13.9 u | 20.7 | 21.4 |
| Popcorn | 14.8 | 6.4 | 13.3 | 16.4 | 19.9 | 18.6 u | 9.4 | 20.9 |
| Potato chips | 40.0 | 52.7 | 45.6 | 38.0 | 42.2 | 47.7 u | 53.9 | 40.7 |

See footnotes at end of table.

## Table C-8. (Continued)

| | All Persons | | | | Children (age 1–18) | | | |
|---|---|---|---|---|---|---|---|---|
| | | | Percent of persons consuming on the intake day | | | | | |
| | Total Persons | Food Stamp Program Partic. | Income-eligible Nonpartic. | Higher-income Nonpartic. | Total Persons | Food Stamp Program Partic. | Income-eligible Nonpartic. | Higher-income Nonpartic. |
| **Added Fats and Oils** | 45.8 | 38.0 | 40.1 | ***48.1 | 30.9 | 25.4 | 29.4 | ***32.8 |
| *Types of added fats/oils, among those eating any* | | | | | | | | |
| Butter | 21.3 | 18.0 | 16.1 | *22.4 | 26.6 | 24.4 | 21.4 | 28.3 |
| Margarine | 31.7 | 32.9 | 31.5 | 32.0 | 34.7 | 31.0 | 35.3 | 35.3 |
| Other added fats | 2.8 | 1.9 | 2.9 | 2.9 | 1.9 | 2.5 u | 1.1 u | 2.1 |
| Other added oils | 2.7 | 3.2 | 1.9 | 2.7 | 0.7 | 0.8 u | 0.8 u | 0.7 |
| Salad dressing | 8.5 | 5.3 | *8.9 | 8.6 | 12.8 | 15.0 | 13.2 | 13.0 |
| Mayonnaise | 3.2 | 3.7 | 5.5 | 2.8 | 3.4 | 2.3 | 6.4 | 3.0 |
| Gravy | 12.4 | 14.4 | 13.9 | 11.8 | 11.7 | 13.3 | 17.7 | 9.6 |
| Cream cheese | 6.7 | 5.5 | 4.7 | 7.3 | 9.0 | 8.5 u | 7.4 | 9.0 |
| Cream /sour cream | 37.7 | 35.6 | 37.6 | 38.4 | 14.4 | 13.0 | 13.9 | 15.2 |

See footnotes at end of table.

## Table C-8. (Continued)

| | Adults (age 19–59) | | | | Older Adults (age 60+) | | | |
|---|---|---|---|---|---|---|---|---|
| | | | Percent of persons consuming on the intake day | | | | | |
| | Total Persons | Food Stamp Program Partic. | Income-eligible Nonpartic. | Higher-income Nonpartic. | Total Persons | Food Stamp Program Partic. | Income-eligible Nonpartic. | Higher-income Nonpartic. |
| **Added Fats and Oils** | 47.8 | 39.2 | 39.9 | ***50.4 | 62.4 | 53.7 | 57.2 | **64.4 |
| *Types of added fats/oils, among those eating any* | | | | | | | | |
| Butter | 18.4 | 17.8 | 13.7 | 18.7 | 23.0 | 8.8 | 15.4 | ***26.0 |
| Margarine | 26.2 | 30.6 | 25.6 | 26.3 | 45.7 | 43.8 | 45.5 | 46.3 |
| Other added fats | 3.2 | 1.7 u | 3.3 | 3.4 | 2.6 | 1.4 u | 4.2 u | 2.4 |
| Other added oils | 3.4 | 3.7 u | 2.2 | 3.5 | 3.4 | 5.4 u | 2.3 | 3.3 |
| Salad dressing | 7.8 | 2.0 | *8.3 | ***7.8 | 4.3 | 1.7 u | 4.2 | 4.3 |
| Mayonnaise | 3.5 | 4.7 | 6.5 | 3.0 | 1.9 | 2.5 u | 1.4 u | 2.0 |
| Gravy | 12.5 | 16.3 | 12.0 | 12.3 | 13.2 | 9.4 | 14.8 | 13.1 |
| Cream cheese | 6.6 | 4.7 | 4.1 | *7.6 | 3.5 | 3.8 u | 2.4 u | 3.7 |
| Cream /sour cream | 47.6 | 44.3 | 45.4 | 48.6 | 40.5 | 41.6 | 47.9 | 39.2 |

Notes: Significant differences in means and proportions are noted by * (.05 level), ** (.01 level), or *** (.001 level). Differences are tested in comparison to FSP participants, identified as persons in households receiving food stamps in the past 12 months.

u Denotes individual estimates not meeting the standards of reliability or precision due to inadequate cell size or large coefficient of variation.

1 "Other raw" and "Other cooked" vegetables include all vegetables not categorized separately. Within these two groups, vegetables in the top quartile of the distribution of Vitamins A or C per 100 grams were categorized as "high in nutrients"; all others are "in nutrients".

"Raw vegetables, high in nutrients include peppers (sweet and hot), broccoli, cauliflower, green peas, seaweed, and snow peas.

Raw vegetables, low in nutrients include onions, cucumbers, celery, radishes, and mushrooms.

Cooked vegetables, high in nutrients include cabbage, peppers, asparagus, cauliflower, brussel sprouts, snow peas, and squash.

Cooked vegetables, low in nutrients include artichokes, onions, mushrooms, eggplant, beets, and yellow string beans.

Source: NHANES 1999–2004 dietary recalls. Excludes pregnant and breastfeeding women and infants. 'Total Persons' includes persons with missing food stamp participation or income. Percents are age adjusted to account for different age distributions of FSP participants andnonparticipants. Tabulations are based on NHANES data containing one record for each individual food reported by respondents. Food choices reflect all individual foods except when foods were reported to be eaten in 'combination' as sandwiches, green salads, and soup. Sandwiches, salads and soups are counted as one food choice.

# Table C-9. Percent of Food Choices From Foods Recommended for Frequent, Selective, or Occasional Consumption - All Persons

| | Total Persons | | | | Food Stamp Program Participants | | | | Income-eligible Nonparticipants | | | | Higher-income Nonparticipants | | | |
|---|---|---|---|---|---|---|---|---|---|---|---|---|---|---|---|---|
| | Foods to enjoy frequently | Foods to enjoy selectively | Foods to enjoy occasionally | | Foods to enjoy frequently | Foods to enjoy selectively | Foods to enjoy occasionally | | Foods to enjoy frequently | Foods to enjoy selectively | Foods to enjoy occasionally | | Foods to enjoy frequently | Foods to enjoy selectively | Foods to enjoy occasionally | |
| **Both sexes** | | | | | | | | | | | | | | | | |
| Daily intake | 22.4 | 20.8 | 56.8 | | 18.8 | 19.1 | 62.0 | | *20.7 | *21.4 | *57.8 | | ***23.2 | **21.2 | ***55.6 | |
| Grains | 14.8 | 47.0 | 38.2 | | 12.6 | 47.2 | 40.3 | | 13.8 | 49.6 | 36.6 | | 15.2 | 46.1 | 38.7 | |
| Vegetables | 26.0 | 28.6 | 45.5 | | 23.8 | 30.9 | 45.3 | | 25.2 | 30.6 | 44.2 | | 26.6 | 27.6 | 45.9 | |
| Fruit | 79.8 | 15.6 | 4.6 | | 79.6 | 15.8 | 4.6 | | 81.5 | 14.5 | 4.0 | | 79.3 | 15.9 | 4.8 | |
| Milk group | 24.4 | 30.4 | 45.2 | | 7.6 | 22.9 | 69.5 | | *14.5 | 28.0 | 57.5 | | **29.2 | ***33.1 | ***37.7 | |
| Meat and meat alternates | 24.1 | 26.0 | 49.9 | | 20.1 | 24.4 | 55.5 | | 22.4 | 26.3 | 51.3 | | 24.9 | 26.5 | 48.7 | |
| Mixed dishes | 18.5 | 27.4 | 54.1 | | 19.9 | 25.7 | 54.4 | | 20.4 | 27.2 | 52.4 | | 17.4 | 27.9 | 54.7 | |
| Condiments, Oils, Fats | 14.6 | 27.9 | 57.5 | | 16.2 | 27.8 | 56.0 | | 13.5 | 29.9 | 56.6 | | 14.4 | 27.5 | 58.2 | |
| Sweets | 0.0 | 5.2 | 94.8 | | 0.0 | 4.2 | 95.8 | | 0.0 | 4.4 | 95.6 | | 0.0 | 5.7 | 94.3 | |
| Beverages | 24.7 | 0.0 | 75.3 | | 20.4 | 0.0 | 79.6 | | 19.8 | 0.0 | 80.2 | | **26.3 | 0.0 | 73.7 | |
| Salty snacks | 0.0 | 13.1 | 86.9 | | 0.0 | 5.5 | 94.5 | | 0.0 | 9.2 | 90.8 | | 0.0 | *15.9 | 84.1 | |
| **Male** | | | | | | | | | | | | | | | | |
| Daily intake | 21.3 | 20.7 | 58.0 | | 18.4 | 19.6 | 62.0 | | 19.9 | 21.3 | 58.7 | | *21.9 | 20.9 | *57.2 | |
| Grains | 14.3 | 47.6 | 38.1 | | 13.6 | 48.6 | 37.8 | | 12.9 | 50.6 | 36.5 | | 14.6 | 46.4 | 39.0 | |
| Vegetables | 24.9 | 29.6 | 45.5 | | 20.5 | 33.7 | 45.8 | | 25.6 | 31.1 | 43.3 | | 25.6 | 28.6 | 45.8 | |
| Fruit | 81.7 | 14.5 | 3.8 | | 82.2 | 14.0 | 3.8 | | 84.3 | 13.5 | 2.2 | | 80.6 | 15.0 | 4.4 | |
| Milk group | 21.4 | 31.8 | 46.8 | | 7.7 | 21.6 | 70.7 | | 12.5 | 29.6 | 57.9 | | **25.3 | ***34.5 | ***40.3 | |
| Meat and meat alternates | 24.0 | 24.7 | 51.3 | | 17.8 | 23.2 | 59.0 | | 22.9 | 23.2 | 53.9 | | 25.0 | 25.2 | 49.7 | |
| Mixed dishes | 17.1 | 27.5 | 55.4 | | 18.6 | 26.9 | 54.5 | | 19.3 | 28.0 | 52.7 | | 16.0 | 27.6 | 56.4 | |
| Condiments, Oils, Fats | 15.8 | 26.7 | 57.4 | | 16.8 | 30.2 | 53.0 | | 14.0 | 29.7 | 56.3 | | 15.6 | 25.2 | 59.2 | |
| Sweets | 0.0 | 5.1 | 94.9 | | 0.0 | 5.2 | 94.8 | | 0.0 | 4.3 | 95.7 | | 0.0 | 5.5 | 94.5 | |
| Beverages | 21.7 | 0.0 | 78.3 | | 18.8 | 0.0 | 81.2 | | 18.1 | 0.0 | 81.9 | | **23.0 | 0.0 | ***77.0 | |
| Salty snacks | 0.0 | 11.4 | 88.6 | | 0.0 | 6.7 u | 93.3 u | | 0.0 | 6.7 | 93.3 | | 0.0 | 13.9 | 86.1 | |
| **Female** | | | | | | | | | | | | | | | | |
| Daily intake | 23.6 | 21.0 | 55.4 | | 19.2 | 18.7 | 62.1 | | 21.6 | *21.5 | ***56.9 | | **24.7 | 21.5 | *53.8 | |
| Grains | 15.2 | 46.3 | 38.4 | | 11.4 | 46.0 | 42.6 | | 14.8 | 48.8 | 36.4 | | 15.8 | 45.7 | 38.5 | |
| Vegetables | 27.0 | 27.5 | 45.5 | | 26.7 | 28.8 | 44.4 | | 24.7 | 30.1 | 45.2 | | 27.6 | 26.3 | 46.1 | |
| Fruit | 77.9 | 16.8 | 5.3 | | 77.6 | 17.2 | 5.1 | | 79.3 | 15.3 | 5.5 | | 77.8 | 16.9 | 5.3 | |
| Milk group | 27.8 | 28.8 | 43.4 | | 7.8 | 23.5 | 68.8 | | **16.8 | 26.2 | 57.0 | | **34.2 | 31.5 | 34.4 | |
| Meat and meat alternates | 24.2 | 27.5 | 48.3 | | 22.2 | 25.4 | 52.4 | | 22.1 | 29.4 | 48.5 | | 24.5 | 28.3 | 47.2 | |
| Mixed dishes | 20.0 | 27.4 | 52.6 | | 20.9 | 25.1 | 54.0 | | 21.3 | 26.7 | 52.0 | | 19.0 | 28.4 | 52.7 | |
| Condiments, Oils, Fats | 13.4 | 29.1 | 57.5 | | 15.8 | 25.8 | 58.5 | | 13.0 | 30.0 | 57.0 | | 13.0 | 30.1 | 56.9 | |
| Sweets | 0.0 | 5.3 | 94.7 | | 0.0 | 3.6 | 96.4 | | 0.0 | 4.5 | 95.5 | | 0.0 | 5.9 | 94.1 | |
| Beverages | 27.9 | 0.0 | 72.1 | | 21.5 | 0.0 | 78.5 | | 21.7 | 0.0 | 78.3 | | **30.3 | 0.0 | 69.7 | |
| Salty snacks | 0.0 | 14.9 | 85.1 | | 0.0 | 5.2 u | 94.8 u | | 0.0 | 10.8 | 89.2 | | 0.0 | 18.1 | 81.9 | |

See notes at end of table.

# Table C-9. (Continued)

| | Total Persons | | | Food Stamp Program Participants | | | Income-eligible Nonparticipants | | | Higher-income Nonparticipants | | |
|---|---|---|---|---|---|---|---|---|---|---|---|---|
| | Foods to enjoy frequently | Foods to enjoy selectively | Foods to enjoy occasionally | Foods to enjoy frequently | Foods to enjoy selectively | Foods to enjoy occasionally | Foods to enjoy frequently | Foods to enjoy selectively | Foods to enjoy occasionally | Foods to enjoy frequently | Foods to enjoy selectively | Foods to enjoy occasionally |
| **Both sexes** | | | | | | | | | | | | |
| Daily intake | 19.0 | 22.7 | 58.3 | 18.3 | 20.5 | 61.2 | 17.2 | ** 23.4 | 59.2 | 19.6 | ** 23.5 | ** 56.9 |
| Grains | 16.4 | 35.1 | 48.5 | 17.4 | 35.8 | 46.8 | 19.3 | 40.2 | 40.5 | 15.2 | 33.8 | 51.0 |
| Vegetables | 26.2 | 29.4 | 44.4 | 22.1 | 35.1 | 42.8 | 24.6 | 31.8 | 43.6 | 27.7 | 27.1 | 45.2 |
| Fruit | 75.2 | 22.6 | 2.2 | 77.9 | 20.8 | 1.3 | 74.3 | 23.4 | 2.3 | 74.9 | 23.1 | 2.0 |
| Milk group | 15.4 | 29.5 | 55.1 | 6.4 | 19.2 | 74.4 | 7.8 | 27.5 | 64.8 | *** 20.6 | 34.2 | 45.2 |
| Meat and meat alternates | 20.0 | 28.3 | 51.7 | 20.2 | 21.5 | 58.3 | 18.1 | 29.4 | 52.5 | ** 20.5 | 30.6 | 48.9 |
| Mixed dishes | 17.9 | 23.6 | 58.5 | 21.8 | 25.6 | 52.5 | 20.2 | 24.9 | 54.9 | 15.4 | 22.9 | 61.7 |
| Condiments, Oils, Fats | 9.1 | 38.1 | 52.8 | 10.6 | 38.4 | 51.0 | 6.3 | 42.4 | 51.4 | 9.6 | 37.1 | 53.3 |
| Sweets | 0.0 | 5.0 | 95.0 | 0.0 | 4.0 | 96.0 | 0.0 | 2.7 | 97.3 | 0.0 | 6.1 | 93.9 |
| Beverages | 8.2 | 0.0 | 91.8 | 9.4 | 0.0 | 90.6 | 7.1 | 0.0 | 92.9 | 8.4 | 0.0 | 91.6 |
| Salty snacks | 0.0 | 14.4 | 85.6 | 0.0 | 10.1 | 89.9 | 0.0 | 4.4 | 95.6 | 0.0 | 19.9 | 80.1 |
| **Male** | | | | | | | | | | | | |
| Daily intake | 18.6 | 22.7 | 58.7 | 18.9 | 20.3 | 60.9 | 16.3 | * 23.2 | 60.1 | 19.1 | 23.6 | 57.2 |
| Grains | 17.2 | 34.2 | 48.6 | 20.1 | 38.4 | 41.4 | 16.9 | 40.2 | 42.9 | 16.4 | 31.3 | 52.3 |
| Vegetables | 25.8 | 30.0 | 44.1 | 20.7 | 39.4 | 40.0 | 25.8 | 32.2 | 42.1 | 27.4 | 26.4 | 46.1 |
| Fruit | 76.4 | 21.3 | 2.4 | 78.8 | 20.2 | 1.0 u | 76.8 | 21.7 | 1.5 u | 75.6 | 21.6 | 2.7 u |
| Milk group | 13.4 | 31.4 | 55.2 | 4.3 u | 20.2 | 75.5 | 5.5 u | 33.0 | 61.5 | *** 18.9 | 35.7 | 45.4 |
| Meat and meat alternates | 19.7 | 28.3 | 52.0 | 20.9 | 20.2 | 58.9 | 19.8 | 28.3 | 51.9 | * 19.4 | 31.2 | 49.5 |
| Mixed dishes | 18.1 | 21.9 | 60.0 | 23.6 | 21.6 | 54.8 | 21.0 | 21.4 | 57.6 | 14.7 | 22.3 | 63.0 |
| Condiments, Oils, Fats | 9.5 | 38.0 | 52.5 | 11.5 | 41.3 | 47.3 | 6.7 | 44.7 | 48.6 | 10.0 | 34.8 | 55.2 |
| Sweets | 0.0 | 4.9 | 95.1 | 0.0 | 2.7 u | 97.3 u | 0.0 | 2.5 u | 97.5 u | 0.0 | 6.3 | 93.7 |
| Beverages | 7.8 | 0.0 | 92.2 | 9.3 u | 0.0 | 90.7 u | 4.4 u | 0.0 | 95.6 u | 9.0 | 0.0 | 91.0 |
| Salty snacks | 0.0 | 13.7 | 86.3 | 0.0 | 9.7 u | 90.3 u | 0.0 | 4.7 u | 95.3 u | 0.0 | 19.6 | 80.4 |
| **Female** | | | | | | | | | | | | |
| Daily intake | 19.4 | 22.8 | 57.8 | 17.7 | 20.7 | 61.6 | 18.2 | * 23.7 | * 58.1 | 20.2 | * 23.3 | * 56.5 |
| Grains | 15.5 | 36.2 | 48.3 | 14.2 | 32.9 | 53.0 | ** 22.4 | 40.2 | *** 37.4 | 14.0 | 36.2 | 49.8 |
| Vegetables | 26.6 | 28.8 | 44.7 | 23.9 | 31.1 | 45.0 | 23.3 | 31.4 | 45.3 | 28.0 | 27.5 | 44.6 |
| Fruit | 74.1 | 23.9 | 2.0 | 77.5 | 20.9 | 1.6 u | 71.9 | 24.8 | 3.4 u | 74.3 | 24.4 | 1.3 u |
| Milk group | 17.5 | 27.5 | 55.1 | 8.7 | 17.8 | 73.5 | 10.7 | 20.4 | 68.9 | ** 22.2 | 32.6 | 45.2 |
| Meat and meat alternates | 20.3 | 28.4 | 51.4 | 19.6 | 22.8 | 57.6 | 16.4 | 30.4 | 53.2 | 21.4 | 30.5 | 48.1 |
| Mixed dishes | 17.7 | 25.5 | 56.8 | 19.7 | 30.5 | 49.8 | 19.6 | 29.1 | 51.3 | 16.0 | 23.4 | 60.5 |
| Condiments, Oils, Fats | 8.6 | 38.3 | 53.1 | 10.2 | 34.4 | 55.5 | 5.5 | 40.0 | 54.5 | 9.3 | 39.2 | 51.6 |
| Sweets | 0.0 | 5.1 | 94.9 | 0.0 | 5.1 | 94.9 | 0.0 | 3.1 u | 96.9 u | 0.0 | 5.9 | 94.1 |
| Beverages | 8.6 | 0.0 | 91.4 | 9.2 u | 0.0 | 90.8 u | 10.6 | 0.0 | 89.4 | 7.9 | 0.0 | 92.1 |
| Salty snacks | 0.0 | 15.4 | 84.6 | 0.0 | 10.6 u | 89.4 u | 0.0 | 3.4 u | 96.6 u | 0.0 | 20.1 | 79.9 |

See notes at end of table.

# Table C-9. (Continued)

| | Total Persons | | | Food Stamp Program Participants | | | Income-eligible Nonparticipants | | | Higher-income Nonparticipants | | |
|---|---|---|---|---|---|---|---|---|---|---|---|---|
| | Foods to enjoy frequently | Foods to enjoy selectively | Foods to enjoy occasionally | Foods to enjoy frequently | Foods to enjoy selectively | Foods to enjoy occasionally | Foods to enjoy frequently | Foods to enjoy selectively | Foods to enjoy occasionally | Foods to enjoy frequently | Foods to enjoy selectively | Foods to enjoy occasionally |
| **Both sexes** | | | | | | | | | | | | |
| Daily intake | 21.0 | 20.1 | 58.9 | 16.8 | 18.1 | 65.1 | * 19.6 | 20.3 | * 60.0 | *** 21.9 | * 20.4 | *** 57.7 |
| Grains | 12.1 | 51.0 | 36.9 | 8.9 | 51.1 | 40.0 | 11.3 | 52.2 | 36.6 | 12.7 | 50.3 | 37.0 |
| Vegetables | 25.9 | 26.8 | 47.3 | 24.5 | 26.9 | 48.7 | 24.5 | 28.3 | 47.2 | 26.3 | 26.3 | 47.3 |
| Fruit | 80.5 | 13.8 | 5.6 | 79.8 | 14.4 | 5.7 | 82.7 | 12.1 | 5.2 | 80.0 | 14.0 | 6.0 |
| Milk group | 24.8 | 30.2 | 45.0 | 6.3 | 24.7 | 69.0 | * 15.9 | 26.7 | 57.4 | *** 29.6 | 32.8 | *** 37.6 |
| Meat and meat alternates | 24.5 | 25.9 | 49.5 | 26.2 | 26.2 | 54.6 | 22.5 | 25.7 | 51.8 | 25.6 | 25.8 | 48.6 |
| Mixed dishes | 17.8 | 27.2 | 55.0 | 17.7 | 25.0 | 57.3 | 19.7 | 25.8 | 54.5 | 17.2 | 28.2 | 54.6 |
| Condiments, Oils, Fats | 15.8 | 26.3 | 57.9 | 18.0 | 26.4 | 55.6 | 15.2 | 27.9 | 56.8 | 15.1 | 26.0 | 58.9 |
| Sweets | 0.0 | 4.9 | 95.1 | 0.0 | 4.4 | 95.6 | 0.0 | 4.3 | 95.7 | 0.0 | 5.2 | 94.8 |
| Beverages | 22.2 | 0.0 | 77.8 | 17.5 | 0.0 | 82.5 | 16.4 | 0.0 | 83.6 | ** 24.2 | 0.0 | ** 75.8 |
| Salty snacks | 0.0 | 11.2 | 88.8 | 0.0 | 3.4 u | 96.6 u | 0.0 | 9.4 | 90.6 | 0.0 | *** 13.4 | 86.6 |
| **Male** | | | | | | | | | | | | |
| Daily intake | 19.8 | 19.9 | 60.3 | 15.7 | 18.9 | 65.3 | * 18.7 | 20.2 | 61.1 | * 20.4 | 20.0 | * 59.6 |
| Grains | 11.4 | 52.0 | 36.6 | 10.2 | 51.1 | 38.7 | 10.9 | 52.5 | 36.6 | 11.6 | 51.7 | 36.7 |
| Vegetables | 24.4 | 28.0 | 47.7 | 18.9 | 28.5 | 52.6 | 24.2 | 28.6 | 47.2 | 25.1 | 28.0 | 46.9 |
| Fruit | 83.3 | 12.3 | 4.4 | 83.5 | 11.6 u | 4.9 u | 86.3 | 11.1 | 2.6 u | 81.9 | 12.9 | 5.1 |
| Milk group | 21.1 | 31.5 | 47.4 | 7.1 u | 22.2 | 70.6 | 12.9 | 28.2 | 58.8 | ** 24.4 | 34.1 | 41.5 |
| Meat and meat alternates | 24.3 | 24.1 | 51.6 | 14.9 | 25.2 | 59.9 | 22.5 | 21.4 | 56.1 | * 26.1 | 23.9 | 50.0 |
| Mixed dishes | 16.4 | 27.8 | 55.8 | 14.9 | 28.0 | 57.0 | 18.6 | 27.8 | 53.6 | 16.2 | 27.7 | 56.0 |
| Condiments, Oils, Fats | 17.6 | 24.8 | 57.7 | 18.0 | 29.4 | 52.6 | 16.1 | 26.8 | 57.0 | 17.0 | 23.4 | 59.6 |
| Sweets | 0.0 | 4.9 | 95.1 | 0.0 | 6.5 u | 93.5 u | 0.0 | 4.5 | 95.5 | 0.0 | 5.0 | 95.0 |
| Beverages | 18.8 | 0.0 | 81.2 | 15.2 | 0.0 | 84.8 | 15.4 | 0.0 | 84.6 | *** 20.1 | 0.0 | *** 79.9 |
| Salty snacks | 0.0 | 9.2 | 90.8 | 0.0 | 3.9 u | 96.1 u | 0.0 | 5.9 u | 94.1 u | 0.0 | 10.8 | 89.2 |
| **Female** | | | | | | | | | | | | |
| Daily intake | 22.5 | 20.3 | 57.3 | 17.6 | 17.6 | 64.9 | 20.6 | 20.5 | * 58.9 | *** 23.8 | 20.9 | *** 55.4 |
| Grains | 13.0 | 49.8 | 37.2 | 7.8 | 51.1 | 41.0 | 11.5 | 52.0 | 36.5 | 14.0 | 48.7 | 37.4 |
| Vegetables | 27.4 | 25.5 | 47.0 | 29.1 | 25.8 | 45.1 | 24.8 | 27.9 | 47.3 | 27.8 | 24.3 | 47.9 |
| Fruit | 77.7 | 15.4 | 6.9 | 76.9 | 16.7 | 6.4 u | 80.0 | 12.9 | 7.1 | 77.5 | 15.4 | 7.1 |
| Milk group | 29.0 | 28.8 | 42.2 | 5.9 u | 26.2 | 67.9 | * 18.8 | 25.6 | 55.5 | *** 36.3 | 31.2 | *** 32.5 |
| Meat and meat alternates | 24.8 | 28.1 | 47.1 | 23.1 | 26.9 | 50.0 | 22.9 | 30.2 | 47.0 | 25.0 | 28.4 | 46.6 |
| Mixed dishes | 19.4 | 26.5 | 54.1 | 20.0 | 22.5 | 57.6 | 20.8 | 23.8 | 55.4 | 18.5 | 28.8 | 52.7 |
| Condiments, Oils, Fats | 14.0 | 28.2 | 57.9 | 18.0 | 24.3 | 57.7 | 14.4 | 28.9 | 56.7 | 12.9 | 29.5 | 57.6 |
| Sweets | 0.0 | 4.8 | 95.2 | 0.0 | 3.1 u | 96.9 u | 0.0 | 4.0 | 96.0 | 0.0 | 5.5 | 94.5 |
| Beverages | 26.0 | 0.0 | 74.0 | 19.1 | 0.0 | 80.9 | 17.4 | 0.0 | 82.6 | ** 29.2 | 0.0 | ** 70.8 |
| Salty snacks | 0.0 | 13.2 | 86.8 | 0.0 | 3.1 u | 96.9 u | 0.0 | 12.3 | 87.7 | 0.0 | 16.4 | 83.6 |

See notes at end of table.

# Table C-9. (Continued)

| | Total Persons | | | Food Stamp Program Participants | | | Income-eligible Nonparticipants | | | Higher-income Nonparticipants | | |
|---|---|---|---|---|---|---|---|---|---|---|---|---|
| | Foods to enjoy frequently | Foods to enjoy selectively | Foods to enjoy occasionally | Foods to enjoy frequently | Foods to enjoy selectively | Foods to enjoy occasionally | Foods to enjoy frequently | Foods to enjoy selectively | Foods to enjoy occasionally | Foods to enjoy frequently | Foods to enjoy selectively | Foods to enjoy occasionally |
| **Both sexes** | | | | | | | | | | | | |
| Daily intake | 36.3 | 21.8 | 41.9 | 33.4 | 21.1 | 45.5 | 36.0 | 22.7 | 41.2 | 36.8 | 21.9 | 41.4 |
| Grains | 29.1 | 45.6 | 25.2 | 29.4 | 47.1 | 23.5 | 28.8 | 40.8 | 30.4 | 30.6 | 46.2 | 23.2 |
| Vegetables | 25.0 | 38.2 | 36.8 | 27.3 | 42.2 | 30.6 | 24.2 | 44.6 | 31.2 | 25.3 | 36.5 | 38.2 |
| Fruit | 85.5 | 11.4 | 3.1 | 86.4 u | 12.4 u | 1.3 u | 90.1 u | 9.4 u | 0.6 u | 84.6 | 11.6 | 3.8 |
| Milk group | 39.7 | 32.6 | 27.6 | 21.0 | 23.7 u | 55.3 u | 19.9 | 35.0 | 45.1 | 44.7 | 34.1 | 21.3 |
| Meat and meat alternates | 29.8 | 20.7 | 49.5 | 15.8 u | 21.1 | 63.1 u | 32.1 | 19.4 | 48.5 | 29.7 | 22.0 | 48.3 |
| Mixed dishes | 24.6 | 34.6 | 40.8 | 34.1 u | 26.9 | 39.0 | 25.6 | 31.1 | 43.3 | 22.9 | 36.3 | 40.8 |
| Condiments, Oils, Fats | 21.2 | 18.5 | 60.3 | 20.1 | 24.2 u | 55.6 | 24.0 | 19.9 | 56.1 | 20.3 | 18.6 | 61.1 |
| Sweets | 0.0 | 8.9 | 91.1 | 0.0 | 5.2 u | 94.8 u | 0.0 | 8.5 u | 91.5 u | 0.0 | 9.9 | 90.1 |
| Beverages | 67.1 | 0.0 | 32.9 | 60.5 | 0.0 | 39.5 | 69.4 | 0.0 | 30.6 | 68.9 | 0.0 | 31.1 |
| Salty snacks | 0.0 | 24.2 | 75.8 | 0.0 | 9.0 u | 91.0 u | 0.0 | 2.4 u | 97.6 u | 0.0 | 27.9 | 72.1 |
| **Male** | | | | | | | | | | | | |
| Daily intake | 34.7 | 21.6 | 43.6 | 35.9 u | 21.3 u | 42.8 u | 31.4 | 24.3 | 44.4 | 35.5 | 21.4 | 43.1 |
| Grains | 29.0 | 46.7 | 24.3 | 22.7 u | 51.8 u | 25.5 u | 27.9 | 42.8 | 29.3 | 31.0 | 45.6 | 23.4 |
| Vegetables | 24.2 | 39.2 | 36.6 | 29.0 u | 42.9 u | 28.1 u | 17.6 u | 45.3 | 37.1 | 24.7 | 38.7 | 36.6 |
| Fruit | 85.4 | 11.0 | 3.6 | 88.4 u | 11.6 u | 0.0 | 90.0 u | 9.4 u | 0.6 u | 83.8 | 11.9 | 4.3 |
| Milk group | 38.2 | 34.4 | 27.4 | 30.8 u | 6.7 u | 62.5 u | 22.3 | 40.8 u | 36.9 | 41.7 | 36.8 | 21.6 |
| Meat and meat alternates | 33.3 | 18.6 | 48.1 | 17.5 u | 32.7 u | 49.8 u | 29.8 | 12.1 u | 58.1 u | 35.0 | 18.9 | 46.2 |
| Mixed dishes | 20.9 | 35.4 | 43.7 | 43.9 u | 23.4 u | 32.8 u | 17.3 u | 40.7 | 42.0 | 18.6 | 36.7 | 44.7 |
| Condiments, Oils, Fats | 20.6 | 17.5 | 62.0 | 27.1 u | 26.1 u | 46.8 u | 19.9 | 20.7 u | 59.4 | 20.1 | 16.6 | 63.3 |
| Sweets | 0.0 | 7.5 | 92.5 | 0.0 | 6.9 u | 93.1 u | 0.0 | 9.4 u | 90.6 u | 0.0 | 8.2 | 91.8 |
| Beverages | 60.3 | 0.0 | 39.7 | 55.3 | 0.0 | 44.7 | 64.4 | 0.0 | 35.6 | 62.0 | 0.0 | 38.0 |
| Salty snacks | 0.0 | 21.8 | 78.2 | 0.0 | 23.3 u | 76.7 u | 0.0 | 0.0 u | 100.0 | 0.0 | 24.8 | 75.2 |
| **Female** | | | | | | | | | | | | |
| Daily intake | 37.6 | 22.0 | 40.4 | 31.7 | 21.0 u | 47.2 u | 39.8 | 21.5 | 38.7 | 38.0 | 22.3 | 39.8 |
| Grains | 29.3 | 44.8 | 26.0 | 33.5 u | 44.2 u | 22.3 u | 29.4 | 39.4 | 31.1 | 30.4 | 46.6 | 23.0 |
| Vegetables | 25.7 | 37.4 | 37.0 | 26.1 u | 41.7 | 32.2 | 29.0 | 44.1 | 26.8 | 25.8 | 34.6 | 39.6 |
| Fruit | 85.6 | 11.7 | 2.7 | 85.2 u | 12.8 u | 2.0 u | 90.2 u | 9.3 u | 0.5 u | 85.2 | 11.4 | 3.4 u |
| Milk group | 41.1 | 31.1 | 27.8 | 13.7 u | 36.3 u | 50.0 u | 17.4 u | 29.4 u | 53.2 | 47.2 | 31.8 | 21.0 |
| Meat and meat alternates | 26.8 | 22.5 | 50.7 | 14.3 u | 11.0 u | 74.6 u | 34.2 | 25.7 | 40.1 | 24.9 | 24.8 | 50.3 |
| Mixed dishes | 27.9 | 33.9 | 38.2 | 29.0 u | 28.7 | 42.3 u | 31.6 | 24.2 | 44.2 | 27.0 | 35.9 | 37.1 |
| Condiments, Oils, Fats | 21.8 | 19.4 | 58.8 | 16.0 u | 23.1 u | 60.9 u | 27.3 | 19.3 u | 53.5 | 20.5 | 20.4 | 59.1 |
| Sweets | 0.0 | 10.1 | 89.9 | 0.0 | 4.0 u | 96.0 u | 0.0 | 7.6 u | 92.4 u | 0.0 | 11.4 | 88.6 |
| Beverages | 73.0 | 0.0 | 27.0 | 64.0 | 0.0 | 36.0 | 73.6 | 0.0 | 26.4 | 75.3 | 0.0 | 24.7 |
| Salty snacks | 0.0 | 26.4 | 73.6 | 0.0 | 4.6 u | 95.4 u | 0.0 | 3.8 u | 96.2 u | 0.0 | 31.0 | 69.0 |

Notes: Significant differences in means and proportions are noted by * (.05 level), ** (.01 level), or *** (.001 level). Differences are tested in comparison to FSP participants, identified as persons in households receiving food stamps in the past 12 months.

u Denotes individual estimates not meeting the standards of reliability or precision due to inadequate cell size or large coefficient of variation.

Sources: NHANES 1999-2002 dietary recalls and MyPyramid Equivalents Database for USDA Survey Food Codes, 1994-2002, Version 1.0, October 2006. Excludes pregnant and breastfeeding women and infants. 'Total Persons' includes persons with missing food stamp participation or income. Percents are age adjusted to account for different age distributions of Food Stamp participants and nonparticipants.

## Table C-10. Healthy Eating Index-2005 (HEI-2005) Scores

| | All persons | | | | | | | |
|---|---|---|---|---|---|---|---|---|
| | Total Persons | | Food Stamp Program Participants | | Income-eligible Nonparticpants | | Higher-income Nonparticipants | |
| | Mean Score | Standard Error | Mean Score | Standard Error | Mean Score | Standard Error | Mean Score | Standard Error |
| **Both sexes** | | | | | | | | |
| Sample size ................ | 16,419 | – | 2,303 | – | 3,577 | – | 9,094 | – |
| Total Fruit .................... | 3.1 | (0.10) | 2.8 | (0.16) | 2.9 | (0.17) | ** 3.2 | (0.10) |
| Whole Fruit ................... | 3.5 | (0.12) | 2.5 | (0.23) | 3.3 | (0.21) | *** 3.7 | (0.12) |
| Total Vegetables .......... | 3.2 | (0.04) | 2.9 | (0.10) | 3.2 | (0.10) | *** 3.3 | (0.04) |
| Dark Green & Orange Vegetables, and Legumes ...................... | 1.4 | (0.06) | 1.3 | (0.13) | 1.4 | (0.10) | 1.4 | (0.06) |
| Total Grains ................. | 5.0 | (0.04) | 5.0 | (0.11) | 5.0 | (0.10) | 5.0 | (0.05) |
| Whole Grains ............... | 1.0 | (0.03) | 0.7 | (0.07) | 0.8 | (0.06) | *** 1.1 | (0.04) |
| Milk .............................. | 6.3 | (0.09) | 5.6 | (0.17) | 5.8 | (0.17) | *** 6.6 | (0.11) |
| Meat & Beans .............. | 10.0 | (0.08) | 10.0 | (0.21) | 10.0 | (0.18) | 10.0 | (0.08) |
| Oils .............................. | 6.3 | (0.09) | 4.7 | (0.15) | *** 5.7 | (0.19) | *** 6.6 | (0.10) |
| Saturated Fat[1] ............. | 3.9 | (0.08) | 3.8 | (0.25) | 4.1 | (0.16) | 3.9 | (0.07) |
| Sodium[1] ...................... | 6.2 | (0.12) | 6.3 | (0.33) | 6.6 | (0.18) | 6.2 | (0.13) |
| Calories from SoFAAS | 7.2 | (0.24) | 5.7 | (0.56) | 6.7 | (0.48) | ** 7.4 | (0.19) |
| Total HEI Score ........... | 57.5 | (0.68) | 51.9 | (1.20) | ** 56.1 | (1.05) | *** 58.4 | (0.64) |
| **Male** | | | | | | | | |
| Sample size ................ | 8,301 | – | 1,099 | – | 1,812 | – | 4,681 | – |
| Total Fruit .................... | 2.9 | (0.11) | 2.6 | (0.21) | 2.7 | (0.18) | 3.0 | (0.10) |
| Whole Fruit ................... | 3.1 | (0.12) | 2.7 | (0.28) | 3.1 | (0.23) | 3.2 | (0.13) |
| Total Vegetables .......... | 3.1 | (0.04) | 2.9 | (0.12) | 3.0 | (0.13) | 3.1 | (0.05) |
| Dark Green & Orange Vegetables, and Legumes ...................... | 1.2 | (0.06) | 1.2 | (0.13) | 1.3 | (0.14) | 1.2 | (0.06) |
| Total Grains ................. | 5.0 | (0.05) | 5.0 | (0.18) | 5.0 | (0.12) | 5.0 | (0.05) |
| Whole Grains ............... | 0.9 | (0.04) | 0.8 | (0.10) | 0.7 | (0.06) | * 1.0 | (0.05) |
| Milk .............................. | 6.2 | (0.10) | 5.7 | (0.25) | 5.9 | (0.25) | ** 6.5 | (0.12) |
| Meat & Beans .............. | 10.0 | (0.11) | 10.0 | (0.36) | 10.0 | (0.31) | 10.0 | (0.12) |
| Oils .............................. | 6.1 | (0.11) | 4.4 | (0.22) | *** 5.6 | (0.27) | *** 6.3 | (0.12) |
| Saturated Fat[1] ............. | 3.9 | (0.10) | 3.7 | (0.29) | 4.1 | (0.24) | 3.9 | (0.10) |
| Sodium[1] ...................... | 6.1 | (0.13) | 6.5 | (0.46) | 6.6 | (0.30) | 6.1 | (0.14) |
| Calories from SoFAAS | 6.7 | (0.26) | 5.5 | (0.77) | 6.7 | (0.57) | 6.8 | (0.21) |
| Total HEI Score ........... | 55.8 | (0.68) | 51.7 | (1.33) | * 55.8 | (1.36) | ** 56.4 | (0.58) |
| **Female** | | | | | | | | |
| Sample size ................ | 8,118 | – | 1,204 | – | 1,765 | – | 4,413 | – |
| Total Fruit .................... | 3.5 | (0.11) | 2.9 | (0.19) | 3.2 | (0.20) | ** 3.6 | (0.11) |
| Whole Fruit ................... | 4.0 | (0.16) | 2.5 | (0.23) | ** 3.6 | (0.26) | *** 4.3 | (0.16) |
| Total Vegetables .......... | 3.5 | (0.05) | 2.9 | (0.11) | ** 3.4 | (0.10) | *** 3.6 | (0.06) |
| Dark Green & Orange Vegetables, and Legumes ...................... | 1.6 | (0.09) | 1.3 | (0.15) | 1.4 | (0.12) | * 1.7 | (0.10) |
| Total Grains ................. | 5.0 | (0.06) | 5.0 | (0.13) | * 5.0 | (0.16) | *** 5.0 | (0.07) |
| Whole Grains ............... | 1.1 | (0.03) | 0.6 | (0.08) | 1.0 | (0.11) | *** 1.2 | (0.05) |
| Milk .............................. | 6.4 | (0.12) | 5.6 | (0.21) | 5.7 | (0.19) | *** 6.8 | (0.16) |
| Meat & Beans .............. | 9.7 | (0.11) | 10.0 | (0.26) | 9.8 | (0.19) | 9.5 | (0.13) |
| Oils .............................. | 6.6 | (0.12) | 4.9 | (0.21) | ** 5.8 | (0.20) | *** 7.0 | (0.14) |
| Saturated Fat[1] ............. | 3.8 | (0.09) | 3.9 | (0.24) | 4.0 | (0.31) | 3.8 | (0.10) |
| Sodium[1] ...................... | 6.3 | (0.13) | 6.1 | (0.43) | 6.5 | (0.22) | 6.3 | (0.17) |
| Calories from SoFAAS | 7.8 | (0.27) | 5.8 | (0.56) | 6.8 | (0.49) | ** 8.4 | (0.28) |
| Total HEI Score ........... | 59.6 | (0.81) | 52.0 | (1.37) | ** 56.6 | (0.95) | *** 61.5 | (0.92) |

See footnotes at end of table.

**Table C-10. (Continued)**

| | Children (age 2–18) | | | | | | | |
| --- | --- | --- | --- | --- | --- | --- | --- | --- |
| | Total Persons | | Food Stamp Program Participants | | Income-eligible Nonparticpants | | Higher-income Nonparticipants | |
| | Mean Score | Standard Error | Mean Score | Standard Error | Mean Score | Standard Error | Mean Score | Standard Error |
| **Both sexes** | | | | | | | | |
| Sample size | 7,583 | – | 1,495 | – | 1,801 | – | 3,682 | – |
| Total Fruit | 3.4 | (0.12) | 3.4 | (0.22) | 3.0 | (0.22) | 3.6 | (0.12) |
| Whole Fruit | 3.1 | (0.14) | 2.7 | (0.26) | 2.7 | (0.20) | *3.5 | (0.20) |
| Total Vegetables | 2.3 | (0.05) | 2.4 | (0.07) | 2.5 | (0.11) | *2.2 | (0.06) |
| Dark Green & Orange Vegetables, and Legumes | 0.8 | (0.05) | 0.9 | (0.16) | 0.8 | (0.10) | 0.8 | (0.08) |
| Total Grains | 5.0 | (0.07) | 5.0 | (0.13) | 5.0 | (0.15) | 5.0 | (0.07) |
| Whole Grains | 0.9 | (0.03) | 0.6 | (0.05) | 0.7 | (0.07) | ***1.0 | (0.04) |
| Milk | 8.4 | (0.16) | 7.8 | (0.26) | 7.7 | (0.41) | **8.8 | (0.21) |
| Meat & Beans | 8.0 | (0.12) | 8.5 | (0.30) | 8.4 | (0.18) | **7.6 | (0.16) |
| Oils | 5.8 | (0.12) | 5.3 | (0.30) | 5.8 | (0.24) | 5.9 | (0.13) |
| Saturated Fat[1] | 4.1 | (0.10) | 3.6 | (0.30) | 4.2 | (0.28) | *4.3 | (0.10) |
| Sodium[1] | 5.4 | (0.12) | 5.2 | (0.33) | 5.0 | (0.23) | 5.6 | (0.16) |
| Calories from SoFAAS | 7.1 | (0.24) | 7.1 | (0.45) | 6.6 | (0.42) | 7.2 | (0.24) |
| Total HEI Score | 55.0 | (0.70) | 53.2 | (1.16) | 53.0 | (1.23) | *56.1 | (0.72) |
| **Male** | | | | | | | | |
| Sample size | 3,824 | – | 758 | – | 920 | – | 1,828 | – |
| Total Fruit | 3.2 | (0.15) | 3.3 | (0.35) | 2.7 | (0.26) | 3.3 | (0.13) |
| Whole Fruit | 2.9 | (0.13) | 2.7 | (0.32) | 2.5 | (0.30) | 3.2 | (0.18) |
| Total Vegetables | 2.2 | (0.07) | 2.3 | (0.11) | 2.3 | (0.14) | 2.1 | (0.07) |
| Dark Green & Orange Vegetables, and Legumes | 0.7 | (0.07) | 0.8 | (0.19) | 0.8 | (0.13) | 0.7 | (0.07) |
| Total Grains | 5.0 | (0.09) | 5.0 | (0.21) | 5.0 | (0.21) | 5.0 | (0.09) |
| Whole Grains | 0.9 | (0.05) | 0.7 | (0.08) | 0.6 | (0.10) | **1.0 | (0.06) |
| Milk | 8.5 | (0.22) | 8.1 | (0.34) | 7.7 | (0.57) | *9.1 | (0.29) |
| Meat & Beans | 8.1 | (0.14) | 8.6 | (0.45) | 8.4 | (0.27) | 7.7 | (0.21) |
| Oils | 5.6 | (0.15) | 5.2 | (0.43) | 6.0 | (0.28) | 5.7 | (0.21) |
| Saturated Fat[1] | 4.0 | (0.14) | 3.3 | (0.34) | 4.0 | (0.35) | *4.3 | (0.18) |
| Sodium[1] | 5.3 | (0.15) | 5.1 | (0.54) | 5.0 | (0.33) | 5.4 | (0.20) |
| Calories from SoFAAS | 7.0 | (0.33) | 7.6 | (0.64) | 6.4 | (0.57) | 7.0 | (0.27) |
| Total HEI Score | 54.2 | (0.91) | 53.5 | (1.80) | 52.1 | (1.62) | 55.3 | (0.73) |
| **Female** | | | | | | | | |
| Sample size | 3,759 | – | 737 | – | 881 | – | 1,854 | – |
| Total Fruit | 3.7 | (0.15) | 3.5 | (0.27) | 3.4 | (0.28) | 3.8 | (0.18) |
| Whole Fruit | 3.5 | (0.22) | 2.8 | (0.36) | 3.1 | (0.31) | *3.9 | (0.30) |
| Total Vegetables | 2.4 | (0.05) | 2.5 | (0.08) | 2.7 | (0.11) | 2.4 | (0.07) |
| Dark Green & Orange Vegetables, and Legumes | 0.9 | (0.07) | 1.0 | (0.17) | 0.9 | (0.14) | 0.9 | (0.10) |
| Total Grains | 5.0 | (0.09) | 5.0 | (0.10) | 5.0 | (0.17) | 5.0 | (0.09) |
| Whole Grains | 0.8 | (0.03) | 0.6 | (0.06) | 0.7 | (0.07) | ***1.0 | (0.04) |
| Milk | 8.2 | (0.16) | 7.6 | (0.34) | 7.8 | (0.35) | *8.5 | (0.23) |
| Meat & Beans | 7.8 | (0.17) | 8.3 | (0.23) | 8.5 | (0.29) | **7.3 | (0.20) |
| Oils | 6.0 | (0.14) | 5.6 | (0.35) | 5.6 | (0.38) | 6.2 | (0.13) |
| Saturated Fat[1] | 4.3 | (0.12) | 3.8 | (0.34) | 4.4 | (0.27) | 4.4 | (0.14) |
| Sodium[1] | 5.5 | (0.17) | 5.3 | (0.35) | 5.1 | (0.26) | 5.7 | (0.22) |
| Calories from SoFAAS | 7.3 | (0.24) | 6.6 | (0.50) | 6.9 | (0.45) | 7.5 | (0.28) |
| Total HEI Score | 56.0 | (0.78) | 52.8 | (1.17) | 54.3 | (1.15) | **57.4 | (0.98) |

See footnotes at end of table.

## Table C-10. (Continued)

| | Adults (age 19–59) | | | | | | | |
| | Total Persons | | Food Stamp Program Participants | | Income-eligible Nonparticpants | | Higher-income Nonparticipants | |
| | Mean Score | Standard Error | Mean Score | Standard Error | Mean Score | Standard Error | Mean Score | Standard Error |
|---|---|---|---|---|---|---|---|---|
| **Both sexes** | | | | | | | | |
| Sample size | 8,836 | – | 808 | – | 1,776 | – | 5,412 | – |
| Total Fruit | 3.0 | (0.11) | 2.5 | (0.17) | 2.9 | (0.18) | 3.1 | (0.11) |
| Whole Fruit | 3.6 | (0.14) | 2.5 | (0.24) | 3.5 | (0.25) | 3.8 | (0.14) |
| Total Vegetables | 3.6 | (0.05) | 3.1 | (0.14) | 3.4 | (0.12) | 3.6 | (0.05) |
| Dark Green & Orange Vegetables, and Legumes | 1.6 | (0.08) | 1.4 | (0.17) | 1.6 | (0.12) | 1.6 | (0.08) |
| Total Grains | 5.0 | (0.04) | 5.0 | (0.13) | 5.0 | (0.13) | 5.0 | (0.05) |
| Whole Grains | 1.0 | (0.03) | 0.7 | (0.09) | 0.8 | (0.07) | 1.1 | (0.04) |
| Milk | 5.6 | (0.09) | 4.9 | (0.20) | 5.1 | (0.16) | 5.8 | (0.11) |
| Meat & Beans | 10.0 | (0.09) | 10.0 | (0.29) | 10.0 | (0.24) | 10.0 | (0.10) |
| Oils | 6.5 | (0.12) | 4.5 | (0.22) | 5.7 | (0.21) | 6.8 | (0.13) |
| Saturated Fat[1] | 3.8 | (0.08) | 3.9 | (0.28) | 4.0 | (0.22) | 3.7 | (0.08) |
| Sodium[1] | 6.5 | (0.13) | 6.7 | (0.43) | 7.2 | (0.22) | 6.4 | (0.15) |
| Calories from SoFAAS | 7.2 | (0.25) | 5.2 | (0.67) | 6.8 | (0.54) | 7.5 | (0.20) |
| Total HEI Score | 58.3 | (0.71) | 51.4 | (1.46) | 57.3 | (1.11) | 59.2 | (0.65) |
| **Male** | | | | | | | | |
| Sample size | 4,477 | – | 341 | – | 892 | – | 2,853 | – |
| Total Fruit | 2.8 | (0.11) | 2.4 | (0.25) | 2.7 | (0.18) | 2.8 | (0.12) |
| Whole Fruit | 3.2 | (0.13) | 2.7 | (0.36) | 3.4 | (0.26) | 3.3 | (0.14) |
| Total Vegetables | 3.3 | (0.05) | 3.0 | (0.18) | 3.2 | (0.16) | 3.4 | (0.06) |
| Dark Green & Orange Vegetables, and Legumes | 1.4 | (0.07) | 1.4 | (0.18) | 1.6 | (0.17) | 1.4 | (0.08) |
| Total Grains | 5.0 | (0.05) | 5.0 | (0.22) | 5.0 | (0.15) | 4.9 | (0.06) |
| Whole Grains | 0.9 | (0.04) | 0.8 | (0.13) | 0.7 | (0.07) | 1.0 | (0.05) |
| Milk | 5.4 | (0.11) | 4.8 | (0.31) | 5.3 | (0.25) | 5.5 | (0.12) |
| Meat & Beans | 10.0 | (0.13) | 10.0 | (0.43) | 10.0 | (0.40) | 10.0 | (0.14) |
| Oils | 6.2 | (0.13) | 4.1 | (0.30) | 5.4 | (0.30) | 6.5 | (0.15) |
| Saturated Fat[1] | 3.9 | (0.11) | 3.9 | (0.35) | 4.1 | (0.31) | 3.8 | (0.13) |
| Sodium[1] | 6.4 | (0.16) | 7.0 | (0.57) | 7.2 | (0.40) | 6.3 | (0.18) |
| Calories from SoFAAS | 6.5 | (0.26) | 4.8 | (0.94) | 6.7 | (0.63) | 6.7 | (0.23) |
| Total HEI Score | 56.4 | (0.65) | 51.0 | (1.67) | 57.1 | (1.44) | 56.7 | (0.59) |
| **Female** | | | | | | | | |
| Sample size | 4,359 | – | 467 | – | 884 | – | 2,559 | – |
| Total Fruit | 3.4 | (0.13) | 2.7 | (0.22) | 3.2 | (0.24) | 3.5 | (0.12) |
| Whole Fruit | 4.2 | (0.18) | 2.4 | (0.26) | 3.7 | (0.34) | 4.5 | (0.17) |
| Total Vegetables | 3.8 | (0.06) | 3.1 | (0.15) | 3.7 | (0.14) | 4.0 | (0.07) |
| Dark Green & Orange Vegetables, and Legumes | 1.9 | (0.11) | 1.5 | (0.20) | 1.6 | (0.15) | 2.0 | (0.13) |
| Total Grains | 5.0 | (0.06) | 4.9 | (0.16) | 5.0 | (0.19) | 5.0 | (0.08) |
| Whole Grains | 1.1 | (0.03) | 0.7 | (0.12) | 1.1 | (0.14) | 1.2 | (0.06) |
| Milk | 5.8 | (0.15) | 4.9 | (0.27) | 4.9 | (0.20) | 6.2 | (0.19) |
| Meat & Beans | 10.0 | (0.13) | 10.0 | (0.36) | 10.0 | (0.22) | 10.0 | (0.17) |
| Oils | 6.8 | (0.17) | 4.7 | (0.32) | 5.9 | (0.25) | 7.3 | (0.19) |
| Saturated Fat[1] | 3.7 | (0.11) | 3.9 | (0.28) | 3.9 | (0.42) | 3.6 | (0.13) |
| Sodium[1] | 6.6 | (0.15) | 6.4 | (0.51) | 7.1 | (0.29) | 6.5 | (0.19) |
| Calories from SoFAAS | 8.0 | (0.30) | 5.5 | (0.73) | 6.8 | (0.61) | 8.7 | (0.31) |
| Total HEI Score | 60.9 | (0.92) | 51.7 | (1.68) | 57.4 | (1.28) | 62.9 | (1.02) |

See footnotes at end of table.

## Table C-10. (Continued)

| | Older adults (age 60+) | | | | | | | |
| | Total Persons | | Food Stamp Program Participants | | Income-eligible Nonparticipants | | Higher-income Nonparticipants | |
| | Mean Score | Standard Error | Mean Score | Standard Error | Mean Score | Standard Error | Mean Score | Standard Error |
|---|---|---|---|---|---|---|---|---|
| **Both sexes** | | | | | | | | |
| Sample size | 3,061 | – | 215 | – | 652 | – | 1,825 | – |
| Total Fruit | 4.6 | (0.11) | 4.1 | (0.55) | 4.1 | (0.27) | 4.7 | (0.11) |
| Whole Fruit | 5.0 | (0.20) | 4.9 | (0.77) | 5.0 | (0.39) | 5.0 | (0.19) |
| Total Vegetables | 4.3 | (0.08) | 3.6 | (0.27) | 4.2 | (0.20) | *4.2 | (0.08) |
| Dark Green & Orange Vegetables, and Legumes | 2.0 | (0.08) | 2.1 | (0.42) | 2.4 | (0.21) | 1.9 | (0.09) |
| Total Grains | 5.0 | (0.07) | 5.0 | (0.26) | 5.0 | (0.13) | 5.0 | (0.08) |
| Whole Grains | 1.6 | (0.06) | 1.3 | (0.29) | 1.5 | (0.11) | 1.7 | (0.07) |
| Milk | 5.9 | (0.14) | 4.9 | (0.38) | 5.7 | (0.23) | *5.9 | (0.18) |
| Meat & Beans | 10.0 | (0.15) | 10.0 | (0.69) | 10.0 | (0.35) | 10.0 | (0.16) |
| Oils | 6.7 | (0.16) | 3.8 | (0.34) | ***6.1 | (0.43) | ***6.9 | (0.20) |
| Saturated Fat[1] | 3.1 | (0.13) | 3.0 | (0.84) | 3.1 | (0.44) | 3.1 | (0.14) |
| Sodium[1] | 6.9 | (0.18) | 7.5 | (0.68) | 6.8 | (0.30) | 6.9 | (0.20) |
| Calories from SoFAAS | 10.8 | (0.15) | 9.8 | (1.02) | 11.2 | (0.32) | 10.9 | (0.18) |
| Total HEI Score | 68.4 | (0.72) | 62.7 | (3.83) | 67.6 | (1.29) | 69.0 | (0.80) |
| **Male** | | | | | | | | |
| Sample size | 1,512 | – | 96 | – | 298 | – | 950 | – |
| Total Fruit | 4.0 | (0.11) | 4.2 u | (0.94) | 4.0 | (0.35) | 4.1 | (0.14) |
| Whole Fruit | 5.0 | (0.18) | 5.0 u | (1.25) | 5.0 | (0.51) | 5.0 | (0.20) |
| Total Vegetables | 4.0 | (0.08) | 3.9 | (0.32) | 3.6 | (0.18) | 4.0 | (0.09) |
| Dark Green & Orange Vegetables, and Legumes | 1.9 | (0.11) | 2.4 | (0.42) | 2.2 | (0.30) | 1.7 | (0.13) |
| Total Grains | 5.0 | (0.08) | 5.0 | (0.24) | 5.0 | (0.18) | 5.0 | (0.10) |
| Whole Grains | 1.7 | (0.07) | 1.7 u | (0.50) | 1.4 | (0.20) | 1.7 | (0.09) |
| Milk | 5.6 | (0.14) | 5.4 | (0.65) | 5.6 | (0.31) | 5.6 | (0.18) |
| Meat & Beans | 10.0 | (0.21) | 10.0 | (1.03) | 10.0 | (0.59) | *10.0 | (0.23) |
| Oils | 6.4 | (0.24) | 3.3 u | (0.80) | 5.5 | (0.68) | ***6.8 | (0.25) |
| Saturated Fat[1] | 3.2 | (0.17) | 1.9 u | (0.87) | 3.5 | (0.65) | 3.2 | (0.18) |
| Sodium[1] | 6.6 | (0.21) | 7.9 | (0.95) | 6.7 | (0.44) | 6.7 | (0.22) |
| Calories from SoFAAS | 10.1 | (0.17) | 9.3 u | (1.16) | 10.4 | (0.50) | 10.3 | (0.23) |
| Total HEI Score | 65.6 | (0.79) | 63.1 | (4.66) | 65.7 | (2.11) | 66.0 | (0.92) |
| **Female** | | | | | | | | |
| Sample size | 1,549 | – | 119 | – | 354 | – | 875 | – |
| Total Fruit | 5.0 | (0.17) | 4.0 | (0.73) | 4.2 | (0.36) | 5.0 | (0.17) |
| Whole Fruit | 5.0 | (0.27) | 4.1 | (0.93) | 5.0 | (0.56) | 5.0 | (0.26) |
| Total Vegetables | 4.6 | (0.13) | 3.4 | (0.33) | **4.8 | (0.32) | ***4.6 | (0.13) |
| Dark Green & Orange Vegetables, and Legumes | 2.2 | (0.11) | 1.9 | (0.49) | 2.6 | (0.29) | 2.1 | (0.11) |
| Total Grains | 5.0 | (0.09) | 5.0 | (0.43) | 5.0 | (0.18) | 5.0 | (0.10) |
| Whole Grains | 1.7 | (0.07) | 1.1 | (0.28) | 1.7 | (0.15) | *1.8 | (0.10) |
| Milk | 6.1 | (0.21) | 4.7 | (0.46) | 5.8 | (0.26) | **6.2 | (0.27) |
| Meat & Beans | 10.0 | (0.18) | 10.0 | (0.90) | 10.0 | (0.48) | 10.0 | (0.20) |
| Oils | 7.0 | (0.19) | 4.0 | (0.45) | ***6.4 | (0.54) | ***7.2 | (0.25) |
| Saturated Fat[1] | 3.1 | (0.17) | 3.6 | (0.82) | 2.6 | (0.47) | 3.1 | (0.19) |
| Sodium[1] | 7.0 | (0.24) | 7.2 | (0.82) | 7.0 | (0.41) | 7.1 | (0.32) |
| Calories from SoFAAS | 11.5 | (0.22) | 10.1 u | (1.20) | 12.1 | (0.30) | 11.6 | (0.25) |
| Total HEI Score | 71.4 | (1.05) | 62.4 | (4.43) | 69.8 | (1.41) | *72.5 | (1.20) |

Notes: Significant differences in means and proportions are noted by * (.05 level), ** (.01 level), or *** (.001 level). Differences are tested in comparison to FSP participants, identified as persons in households receiving food stamps in the past 12 months.

u Denotes individual estimates not meeting the standards of reliability or precision due to inadequate cell size or large coefficient of variation.

– Not applicable.

[1] Calculated as the mean of individual HEI scores, rather than the score of group means to enable significance testing (see Appendix A).

Source: NHANES 1999–2004 dietary recalls and MyPyramid Equivalents Database for USDA Survey Food Codes, 1994-2002, Version 1.0, October.2006. Estimates are based on a single dietary recall per person. 'Total Persons' includes persons with missing FSP participation or income are age adjusted to account for different age distributions of FSP participants and nonparticipants.

## Table C-11. Average Amount of MyPyramid Groups Consumed Per Person

| | All Persons | | | | Children (age 2-18) | | | |
|---|---|---|---|---|---|---|---|---|
| | Total Persons | Food Stamp Program Partic. | Income-eligible Nonpartic. | Higher-income Nonpartic. | Total Persons | Food Stamp Program Partic. | Income-eligible Nonpartic. | Higher-income Nonpartic. |
| Sample size | 16,419 | 2,303 | 3,577 | 9,094 | 7,583 | 1,495 | 1,801 | 3,682 |
| **Total Fruit (cup equiv.)** | 1.03 | 0.84 | 0.92 | ***1.08 | 1.03 | 1.01 | 0.91 | **1.07 |
| Whole fruit | 0.57 | 0.38 | ***0.52 | ***0.61 | 0.48 | 0.42 | 0.40 | **0.53 |
| **Total Vegetable (cup equiv.)** | 1.51 | 1.24 | ***1.41 | ***1.56 | 1.04 | 1.02 | *1.13 | 1.00 |
| Dark green and orange vegetables, and legumes[1] | 0.24 | 0.20 | 0.22 | *0.24 | 0.13 | 0.14 | 0.13 | 0.12 |
| Other vegetables | 1.29 | 1.07 | **1.21 | ***1.34 | 0.93 | 0.90 | *1.01 | 0.90 |
| **Total Grain (ounce equiv.)** | 6.74 | 6.19 | 6.59 | **6.86 | 6.91 | 6.46 | 6.87 | ***7.06 |
| Whole grain ounce equiv. | 0.61 | 0.39 | 0.47 | ***0.67 | 0.51 | 0.36 | 0.39 | *0.59 |
| Non-whole grain ounce equiv. | 6.13 | 5.80 | 6.12 | 6.19 | 6.41 | 6.10 | 6.48 | 6.47 |
| **Total Milk group (cup equiv.)** | 1.71 | 1.43 | 1.52 | ***1.82 | 2.12 | 1.94 | 1.97 | ***2.24 |
| Milk cup equiv. | 1.06 | 0.94 | 0.99 | ***1.11 | 1.48 | 1.40 | 1.40 | 1.55 |
| Yogurt cup equiv. | 0.00 | 0.00 u | 0.00 | ***0.00 | 0.00 | 0.00 u | 0.00 u | ***0.00 |
| Cheese cup equiv. | 0.61 | 0.48 | 0.51 | ***0.66 | 0.60 | 0.53 | 0.55 | *0.64 |
| **Total Meat and Bean (ounce equiv.)** | 5.40 | 5.15 | 5.28 | 5.44 | 4.04 | 4.09 | 4.33 | 3.88 |
| Total lean meat from meat, poultry, fish | 4.41 | 4.39 | **4.28 | 4.41 | 3.37 | 3.59 | *3.65 | **3.17 |
| Total lean meat from meat alternates | 1.00 | 0.76 | 1.00 | ***1.03 | 0.67 | 0.51 | 0.69 | ***0.71 |
| **Oils (grams)** | 16.53 | 11.72 | ***14.52 | ***17.58 | 14.60 | 12.72 | 15.09 | **14.93 |
| **Discretionary fats, added sugars, and alcohol** | | | | | | | | |
| Solid fat (grams) | 47.15 | 46.60 | 45.79 | 47.57 | 47.05 | 46.64 | *49.32 | **46.52 |
| Added sugars (teaspoon equiv.) | 22.64 | 23.80 | 23.71 | 22.44 | 23.89 | 21.62 | 24.60 | 24.40 |
| Alcohol (drinks) | 0.62 | 0.48 | 0.43 | 0.69 | 0.06 | 0.00 u | 0.00 | 0.07 |

See footnotes on next page.

## Table C-11. (Continued)

| | Adults (age 19-59) | | | | Older adults (age 60+) | | | |
|---|---|---|---|---|---|---|---|---|
| | Total Persons | Food Stamp Program Partic. | Income-eligible Nonpartic. | Higher-income Nonpartic. | Total Persons | Food Stamp Program Partic. | Income-eligible Nonpartic. | Higher-income Nonpartic. |
| Sample size | 5,775 | 593 | 1,124 | 3,587 | 3,061 | 215 | 652 | 1,825 |
| Total Fruit (cup equiv.) | 0.96 | 0.72 | *0.90 | ***1.00 | 1.27 | 1.00 | 1.02 | **1.36 |
| Whole fruit | 0.54 | 0.30 | ***0.53 | ***0.56 | 0.84 | 0.61 | 0.67 | ***0.91 |
| Total Vegetable (cup equiv.) | 1.68 | 1.36 | 1.52 | ***1.77 | 1.62 | 1.14 | **1.42 | ***1.67 |
| Dark green and orange vegetables, and legumes[1] | 0.27 | 0.21 | 0.24 | **0.29 | 0.28 | 0.26 | 0.30 | 0.28 |
| Other vegetables | 1.43 | 1.19 | 1.31 | ***1.51 | 1.36 | 0.94 | **1.15 | ***1.41 |
| Total Grain (ounce equiv.) | 6.96 | 6.34 | 6.86 | 7.05 | 5.68 | 5.23 | 5.28 | **5.92 |
| Whole grain ounce equiv. | 0.57 | 0.34 | 0.43 | ***0.63 | 0.86 | 0.60 | 0.70 | *0.93 |
| Non-whole grain ounce equiv. | 6.39 | 6.00 | 6.43 | 6.41 | 4.82 | 4.63 | 4.58 | 4.99 |
| Total Milk group (cup equiv.) | 1.66 | 1.34 | 1.44 | ***1.77 | 1.31 | 0.97 | *1.16 | ***1.36 |
| Milk cup equiv. | 0.92 | 0.81 | 0.84 | *0.97 | 0.95 | 0.69 | *0.92 | **0.98 |
| Yogurt cup equiv. | 0.00 | 0.00 u | 0.00 u | ***0.00 | 0.00 | 0.00 u | 0.00 u | **0.00 |
| Cheese cup equiv. | 0.69 | 0.52 | 0.58 | ***0.75 | 0.33 | 0.26 | 0.23 | *0.35 |
| Total Meat and Bean (ounce equiv.) | 6.16 | 5.80 | 5.90 | 6.26 | 4.81 | 4.48 | 4.56 | 4.89 |
| Total lean meat from meat, poultry, fish | 5.04 | 5.00 | 4.78 | 5.11 | 3.76 | 3.50 | 3.49 | 3.83 |
| Total lean meat from meat alternates | 1.12 | 0.81 | *1.12 | ***1.16 | 1.05 | 0.98 | 1.06 | 1.06 |
| Oils (grams) | 17.99 | 12.62 | *15.11 | ***19.36 | 14.38 | 7.08 | ***11.66 | ***15.39 |
| Discretionary fats, added sugars, and alcohol | | | | | | | | |
| Solid fat (grams) | 50.11 | 49.87 | 47.56 | 50.82 | 37.12 | 35.33 | 34.74 | 37.81 |
| Added sugars (teaspoon equiv.) | 24.73 | 27.83 | 26.74 | 24.12 | 13.53 | 13.11 | 12.33 | 13.66 |
| Alcohol (drinks) | 0.93 | 0.76 | 0.69 | 1.01 | 0.40 | 0.14 | 0.13 | ***0.48 |

Notes: Significant differences in means and proportions are noted by * (.05 level), ** (.01 level), or *** (.001 level). Differences are tested in comparison to FSP participants, identified as persons in households receiving food stamps in the past 12 months.

[u] Denotes individual estimates not meeting the standards of reliability or precision due to inadequate cell size or large coefficient of variation.

[1] Legumes count as meat until a person's meat intake reaches 2.5 ounce equivalents per 1000 kcal, and then count as vegetables (HEI-2005).

Source: NHANES 1999–2002 dietary recalls and MyPyramid Equivalents Database for USDA Survey Food Codes, 1994-2002, Version 1.0, October 2006. Estimates are based on a single dietary recall per person. Excludes pregnant and breastfeeding women and infants. 'Total Persons' includes persons with missing food stamp participation or income. Percents are age adjusted to account for different age distributions of Food Stamp participants and nonparticipants.

# INDEX

## D

## W

## Y

## Z